# Healthy Holidays

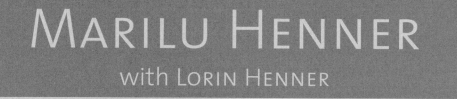

# MARILU HENNER

with LORIN HENNER

# Healthy Holidays

## TOTAL HEALTH ENTERTAINING
## ALL YEAR ROUND

ReganBooks

*An Imprint of HarperCollinsPublishers*

HarperCollins books may be purchased for educational, business, or sales promotional use. For information please write: Special Markets Department, HarperCollins Publishers Inc., 10 East 53rd Street, New York, NY 10022.

FIRST EDITION

Designed by Brenden Hitt

Photographs by Dennis Gottlieb

Printed on acid-free paper

Library of Congress Cataloging-in-Publication Data
Henner, Marilu.
    Healthly holidays : total health entertaining all year round / Marilu
        Henner.—1st ed.
        p.   cm.
    ISBN 0-06-039363-7
    1. holiday cookery.  2. Entertaining.  I. title.

    TX739 .H46 2002
    642'.4–dc21                                             2002031806

    02  03  04  05  06  WBC/RRD  10  9  8  7  6  5  4  3  2  1

To my family and friends,
and to holiday lovers everywhere

# Acknowledgments

Of the seven books I've written, I can honestly say that this book is my favorite. It has been a labor of love from the beginning—interesting, challenging, creative, whimsical, tasty—and a lot of fun to work on because of the following people. Therefore, I would like to thank:

The ever-impressive Judith Regan, who always provides the right balance of expectation and encouragement. Her exceptional and dedicated team at HarperCollins, starting with her unflappable assistant Angelica Canales. Dan Taylor,

ACKNOWLEDGM

# Acknowledgments

Brenden Hitt, and Anthony Velarde, who did a beautiful job making this book look holiday-festive. Kurt Andrews, Tom Wengelewski, Kim Lewis, and Joyce Wong, who made sure that everything tracked and made sense (no easy task with a book this size). Carl Raymond, who always knows how to sell a book, and the irrepressible Paul Olsewski, who always knows how to sell me selling a book. (You are the B.E.S.T.!) I would also like to thank Liz Lauricella and Emily Katz, who helped my incomparable editor, Cassie Jones, do her magic. And thank you, Cassie, for your passion, energy, intelligence, patience, taste, and charm. And most of all, for being the motor on a project that was often unwieldy in its logistics and scope. To the wonderful team who created such delectable food photography and were a blast to work with: Dennis Gottlieb, Marie Haycox, Randy Barritt, Jim Ong, Kelly Kalhoefer, Tina Gehrig, and Barbara Gold. And to Suzanne Unrein, who helped me so much with her great style and artistic flair.

To the fabulous Kalinka, for the gorgeous gown she made for the cover shot. She and her dashing husband, Stan, are always a blast to hang out with. To Michael Gardner, who helped me throughout this process, whether it was in the dressing room or at the photo shoots. To Guy LeBaube for his beautiful cover.

To Alyce de Toledo, Richard Kind, and his cousin Barbara, Bobby Levin, and Robert Forster for their contributions.

A big special thank you to all of my friends and members at Marilu.com who live the THM lifestyle, love to cook, and sent in recipes: Jo Taylor, Jan Davis, Deanna Little, Michelle Flanagan (Kinney), Bev Powell; my wonderful moderators, the fearless Erin Moore, the engaging Suzanne Palumbo, and the unstoppable Susan Romito, a fabulous cook and baker. (You can reach her at susan@loveandsweets.com.) And to the effervescent Mary Beth Borkowski, not only for her recipes, but also for her willingness to help out at a moment's notice. To Lin Milano and her amazing staff at safesearching.com, who help us at marilu.com get the message out. And of course, to the irreplaceable Tonia Raebiger, without whom marilu.com could not be what it is.

To the charismatic Jonathan Waxman of Washington Park (my favorite New York restaurant), a big thank you for his inspired meals and delicious recipes. To Emeril Lagasse and his lovely wife, Alden, for his contribution to Mardi Gras, a holiday made more festive because of his dazzle.

To my lovely sister Christal, her unbeatable husband, Roy Welland, and their incredible boys, Willy and Christopher, who so generously allowed us to set up Book Team East in their apartment. They never complained even as we took over their office, kitchen, telephone, and social life. I couldn't have done this book without you.

To my extraordinary book team (east and west!): Karen Roberts, the rookie on the team, who did the initial research and endlessly shopped for supplies, and also supplied her wicked sense of humor. To Wanjira Banfield, with her dazzling smile, who added the right spark at the end, just when we needed it. She is an asset to any team, and we were lucky to have her. To Patty O'Malley, for her unique knowledge of scents and flavors; Beth Heffner, for her typing, emailing, faxing, and ability to THM great recipes; Elena Lewis, for her dedication, organization and delicious sense of fun; Brent "Magic Fingers" Strickland, for his computer skills and killer charm. His positive attitude and can-do nature are always a delight to work with, even long distance and over the phone. To Inara George, factoid queen and recipe maven, whose elegant presence always makes me feel good about life; Bryony Atkinson, for her unique talents and skills in so many areas, whether it's typing, computers, research, and especially her integrity and musical sense which added so much to this book. To Lynnette Lesko, for her inspired creativity and her ability to think far outside the box. To my niece, Suzanne Carney, an incredible writer and party thrower who added the perfect balance of class and whimsy, and to her out-of-this-world daughter, Charlotte, who hung out and kept all of us (especially my boys!) in line.

To MaryAnn Hennings, culinary goddess, whose ability to take any recipe and make it healthy and delicious is a feat surpassed only by her ability to be a true and loving best friend. (Not to mention the world's greatest hairdresser!) To my niece, Elizabeth Carney, who sees it all and does it all and makes it look effortless. Her natural talent for being able to multi-task, trouble shoot, and keep it all together, even when it's not easy, is what makes her such a brilliant producer. And last, but certainly not least, to Lorin Henner, my brother, my co-author, my buddy, my friend. There are no words to express how incredible I think you are, and how much fun I had working with you on this project. Your talent, creativity, focus, and sense of humor are the cornerstone of this book, and you are the best darn uncle my boys could ever have!

Thank you, team, from the bottom of my heart. I love each and every one of you!

To Dr. Ruth Velikovsky Sharon, the brilliant psychoanalyst, who continues to be a positive and profound influence in my life. I couldn't "do it all" without you.

And to Robert Lieberman, who shares with me the greatest joy I've ever known: our two little guys, Nicky and Joey, who make every day a holiday!

# Contents

# Introduction

INTRODUCTION

**H**ealthy holidays.

It sounds like an oxymoron, right? It's right up there with jumbo shrimp, slumber party, and working vacation. It's kind of like saying "disciplined indulgence." I was telling a friend of mine recently that I was writing a book called *Healthy Holidays,* and he said, "Healthy holidays? Is that even possible?" Well I'm here to tell you that not only is it possible, it's guaranteed if you follow just a few simple rules. After reading this book and enjoying a few healthy holidays of your own, I'm sure you will agree that making your holidays healthy is the best way to enjoy them to their fullest.

I used to see every holiday as an opportunity to completely fall apart. And I actually looked *forward* to falling apart! I would even factor in recovery time, naturally building it into my year. I would plan for those days of indulgence and accept the consequences—extra weight, puffy face, watery eyes, stuffy nose, headache, constipation, and bloating—as though they were supposed to be a natural part of the celebration. (Not to mention a pimple or two within the following week!) To most of us, the essence of a holiday *is* indulgence. And it should be. But *over*indulgence is often the factor that ruins a holiday or party. The suffering usually outweighs the pleasure, not to mention how dangerous it is for our health.

The essence of a holiday is friends and family sharing and celebrating with a meal that usually involves some kind of guilty pleasure, a little naughty and perhaps a little unhealthy, but one that we look forward to because it isn't a part of our everyday routine. In fact, celebrating the holidays is a way of balancing our routine. We work forty-plus hours a week, and a holiday is a way of letting off steam and taking a break from that work. We have been working hard and have been mentally building toward a reward. Holidays are usually celebrated on a weekend, now that most of them have been moved to a convenient Monday, and the main objective is to gather with friends and family, eat a little more, play a little more, and drink a little more. In short: *live* a little more. Sometimes *a lot* more!

Now I don't want you to think that this is a book about avoiding those things we love during the holidays. It's not about being overly disciplined on holidays or at parties—you won't be eating only raw food at your next Thanksgiving dinner. This book is about building a few simple corrective actions right into your holiday routine so that you won't gain weight or be sick, hung over, or forced to diet and detox for days or weeks after the holiday. You're going to build a few of the elements of detox and diet right into your day—and barely notice it.

This is analogous to sound financial planning. If your overall goal is to be financially stable, it's best to budget and have a balanced and secure financial plan. If you overspend during the holidays and blow money carelessly on every vacation, you're likely to go into debt—unless, of course, you are *extremely* wealthy. But you can never reach a point with your health that would be equivalent to a billionaire with his money. You can never be so healthy that it would be possible to eat and drink large quantities of junk and still be healthy and look great. And even though the most affluent people can afford reckless spending, I find it interesting that they usually tend to budget the most. It is one of the main reasons the wealthy *stay* wealthy. And that is the mentality I would like you to adopt regarding your health. I want you to stay healthy and still thoroughly enjoy the holidays—in fact, you'll probably enjoy them more. And you won't need to recover for three days afterward.

People are always going to overdo it. It's human nature to want to contrast working hard with overindulging. But if you can embrace little ways to keep yourself from falling off the deep end, you will also teach your children some healthy habits in the process. Balanced eating during the holidays is a great message to send our kids. We teach them by showing a good example, which plants the seed in their heads that extreme eating habits are *not* a good idea. This is more important than ever today, when there is so much junk food in our children's environment compared to when we were growing up, and so many more opportunities for them to pick up bad habits.

When I was growing up, I would eagerly wait for the holiday season, starting with Halloween. I knew I was going to be sick the day after eating all that junk, but there was no way I was going to skip even one candy corn. And after Thanksgiving dinner, I knew I was going to be full and bloated and sick. It's not just an American tradition to be miserable after every holiday. It's the law! And we don't feel satisfied until we are completely stuffed. It is our goal to actually *become* the turkey.

I remember returning to school every January after Christmas vacation, even when I was as young as fourth grade, realizing "Oh my gosh, my uniform doesn't fit anymore." As a teenager I would always begin a serious diet every January. I know I'm not the only who approached January this way. In fact, most people still do. The average person gains seven or eight pounds between Thanksgiving and New Year's Day, and everyone, at one time or another, attempts to change his or her life beginning in January right after the big holiday sweep. These attempts are called New Year's resolutions.

If you're familiar with my books *Marilu Henner's Total Health Makeover, The 30-Day Total Health Makeover,* and *Healthy Life Kitchen,* you know that one of the most important elements I've strived for in developing the Total Health Makeover (or THM) lifestyle over the past twenty-three years has been to find a way of eating that I could live with every day. So, of course, much of this lifestyle had to be flexible and forgiving, especially during the holidays. I have always been somewhat of a party girl, so it was important for me to find a way of getting through the holidays while still indulging and enjoying myself. To this day, I associate holidays with being a little naughty and eating and partying too much, but now I don't fall apart. And I enjoy the holidays now more than ever!

People always make fun of me for eating what they consider to be a strict diet. They can't believe I have the discipline to never eat meat, sugar, or dairy products. When I dine with friends for the first time, they will often apologize for ordering something that I would not eat myself. What they don't realize is that flavor-wise and satisfaction-wise my diet is identical to theirs. It's just healthier. My taste buds now prefer healthier, better food.

I threw a holiday party once for three hundred people. I carefully went over the THM guidelines with the caterer (no meat, no sugar, no dairy). It was an endless feast with many hors d'oeuvres, entrées, desserts—everything devilish you can imagine. Because the food was so incredible, people said, "Wow, you really broke the rules tonight, didn't you?" They couldn't believe it when I told them that all the food fit within the THM guidelines, and that not one item was served that I would not eat myself. THM is simply a way to eat, enjoy, indulge, and not feel sick the next day.

Have you ever gotten into really great shape, just to fall apart? We get in shape to go on vacation, be someone's Valentine, see our relatives at Christmas, fit into that slinky Halloween costume or tight little black dress. We bust our butts and do whatever we must to get in perfect shape, and then blow it all in one night by going for everything we've been missing. It's all about the entrance. You want to look great for that moment when he, she, or they (whoever you've been dieting for) see you for the first time. Once that moment has passed, you relax and don't stop eating and drinking until the party or holiday is over. You may be thinking, "Oh, big deal! So I gain one or two or ten pounds over the holidays. That will only set me back a few days." Well, I think a few days five to ten times a year *is* a big deal! And it can be a serious setback for your health, your appearance, *and* your career. Even one overindulgent meal does measurable damage to our bodies, especially our arteries. This conclusion was reached after an extensive study conducted in Australia recently. After consuming just *one* meal high in animal fat, around fifty grams, the elasticity of a person's arterial walls and impeding blood flow *drops by 27 percent.* And this lasts for several hours.

It was a pattern for me every Christmas, when I first moved to New York and later Los Angeles, to get in great physical shape before I would go home to Chicago. It was important to me to show that I was doing well on my own in a new city, and I knew I would see old boyfriends, old friends, and my three sisters and two grown-up nieces (you know how female relatives can be). I would arrive and people would see me and say, "Wow! You've lost weight! How'd you do it *this* time?" After that initial presentation was over, it became my personal responsibility to eat my way through Chicago. And for those of you not familiar with that incredible city, Chicago is *made* for eating! The bottom line was I got in great shape so I would look good pigging out.

I was not the only one in my family who got in shape for Christmas. It was funny to observe how everyone worked their tight, hot clothes the first few days, but then the baggier stuff would quickly creep into everybody's wardrobe. By New Year's Day, everyone would be wearing big T-shirts, pajamas, robes, and sweatpants. I always had thin legs no matter how much I overindulged, so I could always wear short skirts or leggings, but my tops would get bigger and puffier as my waistline grew more undefined.

I would return to Los Angeles in January about twelve pounds heavier, but it was not a big deal to me at the time. A recovery period after every holiday was normal. I would always make sure that I had at least one week off from business and major social obligations, because I knew that when I got home, I'd be overweight and constipated and my skin would be broken out. For a week or two I would screen my calls or tell my agent that I had pinkeye or something else until I reached a respectable weight. When it comes to work, it's a shame we can't call in *fat!* We should get seven or eight fat days built into our work schedule per year, and a whole fat week following Christmas.

After many years of research and experimentation, this mentality ended for me, and now it can end for you. On this program you will learn what to eat earlier in the day and what to eat the day after so that your holiday meal will go right though you. There are foods and activities that will keep your body and digestion system functioning most efficiently, and that is the key. It's all about taking out the trash. A little naughty food and drink is not so bad if you rid your body of it quickly and, most important, naturally. As I said, it is building little pockets of discipline into your holiday experience, and that little effort does the trick.

Always keep in mind that health is a total picture. The essence of this book is about celebrating holidays in a healthier way, and that goes much deeper than simply planning what to eat. Food is only one of the elements to consider in planning your holiday. There are many other exciting elements—holiday history, holiday memories, invitations, decorations, toasts, scents, games and activities, calorie-burning exercises, music, movies, party favors, and just about anything else that can spice up a holiday. The idea is to enjoy the holidays the way you did as a child and take some of the attention away from the food. Trust me—it gets far too much attention as it is. It's like George Clooney at a women's yoga class. I keep waiting for him to show up at mine! The point is you never know when someone like George Clooney is going to pop into your day. You've always got to be prepared and look your best. And you can't consistently allow the holidays to set you back and force you into hiding. Let's start a year of healthy holidays together, from New Year's Day to New Year's Eve. I'm sure they'll be the best holidays ever!

# Making Your Holidays Healthier

There is no doubt in my mind that healthy holidays are ultimately the most satisfying and rewarding holidays. I can tell you that they have made a profound difference in *my* family's lives. But what exactly makes a holiday healthy? How do we choose between cranberry sauce and Jell-O, turkey and duck, pecan and pumpkin pie, eggnog and wine? Is animal meat really that bad? What about pastas, cakes, and ice cream? And is it *really* important to exercise on *holidays*? All of this can be confusing, but I'm going to help you sort it out.

# Making Your Holidays Healthier

In the next few pages, I'm going to summarize the essence of this program, which I have been developing for the past twenty-three years, and explain what makes these recipes healthy, or at least healthier than what Americans typically consume during the holidays.

Although the Total Health Makeover program is complex, with lots of variables and subtleties, the core is one very basic principle: *We human beings,* and every other animal for that matter, *should eat the diet our bodies were designed to eat and move our bodies the way they were designed to move.*

Now ideally that would mean living in a lush Garden of Eden (let's call it our THM Utopia) where mealtime would simply involve picking from trees, vines, and gardens stocked with an unlimited variety of fresh, ripe, organic fruits and vegetables full of phytochemicals and dense in nutrients. We would also frequently eat organically grown whole grains and legumes harvested right from the rich soil in our nearby fields. Occasionally we would pull a healthy, vibrant fish right out of the (completely unpolluted) lake or ocean just seconds before preparing it for lunch or dinner and, on very rare occasions, eat a naturally uncaged small mammal or fowl that had never been injected with hormones or antibiotics. And on holidays we would probably enjoy everybody's favorite choices, because holidays have to be *special*! It is essential on holidays for us to look forward to having something we really love and don't have every day.

In our THM Utopia, preservatives, additives, pesticides, processed sugar, caffeine, nicotine, and chemicals don't even exist. Activities involve lots of brisk walks, light jogs, swimming, Pilates, yoga, dancing, tennis, and golf. (Actually this is starting to sound like Sun City.)

Of course, a utopian society like this doesn't exist. We live in the *real* world. But that doesn't mean we shouldn't strive to live as close to this ideal as possible. The saddest fact is that the more "progress" we make in this extremely fast-changing, overly complex, and much too convenient world of ours, the further we get from this idyllic lifestyle. For 99 percent of the last 100,000 years, our *Homo sapiens* ancestors lived much closer to this lifestyle than we do. Don't get me wrong—I'm not looking to trade with them. Some progress has been wonderful. Our ancestors had much more serious problems than we do (starvation, disease, constant danger, and lack of shelter) and, worst of all, no HBO or *Survivor*! But our bodies, which have taken 4.4 million years to evolve, are designed for that Garden of Eden diet and lifestyle, and certainly not the typical fast-food-eatin', crowded, sedentary, corporate cutthroat world that we have been forced to adapt to in an amount of time that is just a fraction of a second relative to our infinite evolutionary timeline.

So how does this philosophy relate to this program? As I mentioned, the essence is to eat, drink, and move in ways that honor the way we humans were designed. Every recipe, beverage, and activity suggested in this book has that goal in mind. And this really can be broken down (for simplification) into two categories: things to *avoid* as much as possible and things to *increase* or *encourage* as much as possible. Let's go back to our THM Utopia for a minute. Notice how everything in the "avoid" list does not exist in our utopia, and everything in the "encourage" list is pretty much the *essence* of our utopia.

| Avoid | Encourage |
|---|---|
| Chemicals | Organic whole foods |
| Caffeine | Water |
| Nicotine | Fruits and vegetables full of phytochemicals |
| Sugar | Legal sweets |
| Meat | Fish, chicken |
| Dairy | Legumes |
| Refined white flour | Natural whole grains |
| Bad fats | Nonhydrogenated natural fats |
| Bloated stomach | Food-combining |
| Inactivity | Exercise |
| Stress | Gusto |
| Erratic sleep | Regular sleep |

Don't get me wrong here. I still want you to enjoy the tastes and pleasures that you associate with the holidays, but now I want you to use whole natural foods and healthier substitutions. You will still be enjoying your holidays because you'll be eating nature's *real* food, and the substitutes for the naughty stuff taste even *better*! And they won't make you sick, bloated, or tired—just satisfied! That is what the recipes in this book are all about—whole real foods and healthy substitutions.

Let's go over each of what I call the health robbers—meat, sugar, and dairy—so you will understand why you should remove them from your holiday meal plan.

## SUGAR

Holidays without sugar? Are you kidding? No Halloween candy, Valentine chocolates, Christmas cookies, or chocolate Easter bunnies? Before you start getting depressed, let me tell you that you will still be able to enjoy ALL your favorite holiday treats, but they just won't be made with the refined, bleached, nutritionless, carbonized, fake-tasting, cooked-in-cow-bones, overly processed white sugar that most people are used to. Americans consume about 136 pounds of refined sugar per person per year, and they really don't have to. All the traditional holiday treats we grew up with can be made with much healthier sweeteners like maple syrup, maple sugar, date sugar, fruit juice, barley malt, raw honey, Sucanat, stevia, Rapidura, raw cane juice, and agave. I call these "legal" sugars. Some are better for you than others, but they are all much healthier than refined white sugar. And I think they taste much better, more real, with more character than refined sugar—especially after you get used to them!

The usual bad rap about refined white sugar is that it adds "empty" calories. I often hear people say, "I don't think sugar is really that bad for you; it's just that it doesn't provide any nutrition." That is *far* from the only problem with sugar. In countless studies, refined sugar has been blamed for hyperactivity, diabetes, hypoglycemia, severe mood swings, decreased brain function, serious digestive problems, yeast infections, obesity, and tooth decay. It depletes your body of all the B vitamins. It leaches calcium from your hair, bones, blood, and teeth, interferes with the absorption of calcium, protein, and other important minerals in the body, and retards the growth of valuable intestinal bacteria. And that's not all! Sugar has a fermenting effect in your stomach. It stops the secretion of gastric juices and inhibits the mouth's ability to digest. (But other than all that, sugar is fine!)

Our bodies have several built-in systems that go into action when we introduce a heavy load of refined sugar into them. Minerals such as sodium, potassium, magnesium, and calcium from our bones are mobilized, and neutral acids are produced in an effort to return the acid-alkaline balance of the blood to a more normal state. Consuming a fairly large amount of sugar each day continuously creates an overly acidic condition, so that more and more minerals are required from within our bodies to create this balance. Eventually so much calcium is robbed from the body, bones, and teeth that decay and weakness result. As I have always maintained, people don't need the calcium from dairy products to strengthen their bones as much as they need to stop eating sugar to avoid the damage it causes to bones.

Brain function is also affected by an excessive consumption of sugar. B vitamins play a key roll in brain function and digestion. Since sugar depletes the B vitamins, calculation, memory, and digestion are all adversely affected by excessive sugar. Notice how difficult it is to concentrate an hour or two after a sugar-loaded treat. I say skip the box of chocolates on Valentine's Day. Don't you want to be extra sharp on Valentine's *night*?

Every single recipe holiday treat in this book (even the chocolate ones) is made with the "legal" sugars I mentioned earlier. All the fun, without all the problems!

## MEAT
### Not Designed for Humans

Humans were meant to be primarily vegetarian. Apes, our closest living relatives from the animal world, are vegetarians. The structure of our skin, teeth, stomach, and bowels and the length of our digestive system are all meant for a vegetarian diet. Somewhere along the way, we overcame our physical limitations and decided to kill other animals for food. Unfortunately, we've become too smart for our own good. Please leave meat for the carnivores. Contrary to what many people believe, we are not carnivores. Our incisors (canine teeth) are not long enough or sharp enough, and our digestive tract is not designed to process meat efficiently.

## Dangerous Process

If you really want the facts about the beef industry, read the book *Mad Cowboy* by Howard Lyman. He tells the story of how he went from owner of a multimillion-dollar cattle ranch business to antibeef activist. You will learn how the practices in the meat industry have gone haywire. Severe competition has forced ranchers to do things to cattle that go way beyond what nature intended: advanced hormone therapy, antibiotic injections, forced feedings, and pesticide sprays.

The concentration of pesticides found in meat is as much as ten times that found in grains, fruits, and vegetables. Chemical and pesticide accumulation in the body is a serious matter. The higher the amount a body consumes and stores, the higher the risk of cancer and liver failure. Cancer growths in animals are much more common than people realize. The butcher cuts them out at the slaughterhouse or supermarket before the meat is sold to the consumer.

Another problem is resistance to drugs. It's become a vicious cycle in the meat industry. Cattle and poultry become more and more immune to the antibiotics and other drugs they are given to control disease, so it becomes necessary to develop even stronger and more dangerous drugs.

Aside from drugs, disease, growths, and cancer (as if that weren't enough!), think about the unsanitary nature of dead animals. When meat is butchered at the slaughterhouse, meat inspectors are forced to work extremely fast. They have only seconds to check inside the dead carcass for grubs, parasites, abscesses, and disease. Meat inspectors must inspect on average three hundred carcasses an hour. That's only seconds per carcass!

The fast-food and meat-packing industries are quite powerful and have great influence on Capitol Hill. That is why efforts to stop the dangerous and questionable practices in both industries are usually thwarted. The Physicians Committee for Responsible Medicine (PCRM) is one group that has been pressuring the U.S. government to make a greater effort to protect its citizens from diseases like mad-cow, hoof-and-mouth, and Creutzfeldt-Jakob disease (CJD), which is the equivalent of mad-cow in humans. The diseases are believed to spread as a result of feeding contaminated meat and bonemeal to uncontaminated animals, as well as through combining contaminated products.

## The Cold Hard Facts About Meat-Eating

Meat eaters, especially red-meat eaters, are three times as likely as vegetarians to suffer from heart disease and breast cancer. Meat eating stresses the liver and kidneys, two important detoxifying organs. It can also deplete calcium, which adds to the risk of osteoporosis, and the uric acid in meat can accumulate in our joints, inflaming arthritis.

People who eat red meat five or more times a week increase their risk for colon cancer by 400 percent compared to people who eat no meat or eat it less than once a month. Women who eat beef, lamb, or pork as a daily staple are two and a half times more likely to develop colon cancer than women who eat meat less than once a month. The substitution of other protein sources such as beans and lentils is known to reduce the risk of colon cancer. Prostate cancer is another risk. Meats are high in animal fat, which is hard for us to digest and therefore stays in our bodies longer.

# Making Your Holidays Healthier

The American meat-eating habit is killing us. "Bad" cholesterol (low-density lipoproteins, or LDLs) in the diet comes exclusively from animal products. Cholesterol-clogged arteries are the main cause of about 50 percent of American deaths from heart disease and strokes. Vegetarians rarely have problems related to cholesterol. As Neal Barnard, M.D., president of the Physicians Committee for Responsible Medicine, said, "The beef industry has contributed to more American deaths than all the wars of this century, all natural disasters, and all automobile accidents combined."

## DAIRY

If you can only give up one item from the "avoid" list, *please* make it dairy products. It will change the way you look and feel and add years to your life. I have been on an antidairy campaign for more than two decades now. You will not find any standard dairy products used in any of these holiday recipes. I use only dairy substitutes made with soy or rice. Why do I feel this way about dairy?

Let's start with milk, since it's the foundation of dairy. We all grew up with this very popular beverage, and many still feel comforted by it. Americans are usually surprised to find out that most people on this planet have never drunk a glass of milk in their entire lives, and if they did, most would get very sick. Since childhood we have been led to believe that milk is a perfect food, but all the most credible studies over the last twenty-five years prove quite the opposite. Dairy products play a major role in the development of heart disease, diabetes, depression, cancer, allergies, sleep disorders, kidney stones, mucus production, hemoglobin loss, mood swings, irritability, and arthritis—even in *children*.

I was never passionate about drinking milk, but I can't say the same about eating cheese. I used to love it, especially Jarlsberg and Brie. In fact, I loved cheese so much that I used to buy "cheese ends" at Zabar's regularly when I first moved to New York. The guy in the cheese department used to put aside select pieces for me the same way people save choice bones for their dog. Years later, a nutritionist suggested (based on my family history and resemblance to Miss Piggy) that I give up dairy completely! (Or perhaps he got a 911 call from the staff at Zabar's.) Anyway, I did give it up, and *everything* changed. My lungs, kidneys, and sinuses began functioning better than at any other time in my life, and I had bone structure I never even knew I had. My Muppet face was gone forever. Unfortunately, less than three months after giving it up (How pathetic! I couldn't go the distance. That's how addicted to dairy I was!) I decided I had to have a night, just *one* shameless, passionate night of pleasure with my love, my hunk, my Jarlsberg! I was too embarrassed to go to my regular cheese dealer, so I went to Zabar's nearby competitor, the Fairway Market. I ate three big bites of it and thought, "Oh my God! This is like eating my shoe!" It was disgusting! The smell was funny (like feet) and the consistency was weird, not at all like the Jarlsberg I remembered. I remember lying in bed that night, writhing with stomach pain, with the smell of Jarlsberg still on my lips and sticky fingers. I made a deal with God that if he'd just let me digest this sludge, I would never eat dairy again! And I didn't have dairy after that until I went to Europe in 1982. (I figured God made exceptions for Italy!) After two of three days of eating cheese, I thought, "This just isn't me anymore. Who do I think I am to be eating like this just because I'm in Europe?"

There are two major problems with dairy:

1) It is not designed for human consumption.
2) The current techniques used to manufacture dairy products (udder to butter, so to speak) are not only appalling, they can be deadly.

## Not for Human Consumption

I'm always telling people that the only thing milk is supposed to do is turn a fifty-pound calf into a three-hundred pound cow in six months. Although it is still common practice, cow's milk should not even be given to infants, let alone adults. Have you ever wondered what the difference is between cow's milk and human breast milk? They are quite different. In fact, the milk of every mammal is unique. Each is perfectly designed to develop its own offspring most efficiently. Cow's milk is much richer in protein than human milk, four times, in fact, and has five to seven times the mineral content. You might be saying, "Great! Even better!" But it is *too much* protein and *too much* mineral content for humans, and it is extremely deficient in the essential fatty acids that are abundant in human milk. Cow's milk is considerably deficient in linolenic acid, and skimmed cow's milk has none. These fatty acids are the building blocks for neurological development and delicate neuromuscular control in humans. It is now fairly well known that breast-fed babies grow up to have IQs an average of 7 points higher than cow's-milk-fed babies.

Cow's milk is designed to build massive skeletal and muscle tissue in a very short amount of time. So if you plan on doing a lot of plowing in your life (and you can't afford a tractor), then by all means drink up. Nature has pretty much given us everything we need to build and sustain our bodies perfectly as long as we stay with the right foods. It's when we veer from the foods nature intended that we get ourselves into trouble. That's what leads to allergies, discomfort, and eventually tissue and organ breakdown and disease. Cow's milk *is* a perfect food, but *only* if you're a *baby calf.* Not only does a baby calf have four stomachs, it also has nine feet of intestines, as opposed to humans, who have twenty-seven feet and only one stomach. Longer intestines are designed for slower, less aggressive digestion. Our digestive enzymes are not capable of breaking down a food that is designed to nurse the offspring of another species. Our stomachs don't even recognize dairy as a food, and everything we eat with it has a difficult time being digested.

## Appalling Practices in the Dairy Industry

That argument alone would be a strong one, even if cow's milk were pure. But it no longer is pure. In fact, it is far from it. The kind of milk we grew up with no longer exists. Fifty years ago the average cow from the top dairy companies produced an average of 2,000 pounds of milk per year. Today the average cow produces about 50,000 pounds per year because of steroid use, hormone therapy, and force-feeding plans. With the added bovine growth hormones, or BGH, there's also a marked increase in mastitis. The BGH tends to enlarge the cow's udders to such an extent that they drag on the ground. The cows frequently step on them, causing severe pinching and bleeding, which leads to mastitis, making antibiotic therapy necessary. So we end up with a product that lacks the fatty acids essential for brain tissue growth and contains a significant amount of growth hormones and antibiotics.

# Making Your Holidays Healthier

There's more. Blood is found in nearly all cow's milk. The USDA actually allows one-thirtieth of an ounce of white blood cells (better known as pus cells) per milliliter of milk. FDA inspectors also maintain very loose standards. They use a detection method that uncovers only two of the thirty or so drugs found in milk. Infections on a cow's udders are common. These require ointments and antibiotics. Penicillin, one of the antibiotics used, is commonly found in samples of cow's milk. Insulin-like growth factor (IGF), found in cow's milk, has been associated with breast, prostate, colon, and lung cancer. Hundreds of studies have confirmed that cow's milk and dairy products are linked to heart disease. In many studies, milk and milk products have been found to have a greater connection to heart disease than even heavy animal meats such as beef and pork. Greenland Eskimos eat a high-fat, high-protein diet yet have a very low incidence of heart disease. This is probably due to the fact that they rarely drink milk.

## Dairy and Saturated Fat

Making butter requires 21.2 pounds of milk for each completed pound of butter. One quart of milk weighs 2.15 pounds. The fat found in dairy products is animal fat, which is high in cholesterol. Whole milk and anything made from whole milk is very high in saturated fat, which can increase your cholesterol level. *Saturated* is a chemical term that means the fat molecule is completely covered with hydrogen atoms. Without those atoms, the fat is unsaturated. Saturated fats stimulate your liver to make more cholesterol. Most animal products contain substantial amounts of saturated fat. Lose dairy, and you'll lose fat.

## The Truth About Calcium in Cow's Milk

Okay, what about all the wonderful things we've heard about milk all our lives, such as that it's a great source of calcium and keeps our bones strong. Well, although millions of dollars are spent every year photographing celebrities with white mustaches proclaiming the virtues of milk, the truth is that the calcium in cow's milk is much coarser than that in human milk, and the human body does not adequately absorb it. Also, all the processing of dairy products reduces the amount of calcium they supply, so it becomes very difficult to use pasteurized, homogenized, or other processed dairy products as a good source of calcium. In fact, cow's milk is so denatured that most of the calcium has been removed and needs to be replaced.

You may as well find a better, less mucus-forming calcium carrier, like calcium-fortified organic orange juice or Original Enriched Rice Dream. The calcium found naturally in food is always better than calcium added in processing, and most of us can get enough calcium through the foods we eat. We don't need to get it from milk, especially if we stop eating sugar, which literally leaches calcium from our bones. Spinach, broccoli, and all other green leafy vegetables contain calcium. Soybeans, tofu, nuts, and sesame seeds are also excellent sources of calcium. So are salmon and sardines. Even concentrated fruits like dates, figs, and prunes offer enough calcium for your body's needs. Cows get their calcium from eating grass in the fields where they graze. They certainly don't get it from eating pizza. Next time you go to drink a glass of milk, think of it as cow breast milk (or better yet, my favorite phrase for it—bovine slime). My slogan on one of my book tours was "Get rid of bovine slime, get rid of bovine butt."

I have been begging people for years to rethink the whole dairy issue. Of the ten steps I took to change my health, I can honestly say that giving up dairy was the most difficult, but it was definitely the step that most improved my health and the health of my family.

## ALCOHOL

It is hard to talk about holiday and party planning without mentioning alcohol. Alcohol and parties seem to go together like chips and salsa. The last thing I want to do in a book about healthy holidays is to encourage the use of alcoholic beverages, but let's be realistic: some people won't even attend a party that threatens to ban alcohol. So I'm suggesting that if you want to include alcohol, you serve it in the most responsible way possible.

All alcoholic beverages have toxins that cause hangovers, but you can lessen their severity by being more selective with your "poison." Some toxins are by-products of fermentation and distillation, which are called *congeners;* and some toxins come from the drink itself, especially from the sugary flavor additives. You reduce the likelihood of a hangover by reducing the toxins, especially the congeners. The more congeners an alcoholic beverage contains, the greater the severity of the hangover. Alcoholic beverages have varying levels of congeners. Cheap spirits, wines, champagnes, and especially dark drinks like whiskey, scotch, bourbon, port, and brandy have lots of congeners, and high-quality (especially light-colored), triple- or quadruple-distilled vodkas and gins have the least. The more rigorous the distillation process, the more congeners are removed. Premium sakes (Japanese rice wines) are also low in congeners.

Sugary drinks are a double whammy. They not only have toxins, they also disguise the alcohol content, leading to excessive consumption and therefore more congeners. Obviously, stay away from mixed drinks with a high sugar content: triple sec, Cointreau (sorry, *Sex and the City* fans, no Cosmopolitans—instead, try my all-natural THM Cosmopolitan), and anything else that's sloe, comfortable, slippery, or screaming.

You may want to consider drinking beer instead of hard liquor or wine. The alcohol content is lower, and the increased volume will make you feel full and perhaps more satisfied. Dark beers have more congeners than lagers, and lite beers have the least. The level of congeners in lite beer is as low as in vodka and gin. The level of congeners in wine is in the middle range; red wine has more congeners than white wine. Cheap booze usually has more congeners than expensive name brands, so a good red wine will probably cause less pain than a cheap white wine.

Tequila is very low in congeners, but it is usually consumed in shots or mixed with cheap, sweet ingredients such as high-fructose-sweetened lime juice or triple sec, so it's likely to give you a hangover anyway. Mixing different types of drinks can also be a problem. This presents different types of congeners to our system, and we have a difficult time processing them.

Encourage your guests to drink two glasses of water for every glass of alcohol, and as a rule of thumb for anyone, no more than two at a time and no more than five a week.

# Making Your Holidays Healthier

## Congener level comparisons:

| | |
|---|---|
| Vodka | ½ |
| Sake | ½ to 1 |
| Beer | ½ to 2 |
| Gin | 1 |
| Wine | 2 to 4 |
| Scotch | 4 |
| Brandy/Rum | 6 |
| Bourbon | 8 |

Now that we have talked about the major holiday health robbers, let's talk about the five easiest ways to make your holiday healthier.

## WATER

Water is essential to life itself. Drinking fresh water frequently and consistently is the key to good health. If you are not hydrating yourself regularly throughout the day, your whole system will not function properly and, over time, will break down. Severe dehydration in just one afternoon can kill a person, even a healthy young adult. Blood carries nutrients, oxygen, and energy to body cells through the bloodstream. It also carries and excretes waste products from the body. It is the transportation and sanitation system of your body. Nutrients, proteins, and waste products cannot get where they need to go without a sufficient amount of water to take them there. You are constantly sweating and urinating and eliminating water, so you must constantly replenish it. Our planet sustains life because of water. It cannot survive without water, and neither can we.

I recommend drinking a daily minimum of eight 8-ounce glasses of water (and water only). Keep in mind that more may be needed depending on your size, how much exercise you've been doing, and how much caffeine, alcohol, and other dehydrating substances you have consumed.

## BETTER-QUALITY FOOD

Just as the severity of a hangover from alcohol will be determined by the quality of your drink, so will your food hangover the day after a holiday binge (or any meal, for that matter) be determined by the quality of your food. Therefore, try to eat fresh, organic, whole foods whenever possible. When people tell me organic is more expensive, I always tell them, "There is nothing more expensive than bad health, especially when you consider sick days, doctor bills, medication, and so on. Besides, organic foods taste better, so you throw less of it away, thereby spending less in the long run. And if we all start buying and demanding better-quality food, the price will go down."

People tend to overeat bad food because their bodies are starving for nutrition and are just not getting it from the poor-quality processed fast and junk foods most people choose. There are millions of people stuffing their faces and literally starving their bodies. By choosing higher-quality, nutrient-dense foods, these same people would end up eating less and satisfying their bodies more. As I always say, "If you improve the quality of your food, the quantity takes care of itself." Read labels to make sure that even the snacks you eat have as few chemicals as possible.

## WETTER FOOD BEFORE, DURING, AND AFTER

As we've already said, holidays are meant for overeating. Quite often you eat certain dishes on that day only, and your taste buds salivate weeks before just thinking about that special Thanksgiving stuffing or Valentine's chocolate or that scrumptious Fourth of July fruit cobbler. You don't have to give up your favorites when pursuing a healthier holiday. You just have to know what to eat with them so that they go right through you. If you've read my first book, *Marilu Henner's Total Health Makeover,* you are probably familiar with the chapter I wrote called "What's the Poop?" It's devoted entirely to the human digestive system, a complicated, intricate, beautifully designed system that works most efficiently, like any other well-oiled machine, when it is fed properly.

We all know about fruits, proteins, and starches, but did you know that food could also be classified into two other main categories—concentrated foods and what I call wet foods? Wet foods are foods like fruits and vegetables that have a high water content and help "move along" the more concentrated foods that most of us eat. Concentrated foods are the heavier, denser proteins, starches, fats, and processed foods that are usually the centerpiece of the meal. Wet foods are usually more yin (expansive), and concentrated foods are more yang (contracted).

If you can begin every day with fresh fruit, you kick-start your metabolism and give yourself a nice wet food base, and you won't believe how much lighter and cleaner you will feel throughout your day. If you make sure you eat some raw fruit and/or vegetables during the day (five servings is the magic number), I guarantee you will lose weight, and your stomach will shrink because it won't be overly taxed with concentrated food.

Plan on serving two or three wet food dishes at every holiday meal. This includes salad and cooked and raw vegetable dishes. Don't overload any of them with heavy dressings and sauces, which are also considered concentrated foods because of their high fat content. Believe me, your body loves a combination of wet and concentrated foods.

You know how a garbage disposal works best if you run the water with it? When you put food in a garbage disposal and turn it on, the food will be chopped up and churned but won't really dissolve and disintegrate efficiently unless you run the water as well. Your stomach works much the same way. The concentrated food you eat will get digested, but not as efficiently as when you also eat wet foods. Don't assume that drinking water with your meals does the job as well. It doesn't. Wet food stimulates the digestive juices, while water dilutes them. If you must drink with your meal, sip rather than gulp.

## FOOD-COMBINING

Proper food-combining as an eating strategy is a wise choice at *every* meal throughout the year, but it is especially smart during the holidays. The principle behind food-combining is to make the most of your digestive chemistry in order to process your food most efficiently. Sounds wonderful, doesn't it? It is! The holidays are a time when we need our digestive system working with maximum precision because there is so much potential for banquet and buffet overload. The beauty of using a food-combining strategy is that you can actually eat *more* because your body is processing all that food so well.

Here's why it works. Food-combining is based on sound physiological principles of digestive chemistry. Some foods are compatible when digested together, and some are not. Not all foods are digested in the same way. Starchy foods require an alkaline digestive environment, which is supplied initially in the mouth by the enzyme ptyalin, and protein foods require an acid environment for digestion (hydrochloric acid). When protein and starches are eaten together, digestion is impaired. The body gets confused and cannot manufacture the necessary enzymes required for proper digestion. Undigested food will just sit in the stomach for hours, rotting. This creates toxins in the bloodstream. Some digestion does take place, but only partially through bacterial action, which causes fermentation that then causes such side effects as gas, bloating, and abdominal pain.

Bacterial digestion creates another serious side effect: poisonous by-products such as ptomaine and leucomaine. Bacterial fermentation of starch can also result in toxic by-products like acetic acid, lactic acid, and carbon dioxide. Proper food-combining helps the body digest enzymatically, which produces essential amino acids that repair and maintain the body. To simplify all this, imagine your stomach as a beaker. When you eat a protein (fish, chicken, meat, eggs, dairy), your mouth sends a signal to the brain to put an acid base in the stomach to digest the protein. When you eat a starch (bread, potatoes, rice, pasta, grains), your mouth sends a different signal to the brain, to send an alkaline base to digest it. But acid and alkaline neutralize each other! When you eat proteins and starches together, everything gets neutralized and nothing (or very little) gets digested. And we derive absolutely nothing from undigested food. In fact, food that is left undigested simply rots in our stomachs. This rotting causes a toxic response by turning into poison and alcohol. We're so used to feeling lousy after a meal (stuffed, bloated, and gassy) that unless we feel that way, we don't feel we've eaten enough.

So what does all this mean? It means you should avoid fish with rice; chicken with potatoes; turkey with stuffing; pasta with chicken, fish, or clams; and turkey, chicken, or fish between two slices of bread (yep, no sandwiches). And you should avoid fruit with vegetables and fruit with proteins. There are a few other combinations to avoid, but you get the idea. Check the chart on page 13 for all the rules.

I know this information must be a little hard to swallow (or should I say *digest*?) because these are the food combinations we've eaten all our lives, but keep in mind that this is only the bad news. The good news is that you can still eat all those wonderful foods; you just shouldn't eat them together. It's really very easy once you get the basics down. Proper food-combining ultimately enhances the nutritional value of well-digested food. It's one of the best ways to keep our body sanitation system working properly, which keeps our weight under control and sets the stage for more overall energy. You will realize how wonderfully food-combining works firsthand once you try it for a while.

# The Basic Rules of Food-Combining

1. Do not eat proteins and starches together. Your body requires an acid base to digest proteins and an alkaline base to digest starches. Both proteins and starches combine well with green, leafy vegetables and nonstarchy vegetables, but they do not combine well with each other.

2. Do not mix fruit with proteins, starches, or any kind of vegetable. Fruits digest so quickly that by the time they reach your stomach, they are already partially digested. If they are combined with other foods, they will rot and ferment. Eat fruit only with other fruit.

3. Melons digest faster than any other food. Therefore you should never eat melons with any other food, including other fruits. Always eat melons by themselves.

4. Do not mix acid and/or subacid fruits with sweet fruits at the same meal. Acid fruits, such as grapefruit, pineapple, and strawberries, can be mixed with subacid fruits, such as apples, grapes, and peaches, but neither of these categories can be mixed with sweet fruits, such as bananas, dates, or raisins.

5. Eat only four to six different fruits or vegetables at one meal.

6. Fats and oils combine with everything (except fruits) but should be used in limited amounts because while they won't inhibit digestion, they will slow it down.

7. Eat legumes like soybeans (edamame) when you improperly combine proteins and starches. Legumes act as a digestive bridge between the two food groups and become a bit of a fix-it device. However, don't rely on this for every meal.

8. Wait the following lengths of time between meals that don't combine:
   a. Two hours after eating fruit.
   b. Three hours after eating starches.
   c. Four hours after eating proteins.

# Making Your Holidays Healthier

CHART 1

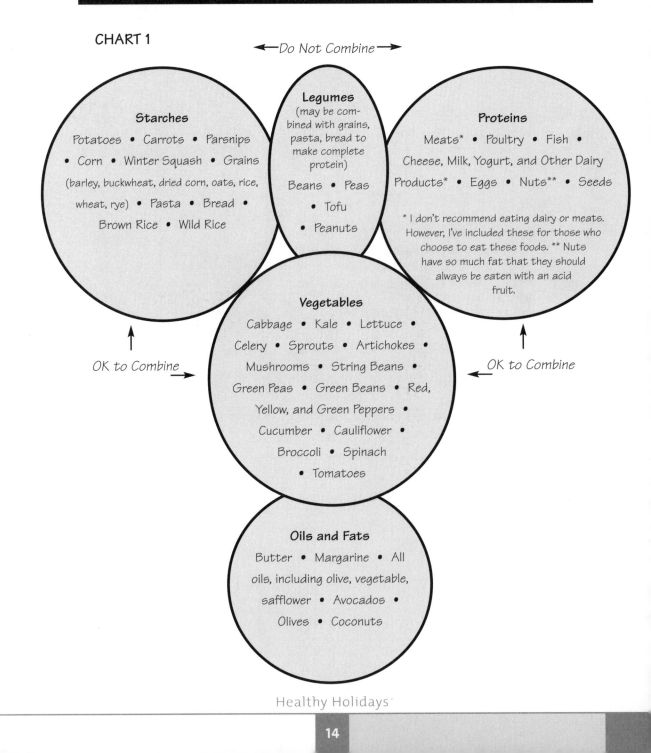

←— Do Not Combine —→

**Starches**

Potatoes • Carrots • Parsnips • Corn • Winter Squash • Grains (barley, buckwheat, dried corn, oats, rice, wheat, rye) • Pasta • Bread • Brown Rice • Wild Rice

**Legumes**
(may be combined with grains, pasta, bread to make complete protein)

Beans • Peas • Tofu • Peanuts

**Proteins**

Meats* • Poultry • Fish • Cheese, Milk, Yogurt, and Other Dairy Products* • Eggs • Nuts** • Seeds

* I don't recommend eating dairy or meats. However, I've included these for those who choose to eat these foods. ** Nuts have so much fat that they should always be eaten with an acid fruit.

**Vegetables**

Cabbage • Kale • Lettuce • Celery • Sprouts • Artichokes • Mushrooms • String Beans • Green Peas • Green Beans • Red, Yellow, and Green Peppers • Cucumber • Cauliflower • Broccoli • Spinach • Tomatoes

OK to Combine →

← OK to Combine

**Oils and Fats**

Butter • Margarine • All oils, including olive, vegetable, safflower • Avocados • Olives • Coconuts

CHART 2

← OK to Combine →

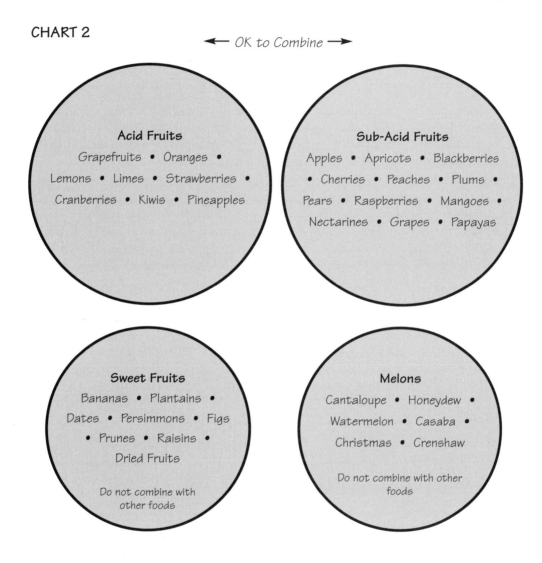

**Acid Fruits**

Grapefruits • Oranges • Lemons • Limes • Strawberries • Cranberries • Kiwis • Pineapples

**Sub-Acid Fruits**

Apples • Apricots • Blackberries • Cherries • Peaches • Plums • Pears • Raspberries • Mangoes • Nectarines • Grapes • Papayas

**Sweet Fruits**

Bananas • Plantains • Dates • Persimmons • Figs • Prunes • Raisins • Dried Fruits

Do not combine with other foods

**Melons**

Cantaloupe • Honeydew • Watermelon • Casaba • Christmas • Crenshaw

Do not combine with other foods

# Making Your Holidays Healthier

## EXERCISE

My THM journey began after my mother died of complications from arthritis in May 1978. By 1987 I had permanently given up meat, sugar, and dairy and had lost a significant amount of weight. (My all-time high was 174.) But there was one key component still missing . . . exercise. Sure, I exercised one or two times a week. But starting the day after Thanksgiving that year, I decided to make the commitment to break a sweat every day for at least ten minutes—and that's when the program finally came together for me. Within three weeks I had finally dropped those last eight pounds that had been stubbornly clinging to my thighs, butt, and cheeks since a parish bake sale I went to in third grade. I hadn't been able to drop those eight little sandbags no matter how disciplined my diet had been. I was thrilled with my new break-through, but I was now nervously facing Christmas and all the fun food I normally looked forward to every year while visiting my family in good old Chi Town. I knew this was going to be a challenge: subzero weather and two thousand miles from my exercise routine. Determined not to let anything stop me, I decided to use every potential exercise opportunity that conveniently came my way. I jogged to the supermarket, ran up and down the stairs at my sister's house, and did squats while watching *It's a Wonderful Life*. I didn't get obsessive with this, mind you; I just did enough to make a difference. It was the first Christmas that I didn't gain weight—in fact, I lost two pounds. I hadn't held back on enjoying the whole holiday, and I was able to go right to work when I got back without my usual postholiday crash diet. In fact, on January 7, 1988, I went to a screening and met the head of a fantastic agency who asked to represent me. I switched agencies and changed my life. That began a consistent working streak that hasn't stopped to this day. I would never go into hiding and allow my career to take a backseat to my backside. Between December 2 and February 11, I lost thirteen pounds, a time when I usually put on ten to fifteen.

There is no doubt in my mind that if you can find convenient little ways to break a sweat every day or at least five times a week, it will make a huge difference in how much weight you put on during a holiday period.

## MAKING YOUR HOLIDAYS SPECIAL

My father always said that there were three elements to every event: anticipation, participation, and recollection. Anticipation is the preparation and buildup, participation is being in the moment and enjoying the event itself, and recollection is talking about it in the days that follow, especially the morning after. Monday morning quarterbacking after an event is a tradition in my family. We love it—talking about the people who were there, how much fun it was, and what we should do or not do the next time. My family ran a dancing school out of our three-car garage, so the house was always full of people. Holidays were a great excuse to either throw a huge party for friends and dance students or to celebrate just within the family. Our family (with six kids and two parents) was big enough to be its own party.

## My Parents Threw the Best Parties

The parties my parents hosted are among the most vivid memories of my childhood. I picture my mom on the dance floor having a great time, partnered, at one time or another, with nearly every person in the room. And I always see my dad off in some corner surrounded by women with their heads thrown back in laughter. My parents were the best guests at their own parties. I learned from their example to be extra prepared as a host so that I could be a fun guest myself.

And I can remember every stage of the three party elements—anticipation, participation, and recollection. The anticipation part was really exciting. The house would be cleaned, shopping lists made, and everyone had the feeling "Oh my gosh, it's just a few days till the Christmas party"—or the Halloween record party—or the Fourth of July Sand-lo Beach party. My mother made list after list for preparation. Throughout my life, I've kept notebooks on everything, and I'm pretty sure I know where I got my obsession for lists and record keeping.

Participation was always a blast! After waiting for so long, the event was upon us and we were ready to throw ourselves into it with full gusto. Every cell was standing at attention and every sense was on fire taking in the event and enjoying it at full throttle. Because I was so mindful of what was happening, the sights and sounds and smells of those holiday events are with me to this day.

My father always said, ". . . and the greatest of these is recollection" when talking about the three parts to every event. No question about it. Rehashing events and reliving them again and again is what makes a memory stay forever. In fact, to this day every one of my five siblings and I can remember our family's holiday parties in such specific detail that you would think they happened last month rather than several decades ago.

My parents always thought "outside the box," which is the key to successful and exciting holidays. That is what I'm hoping to inspire in this book. I am presenting a list of suggestions for every holiday so you can mix and match ideas and create the blend that works best for you.

## Carrying on the Henner Tradition

I have always felt it was my responsibility to carry on the Henner party-hosting tradition with every group I've ever been involved with. Whether it was college dorm life at the University of Chicago, the TV world of *Taxi* and *Evening Shade,* or life on Broadway with *Grease, Chicago,* and *Annie Get Your Gun,* I was there hosting the party. For example, whenever people ask, "What was your experience on *Taxi* like?" I always say, "Let me put it this way: we made a hundred and twelve shows, and we had a hundred and twelve parties." I collected money every week from my castmates and took on the responsibility of working with the caterers, picking the music or hiring a band, arranging tables to make room for the dance floor, and organizing any other activities that I thought would spice things up. I'm a natural at this. (I was the banker in Monopoly, too!)

It was the same story when I played Roxie Hart in *Chicago* on Broadway in 1997 and 1998. My favorite party was when I took the entire company on a boat trip that circled Manhattan. It was wild. It may have been the best party I've ever thrown. After a Sunday matinee, everyone got foxed out and revved up for the party. It was the cast, crew, musicians, everybody—about 180 people on a huge boat three levels high. Once I made sure that everyone had a comfortable place to sit and enough to eat and drink, I got on the dance floor and stayed there until the party was over. We were still partying at four in the morning (after being together nearly sixteen hours) because it was the kind of party you simply didn't want to end. I could barely walk the next day. Thank God we didn't have a show that Monday!

## How to Be a Good Host

### Preparation Is Key

A good host is well prepared, yet spontaneous. That almost sounds like a contradiction, but it's not. It is important to have all your bases covered but to be flexible. Things are going to come up all the time. People will cancel or show up with an extra person, or arrive late not knowing it's a sit-down dinner. Some food may get burned or not turn out right. You have to be good with plan B, because plan B is what usually happens. It is always a good idea to plan creatively and design fun and exciting options that allow you to change course when you need to as the party progresses. Believe me, there is nothing better than a host who can read the room, assess the situation, and go with the flow. One of the best examples of this is the way Billy Crystal hosts the Oscars. He prepares hundreds of jokes beforehand but uses only about 10 to 20 percent, depending on what works best at each moment. He is an extremely talented comedian, but it is his careful preparation that makes him Oscar's best emcee. Also, the more prepared you are, the more you can relax and enjoy the party with your guests. Don't ruin the party by scrambling around at the last minute with a frazzled attitude. A good host enjoys her own party, and guests take their cues from the host. The more relaxed and laissez-faire you are, the more you will communicate that to your guests. Conversely, they will be tense if the host is harried, nervous, upset, or has some kind of drama going on. Guests will feel as though they have walked into someone else's nightmare. They will be thinking, "Well, she really wants me to have a good time so I better appear to enjoy myself even though she's making me feel nervous." That's inhibiting for your guests, because no one wants to feel disconnected. My most successful parties have been the ones I've enjoyed most myself.

### It's Not About You

Try to see the party from your *guest's* point of view. What kind of party would you have a good time at? It's not about impressing your guests and showing off, it's about creating an environment that's conducive to a great time. Always keep this in mind as you organize and decorate. For example, you should not have anything around that is really precious and fragile. It's risky for your valuables and confining for your guests. Just the way you child-proof your home for your kid's safety, you should guest-proof your house for a fun party. It's hard to boogie on down when you're surrounded by Waterford crystal!

### The Bathroom

It goes without saying that you should provide fresh, clean guest towels and fresh soap. Have you ever been in someone's bathroom where the towels were so pristine and so perfectly matched that you chose to dry your hands with toilet paper instead so that you wouldn't spoil anything?

That's okay. It's better to create an environment that's too perfect than one even slightly messy when it comes to the bathroom. I will often supplement the guest towels with some nice-looking disposable paper hand towels. Also, make sure there is an extra roll of toilet paper that is easy for your guests to find. You don't want one of your guests having to cry out for necessities while they're in the middle of their business, or worse, being creative with some of the products under the sink.

Now that we have gone over some of the broader strokes of holiday party celebrations, let's get into the specifics of what you will find in each holiday chapter.

# How to Use
# This Book

As you have already discovered, this book is not just about healthy recipes. Making your holidays healthier involves the total picture for each specific holiday. My goal has been to cover as many bases as possible to create a totally healthy holiday experience.

## LOTS OF OPTIONS

Holiday books usually present one perfectly organized example with every party element and category designed to fit together like an elegant furniture showroom layout at Macy's.

# How to Use This Book

Most of the guesswork has been taken out. The reader only needs to copy the one given party plan seen in the photo and prepare the menu listed. I often look at these lovely books and say to myself, "This sounds great, but I don't know if I like all this food. I only like a few of these dishes." Or "I don't have that kind of layout in my dining room." Or "I don't think this will work well for the group of people I've invited." It's kind of like those mobiles that hang over an infant's crib. Mobiles must maintain a certain balance. If you remove any one piece, the balance is thrown off. With those kinds of books you often think, "Gee, if I leave that dish out, will this meal still work?" If you want to present a precise dinner party or holiday, then those kinds of books are ideal. However, if you want to do most of the choosing yourself, using your own personal style and creativity, then you should find this book helpful.

I want to give you as much information and as many options and varying elements as possible so that you can mix and match and plan your own holiday, taking into consideration your particular surroundings, situation, personality, and style. I don't want to give you a fixed menu with perfectly matched table settings. This book is packed with tons of different categories so you can create your own healthy holiday picture. Using this book should feel like selecting from a buffet table of party options. These samples and options come from things I've done myself, seen at parties I've attended, or found with my research team. And after you've thrown one Valentine's Day party (for example), perhaps next year you'll want to throw a completely different party. You'll be able to do just that using this same book. Think of this as your healthy holiday reference library. The idea is to spark your imagination and be a springboard for finding what you like. You can even mix and match suggestions from various holidays to create your own "perfect" version of any holiday.

## Making Holidays Healthier

Every holiday has its pitfalls that challenge our health and belt buckle, those little land mines that I'll help you avoid. For example, for Valentine's Day it's sugar, for Thanksgiving it's bad food-combining and overeating, and for Saint Patrick's Day it's drinking. Even if you don't use any of my recipes, you will certainly want to read the beginning of each chapter just to be aware of each holiday's warning signs. They will help you be better prepared to make those minor changes that can make an enormous difference in the way you will feel. I've been developing these little "adjustments" since Christmas 1978, the year my sister JoAnn served a huge roast beef with tons of creamy, buttery gravy and Yorkshire pudding. It was the first Christmas after my mother died, and I remember feeling it was time for my family to rethink the way we had been eating, especially during the holidays. It was around the time I started doing research about meat, sugar, and dairy, and the connection to our family's health problems was becoming clear to me.

What you eat and drink earlier in the day and what you eat and drink the following day can help your big holiday meal go through your digestive system faster and more efficiently. As I always say about digestion, something goes in, something gets processed, and something goes out. The more efficiently this works, the better. And this is really the core point of this book: You are not giving up the fun things you look forward to on holidays. You are simply building a few corrective actions right into your holiday routine that can counterbalance anything devilish or excessive that you've consumed. I have tailor-made these "corrective actions" based on the theme of the holiday, what you are likely to eat on that particular holiday, and which season the holiday is in. You will see that pure spring water plays a key role in this section. Think of pure water the same way you think of oxygen and blood. In fact, plentiful consumption of pure water adds oxygen to your blood and over time keeps your blood flowing more freely and efficiently, which significantly helps lower the risk of cardiovascular disease. Drinking large quantities of water is also the best preventive measure to reduce the effects of a hangover. I'm very big on water, and I'll mention it repeatedly in this section, along with other great tips.

## THE CATEGORIES

Now that you know that this book contains an assortment of options, let me go through each category to explain what they mean, what to expect, and how to use them.

## History, Facts, and Folklore

I start each section with the history of the holiday: how it originated and evolved, with a special focus on obscure, cool facts that we didn't necessarily learn in junior high. I have also kept an eye out for historical facts that have a healthy twist, perhaps something our ancestors did that could give us a healthier perspective on how we can appreciate that holiday today. It's a way of getting back to the basics. I'm sure the Pilgrims didn't serve green bean mushroom soup and onion ring casserole at the first Thanksgiving in 1621. In fact, they served berries, watercress, and fish, which is much closer to the THM lifestyle.

## Henner Holiday Traditions and Stories

My family has always embraced the holidays with passion. I want to share with you some of my favorite stories about my growing up and the traditions that have carried over to the present with my own children, along with some new ones that we've started.

## Recipes

There are several recipes per holiday for you to mix and match. They contain no meat, no refined sugar, and no dairy products. They call for pure, natural whole foods when practical and organic ingredients whenever possible. The only animal proteins used are primarily fish, some chicken, and eggs (mostly egg whites).

Every menu will contain a balance of simple wet foods (whole vegetables and fruits) and concentrated foods (fish, chicken, whole grains, and legumes). You can mix and match any of the recipes, but it's best if you check the food combining chart on page 14 for the best food combinations for optimal digestion. For example, when you eat a protein and starch at the same meal, it is important to also add a legume. Legumes will balance your digestive juices and convert the meal into a complete protein for a more efficient use of nutrients. Proper food-combining is one of the best tricks for enjoying the holidays (and the naughty foods that go with it), allowing you digest food quickly and not have that usual bloated feeling after holiday meals. Food combining has kept my weight stable through many holidays in the past twenty years. If you haven't experimented with food combining yet, you'll see what I mean—and love it!

# How to Use This Book

The recipes are all color coded according to the rainbow theory. If you're familiar with my book *The 30-Day Total Health Makeover,* you know that I based the weeks of the program on the colors of the rainbow. The colors refer to the fluctuating cycle a person goes through with their lifestyle habits—from very strict (purple) to extremely indulgent (red). I used only the colors purple, blue, green, and yellow because in orange, you're a party animal, and in red, you're either lying on the floor with drool coming out of your mouth, or you're in Las Vegas (or in Italy, my favorite place to be in red!).

The recipes in this book are color-coded from purple to yellow:

- *Purple:* The recipes are simple, uncomplicated, low-fat, and spa like, and they are perfectly food-combined. They use easily digested ingredients.
- *Blue:* The recipes use simple ingredients but are slightly more complicated than purple. They use some legumes and have a slightly higher fat content.
- *Green:* These recipes feature more complicated ingredients, with some food mis-combinations and a higher fat content than blue.
- *Yellow:* Here you'll find the most complicated ingredients, more food mis-combinations, and a higher fat content than green.

You can find out more in *The 30-Day Total Health Makeover.*

## Party Ideas

I provide several options for every holiday. Just remember to use them as a springboard for your own imagination. Consider that any party can be made large or small; you don't need a big party to do something special for you and your kids.

## Invitations

Invitations are the key to starting your party on the right foot. They set the tone and are your guests' main reference to check and recheck for information, so they *must* be accurate. You don't want a lot of telephone calls back and forth for double-checking. Even if you are having a small dinner party, it's nice to send out some kind of little invitation with the specifics on it.

Invitations should give your guests an idea of what the party will be like, and should definitely grab attention. Make sure they contain the following: what kind of party it's going to be, what the occasion is, whom it's for, where it will be, the date and time, what the guests should bring, precisely whom you are inviting, and—without insulting anyone—who is not invited (like children, extra guests, and so on). For example, you may simply write *Mr. and Mrs. Jones.* By omitting "and family" you are politely letting them know that their children are not invited. Other elements to consider are valet parking (important if you live in Los Angeles) and dress code (*especially* important if you live in Los Angeles). Few things make a guest more uncomfortable than being overdressed or underdressed at a party. If it's business attire, dressy casual, black tie, costume only, lingerie, or toga, they need to know.

One footnote: invitations are also your best shot at campaigning for attendance. One of the best invitations I've ever seen was for my brother Lorin's wedding. It was designed as a children's activity book, with crossword puzzles, mazes, dot-to-dots, and jumbles, and it came with a box of personalized crayons. You had to solve the puzzles to get the who, what, when, and where information for the party. It opened with a maze where you had to move the engagement ring from his hand to his fiancée's finger. Of the 140 people invited, 147 people attended. I think the reason they had more than 100 percent attendance was that the invitation sent the message that this was going to be a really fun event—not to be missed. If Lorin and Lynette ever get divorced, it would be just like them to send out activity books to help them divide their assets.

## Decorations

Decorations create an instant atmosphere and can totally make or break a party. They have the same impact on your guests that a Broadway set has on the audience when the curtain rises. It immediately puts them in the mood and tells them what kind of experience they're going to have. There are endless possibilities here. It's always fun when you walk into a party and have an instantly festive "I'm definitely going to have fun at this party" feeling from the atmosphere. If decorations are done right, the guests know that the host put a lot of time and thought into creating a perfect atmosphere and that they are in the middle of a special event. Decorating your party or table is your opportunity to create an atmosphere that will make your guests feel special.

I went to a forties film noir detective theme party once. Not only were all the guests dressed in that period and style, but the decorations were perfection, with antiques, magazines, and advertisement and movie posters from that period strewn everywhere. And thrown in for good measure were forties-style hatcheck girls with Veronica Lake hairdos handing out penny candy from the large cigar boxes hanging around their necks. Walking into that party felt like stepping back in time. I think people actually behaved differently—they really got lost in the moment. It was fantastic!

Lighting is very important, too. Well-placed candles burning at eye level will put a glow on your guests' faces and make everyone feel good about the way they look. That is why people often pick restaurants more for atmosphere and lighting than for food (especially on a date). And whatever you do, avoid harsh overhead lighting. Nothing will make your guests look more garish and hard (and unhealthy!) than bad overhead fluorescent lighting.

Decorations are also a great opportunity to get children involved in the party. Many times I have put out a craft table full of paint, brushes, crayons, paper, frames, beads, jewels, buttons, feathers, glitter, string, and glue, and the kids have created their own decorations.

Seating is a big deal in Los Angeles. Most big parties are divided by table numbers. People arrive, find out which table number they're at, and then sit—very simple. It's really fun as hostess to plan ahead by arranging, dividing, and mixing different seating combinations to create the best chemistry for couples, kids, singles, snobs, intellectuals, and artists. But even if you are throwing a small party, you can prepare a seating plan. It adds excitement to the party when you are creative and try different themes rather than numbers. When my sister Christal got married, she and her fiancé, Roy, hosted an elegant wedding in France for thirty-two people. Both are bridge champions and, in fact, met playing bridge. Instead of using table numbers, they divided their guests into four tables of bridge suits (spades, hearts, diamonds, and clubs). It was so clever, and no one felt slighted for being at table number four instead of table one. The bridal table was, of course, hearts. I've also been at parties in Los Angeles and New York that did variations on this. I went to one political fund-raiser on forest conservation where the guests were seated at the birch table, the walnut table, the oak table, and so on. So you can always do something like that to add a Hollywood touch to your table seating.

## Scents

Few hosts use holiday potpourri, oils, candles, or other scents to enhance the impact of their parties. This is a sadly missed opportunity. Scents stimulate like music. Together they can be a turbocharged double whammy to the senses, creating an exciting atmosphere and the proper mood. I think people have gotten a little lazy in terms of using all their senses. Think of your healthy holiday as a total experience that incorporates all the senses, not just taste. You can't get fat from seeing, hearing, smelling, or touching—*only tasting*! There are several fragrance style options available, including candles (pillars, votives, candle jars, tea lights, tapers), wax melt burners, room fragrance sprays, light bulb rings with fragrance oil, oil burners, potpourri burners, open bowls of potpourri, and terra cotta oil pots. For every holiday you'll find lots of scented options to play with. Just go to your nearest soap, oil, and candle shop and experiment.

## Toasts

I wanted to include a section on toasts because I have been to far too many parties where I have heard people stumble for what to say. In order for toasts to be exciting, the speaker *must* put some thought into them. It is always better when the toast is specific to the event, as opposed to a generic one taken from a book of toasts. Ideally a toast should focus on what the occasion is all about, personalize that focus, and connect and inspire everyone in some way. In the "toasts" sections for each holiday, I give some examples, but more important, I sometimes give you suggestions to help you create your very own personal and compelling toast.

It is always best to have a specific story in mind when talking about the event or guest of honor. Don't worry if your story is too intimate. I know from being an actress that funnily enough, the more specific and personal you are, the more people will relate. Remember the saying "God is in the details?" It means that the best is the specific. If you follow this rule, your toast will be exciting and original because it will be coming from your heart.

One of my favorite toasts is one that is very popular in show business circles. One person starts and tells a little something about his or her own experience or relationship to the main theme, be it holiday, anniversary, birthday, graduation, or wedding. When he is finished toasting, he then passes it to any person of his choosing who looks eager enough, and that person then says a few words, and so on. Some people won't want to get involved, and that's fine. Guests should never be forced. And remember, as host, that you must step in before this gets boring. I've seen this work really well at anniversary parties (as at *Chicago*'s first anniversary party), but it can work for almost any holiday or party.

## Activities and Games

Whether it's a game of cut-throat charades on Thanksgiving, killer Pictionary at Christmas, or a sudden death winner-take-all Academy Awards pool, my family has always been intense about holiday games and activities. Holiday activities are one of the best ways to take the focus away from the food, plus you may even burn a few calories. As I said earlier, people often do nothing on holidays except make themselves sick with food and alcohol, so why not add activities and games to help burn up the food and stimulate your guests' minds? It's a shame that people rarely play games together anymore. The only games people play are at the computer. Our lives have become so convenient that nobody takes time out to be clever anymore and use a little mental strategy. I think we desperately need to return to real games with real people. For each holiday I give activity suggestions that have something to do with the holiday itself, which will add to your overall appreciation for each holiday.

## Prizes, Gifts, and Party Favors

People love getting little prizes and party favors. I think it goes back to our breakfast cereal and Cracker Jack days. You can make them as simple or as extravagant as you want. You can give prizes out to the people or team that wins the games and/or give them out to everyone as parting gifts. At Nippersink Manor, the summer resort we stayed at every year as kids, they used to give out cheap little three-inch plastic trophies for winning events like ping-pong, shuffleboard, or volleyball. These trophies always became the most coveted souvenir of our stay. Even my father got obsessed with collecting as many little trophies as possible.

My niece Elizabeth had one of the most perfect party favors at her wedding. She placed small, elegant sterling silver picture frames as name cards at each guest's table setting, along with a Polaroid camera on each table for the guests to play with, and voila—instant party favor! Every guest got a beautifully framed souvenir photo of whatever they chose to snap at the wedding. If you buy things like that in bulk, they don't cost much, and you can use something a lot less expensive than sterling silver, even for a wedding. People are just as happy with plastic. It's the fact that they're getting their own little gift that counts. This is really a fun category to plan and presents lots of opportunity for creativity.

Even the jaded Hollywood crowd shares my family's love of party favors. The most coveted prize after an awards show is not the award itself but rather the gift bag that everyone takes home. This is usually a large shopping bag filled with assorted goodies, from shampoos to T-shirts to CDs to gift certificates. Or at the major events, all of the above plus a watch or Filofax or Tivo. I am always amazed at the way women will painstakingly spend time and a lot of money on the perfect evening bag, only to look like a bag lady by the end of the evening.

## Music

Music is even more important for creating the proper mood than decorations. When you turn the corner from Thanksgiving and start playing Christmas music, it immediately gets you into that wonderful Christmas spirit. Why not use music to get in the spirit for *all* your favorite holidays? You don't even have to wait for the party. Listen as you are preparing and planning. The right music can be your theme and the metronome that sets the pace.

Whenever I act in a play, movie, or TV show, I get myself in the mood by listening to music. You can get yourself primed before Valentine's Day, Halloween, or even a Fourth of July picnic. And when it comes to the party itself, music is the perfect tool for instantly putting your guests in the right frame of mind the moment they arrive. During the Michael Jordan era, the Chicago Bulls played their dramatic, pulsating theme music as they introduced the players before games. It would immediately ignite and unite the fans and players. I have no doubt that this ritual was one of the ingredients that led them to six world championships. Nearly every other team has copied this since. Music is also a great catalyst for simply making people move. If you want your guests to dance, make sure you choose music that compels them to get on the dance floor (Motown always works). I have compiled a huge list in the "Music" section for every holiday, so you'll have a lot to choose from.

## Movies

Movies are usually best to watch before rather than during the holiday or party. They're great for getting you in the mood and teaching you a little something about the holiday. This past Fourth of July my sister Christal and I took our four boys to Philadelphia. Before we left, we rented the musical *1776* so that the boys could learn why we celebrate Independence Day in the first place. I had no idea Ben Franklin could sing and dance so well! Anyway, I have listed as many movies as possible to give you more than enough options and to perhaps remind you of films you've seen that you may want to see again. And because it is so easy to get inexpensive DVDs these days, consider giving DVDs as parting gifts. It's a nice touch for someone to leave your Saint Patrick's Day party with a copy of *Ryan's Daughter*. You can also have an assorted basket of DVDs pertaining to the holiday and raffle them off or give them out as prizes for any games that are played at the party. One final note: movies can spark lots of party ideas beforehand, too. They do more than just put you in the mood.

## Exercise and Calorie Chart

Besides eliminating the big three (meat, sugar, and dairy), the single most important factor in a healthy holiday is incorporating some kind of exercise in your day, even if it's just walking around the block, jogging on a treadmill, or playing tag with your kids. The point is to do something physical every day, and *especially* on holidays. Just getting that extra oxygen in your blood and elevating your body temperature makes a huge difference. And exercise does so much for your mental well-being, too. I'm so used to getting that little euphoric boost every day that I actually feel a little less energetic when I *don't* exercise. I'm staying in New York while I write this book, and I start my day with a wonderful jog/walk through Central Park. It's the perfect kick-starter and energy-lifter. Human beings are wonderfully designed animals that need to move and *love* to move. You wouldn't leave your dog inside all day and stuff him full of junk food, yet people think nothing of doing that to themselves every day. In every exercise section, you'll find movement and activity suggestions that are connected with each holiday, along with a chart showing how many calories those holiday activities burn.

## Ethnic Traditions

Other cultures have rich holiday traditions that we may not be familiar with, and that's why I wanted to include them, especially for the most popular holidays. Celebrating holidays like Chinese New Year, Bastille Day, and Cinco de Mayo is a great opportunity to learn about and experience other cultures, but here you'll also learn how familiar holidays like Christmas and New Year's are celebrated in other parts of the world. It's a chance to celebrate in somebody else's shoes for a change. And these other traditions are often healthier than ours, so they're worth exploring for that reason alone.

## For the Kids

Kids are a great inspiration for celebration. One of the things I love most about being a mom is seeing the holidays through my kids' eyes. They view the holidays in a completely different way, and their viewpoint changes every year. This section is full of fun facts, holiday history, party suggestions, games, prizes, and decorations with the focus totally on kids.

## For Couples

This section is devoted to intimate holidays for two. Holidays don't have to be celebrated with lots of people at a party, and all couples, especially those who have been together a long time, are always looking for fun ways to keep that spark alive. You can also celebrate the day before the actual holiday so that you will you have your own time together. Think of it this way—if you can't be naughty with your food, you might as well be naughty with your partner.

# The Holidays

# New Year's Day

If you are like most people, you woke up on New Year's Day and said to yourself, "I am *never* going to do *that* again!" Let me guess. You had a pounding headache, bloated stomach, and a moaning partner in the same condition (hopefully someone you had known more than twenty-four hours). And then, to completely deflate your ego, you got on the scale and the scale said, "*Get off*!" The national average weight gain between Thanksgiving and New Year's is eight pounds. So how did *you* do this year? More important, are you feeling that strong resolve to do something about the state of your self/body/relationship/life? Well then, this is the perfect day to start over—a whole new slate, a whole new you. Why not spend the day renewing your soul and detoxing your body with some of the rejuvenating rebuilding plans I have in store for you, your partner, your family, and your friends?

New Year's Day is the perfect opportunity to start a detox program and begin a journey toward refining your taste buds, but first you have to come down from overdoing it the night before. If you are like most people, you'll be craving savory, salty, concentrated yang food like lox, tomato juice, a Spanish omelet, or bacon, but giving in to those cravings may only prolong the yin/yang cycle. You have most likely been in this mess before, perhaps *last* year on the same day. What can you do to avoid feeling this way ten to twenty more times this year, on the other holidays? You may have a lot of great resolutions that you're determined to keep, but how many did you keep from last year, and how many are just repeats from the last five or ten years that never succeeded?

You know what? It doesn't matter. This is the first day of the rest of your life—and a great time to break that cycle. Just say to yourself, "This is the year it's all going to come together. I'm going to finally get healthy and be the fabulous person I'm meant to be!"

Here are three steps you can take to make your resolutions stick:

1) *Awareness.* Evaluate your past successes and failures. Examine why you were so committed last New Year's, only to find yourself ten pounds heavier and watching videos alone on Valentine's Day. What was it that triggered your giving up?

2) *Discipline.* The first couple of days, you have to force yourself to get that discipline muscle in gear. Most habits take about four days to kick in, whether it's morning exercise or flossing your teeth before bedtime.

3) *Practice.* Be diligent and keep reminding yourself how important this is—until you own it.

And finally, this is not a step, but a recommendation. Choose resolutions that are *attainable.* Don't go for ten resolutions at once. After one fails, the rest usually fall apart, too. Make two or three or even one that you can easily incorporate into your life. Consider making one simple resolution per holiday. By the end of the year, you will be looking and feeling great!

A good checklist for choosing resolutions is the "avoid/encourage" chart in our THM Utopia example on page 3. If you are not sure which resolution to start with, let me choose for you. For New Year's Day, I recommend a new awareness of water. We have already talked about how essential abundant fresh water is for health and well-being, and New Year's Day is a major dehydration day, following the previous evening's activities of drinking alcohol, eating salty foods, and sweaty dancing. Starting today, as one of your New Year's resolutions, I want you to always have water nearby. Create a place for your water bottle, whether it's next to your computer or your bed, on your kitchen table, or any other place that's part of your day. Always buy water in several sizes—gallons, liters, and small bottles—and refill them whenever possible. Small bottles are important so you can carry them anywhere. Make a conscious effort to think about and drink water throughout your day. After a while it will become a natural part of you, and you'll become a more vibrant, hydrated animal. Also, try to drink between meals rather than during, so as not to dilute your digestive juices. And frequently choose high-water-content foods: wet, juicy fruits and vegetables.

## HENNER HOLIDAY TRADITIONS AND STORIES

When I was in first grade, my family became obsessed with an album by the MacGuire Sisters called *The Children's Holiday*. It had eleven songs representing each of the major holidays, from New Year's Day to Christmas. I became a celebrity in my grammar school when I was recruited by the principal to go from classroom to classroom every holiday to teach the appropriate song for the school's assembly. I was the Maria Von Trapp of St. John Berchmans. My first taste of fame, and I was only six!

Those songs so completely scored my childhood that to this day I remember every lyric, although I haven't heard the album in decades. (I'll hear it soon enough, though, because my brother Lorin recently found a copy on eBay! Now all we need is a turntable.)

As a child, I used to love to start my New Year singing the "Happy New Year Song," the first song on the album. My children know most of these songs because I recently taught them at *their* school, too. Maria Von Trapp is back! I taught the Columbus Day, Halloween, Thanksgiving, Christmas, New Year's, Valentine's Day, April Fool's, and Mother's Day songs (pretty much my repertoire from first grade). If you ever get your hands on a copy of this treasured album, hang on to it for dear life, or copy it onto a cassette tape and then start a bidding war on eBay!

## RECIPES
# Miso Soup with Spring Greens

Serves 8 (blue)

2¼ cups dried kombu or other shredded seaweed (about 1 ounce)

1 cup yellow miso (soybean paste)

1 teaspoon olive oil

2¼ cups peeled, shredded organic daikon radish or sliced radishes

⅓ cup shredded carrot

4 tablespoons chopped organic green onions, white parts only

2 bunches organic watercress, trimmed

4 tablespoons chopped green onion tops

In a large saucepan over medium-high heat, combine the kombu and 8 cups water; bring to a boil. Reduce the heat and simmer 1 minute. Drain in a colander over a bowl, reserving the liquid. Discard the kombu. In a small bowl, combine ¼ cup of the reserved liquid and the miso, stirring with a whisk. In a large sauté pan over medium heat, heat the oil. Add the daikon, carrot, and onion whites; cook 3 minutes, or until the daikon and carrot are tender. Add the miso mixture and bring to a boil. Reduce the heat and simmer 5 minutes. Add the watercress and cook 1 minute, just until wilted. Sprinkle with the green onion tops. Serve hot.

New Year's Day

## Sautéed Bok Choy and Cucumber

Serves 6    (purple)

- 2 6-inch organic English cucumbers, peeled
- 2 6-inch heads organic baby bok choy
- 2 teaspoons olive oil
- 1/4 teaspoon ground pepper
- 3 tablespoons chopped organic dill

Halve the cucumbers lengthwise and scoop out the seeds. Cut the cucumbers crosswise into 1/2-inch-thick pieces. Slice the heads of the bok choy—leaves, stems, and all—crosswise into 1/2-inch-thick pieces. Coat a large frying pan with nonstick cooking spray. Place over medium-high heat and add the olive oil. When the oil is hot, add the cucumbers and pepper and sauté 5 to 7 minutes, or until the cucumbers are slightly soft on the outside and still crunchy on the inside. Turn the heat to high and add 1/4 cup water and bok choy. Continue cooking for 2 to 3 minutes, stirring and tossing a few times, until the bok choy is wilted and tender and most of the liquid has evaporated. Stir in the dill and pepper.

## Asian Greens   Serves 4    (blue)

- 4 tablespoons light sesame oil
- 3 tablespoons white hulled sesame seeds
- 1/2 teaspoon red pepper flakes
- 4 teaspoons peeled, minced organic gingerroot
- 2 organic garlic cloves, minced
- 2 pounds tender organic Asian greens (baby bok choy, watercress, or tatsoi), coarsely chopped
- 2 tablespoons naturally brewed soy sauce
- 4 teaspoons rice vinegar

In a wide, heavy sauté pan or wok, warm the oil over medium heat. Add the sesame seeds and pepper flakes and stir until the seeds pop and become fragrant, about 2 or 3 minutes. Add the ginger and garlic and sauté for 1 minute. Add the greens and 1 tablespoon soy sauce, raise the heat to high, and cook 1 minute. Uncover and sauté for 1 to 2 minutes more, until the greens are tender. Stir in the remaining 1 tablespoon soy sauce and the vinegar. Serve immediately.

# Crunchy Salad with Sesame Vinaigrette

Serves 4    (blue/green)

1 cup shredded organic purple cabbage

1 cup shredded organic green cabbage

½ cup shredded organic daikon radishes

2 cups shredded organic carrots

1 cup organic sunflower sprouts

1 cup organic pea shoots

3 tablespoons organic mint leaves

¼ cup rice vinegar

1 tablespoon honey

¼ cup sesame oil

2 tablespoons walnut oil

2 tablespoons canola oil

Kosher salt

Freshly ground black pepper

1 tablespoon boiling water

2½ tablespoons sesame seeds

In a large salad bowl, combine the cabbages, radishes, carrots, sprouts, pea shoots, and mint leaves and toss thoroughly. To make the sesame vinaigrette, in the bowl of a small food processor, place the vinegar, honey, oils, and salt and pepper to taste and blend for 30 seconds. Add the boiling water and process for an additional 10 to 15 seconds. Sprinkle in the sesame seeds. (The vinaigrette will keep in the refrigerator for a week.) Toss 4 tablespoons of the vinaigrette with the salad and serve.

## Japanese Chicken Salad Serves 5 (green)

2 organic chicken bouillon cubes

1 pound skinless, boneless chicken breasts

1 2-inch piece organic ginger, peeled and
   sliced

¼ cup Sucanat

¼ cup white wine vinegar

2 teaspoons vegetable oil

¼ teaspoon salt

¼ teaspoon black pepper

12 cups torn organic romaine lettuce

½ cup chow mein noodles

⅓ cup sliced organic green onions

¼ cup toasted sliced almonds

2 tablespoons toasted organic sesame seeds

In a large, heavy saucepan over medium-high heat, combine 2 cups water and the bouillon cubes and stir until the cubes dissolve. Add the chicken and ginger and bring to a boil. Reduce the heat to low and simmer 20 minutes, or until the chicken is cooked through. Cool the chicken in the broth; discard the broth. Shred the chicken with two forks. In a small mixing bowl, whisk the Sucanat, vinegar, oil, salt, and pepper. In a large bowl, combine the lettuce, noodles, onions, almonds, and sesame seeds. Add the chicken and dressing, tossing to coat. Serve immediately.

## Chanterelle and Shiitake Frittata

Serves 4 (purple/blue)

9 organic egg whites

3 organic eggs

½ cup organic chanterelles, cleaned and
   chopped

½ cup organic shiitake mushrooms, cleaned
   and chopped

Kosher salt

Freshly ground black pepper

¼ cup small, whole organic sage leaves

2 cups organic mixed greens, trimmed,
   washed, and dried

Preheat the oven to 375°F.
   In a large bowl, whisk the egg whites until frothy. In another large bowl, whisk the eggs until foamy. Fold the egg whites into the eggs. Add the chanterelles and shiitake mushrooms and season to taste with salt and pepper. Coat a nonstick ovenproof skillet with cooking spray and heat over a medium flame. Add the egg mixture, sprinkle the sage leaves on top, and cook for about 4 minutes, or until the edges are set. Transfer to the oven and cook for 4 to 6 minutes, until set and golden. Cut into wedges and serve over the mixed greens.

# Asian Grilled Salmon  Serves 8  (purple/blue)

*MaryAnn Hennings*

- 8 tablespoons olive oil, plus more to coat the grilling rack
- 4 pounds salmon, boned, skin on
- 4 tablespoons Dijon-style mustard
- 6 tablespoons tamari sauce
- 2 to 3 garlic cloves minced

Light the grill and brush the grilling rack with oil to keep the salmon from sticking. While the grill is heating, lay the salmon skin-side down on a cutting board and cut it crosswise into 8 equal pieces. In a small bowl, whisk together the mustard, tamari, 8 tablespoons olive oil, and the garlic. Drizzle half the marinade onto the salmon and set aside for 10 minutes.

Place the salmon skin-side down on the hot grill; discard the marinade the fish was sitting in. Grill for 4 to 5 minutes, depending on the thickness of the fish. Turn carefully with a wide spatula and grill for another 4 to 5 minutes. The salmon will be slightly raw in the center; it will keep cooking as it sits. Transfer the fish to a flat plate, skin-side down, and spoon the reserved marinade on top. Allow the fish to rest for 10 minutes. Remove the skin and serve warm, at room temperature, or chilled.

# Broiled Salmon Sandwich with Wasabi Mayonnaise  Serves 4  (green)

- 1 1-pound salmon fillet, skinned
- ¼ teaspoon salt
- ¼ teaspoon black pepper
- ½ teaspoon wasabi powder
- ⅓ cup Vegenaise
- 3 organic scallions, minced, white and green parts
- 1 teaspoon low-sodium tamari sauce
- ¼ teaspoon dark sesame oil
- 4 leaves organic curly lettuce
- 8 1-ounce slices multigrain bread

Preheat the broiler. Sprinkle the fish with the salt and pepper. Place the fish on a broiler pan coated with cooking spray and broil 4 minutes on each side, or until the fish flakes easily when tested with a fork. Cut the fish into 1-inch pieces. Cool.

In a small bowl, combine the wasabi and ½ teaspoon water. Add the Vegenaise, scallions, tamari, and oil and stir to combine. Add the fish and toss gently. Arrange a lettuce leaf over each of 4 bread slices. Divide the fish mixture evenly over the lettuce and top with the remaining bread slices.

## Tuna Steaks with Wasabi Whip

Serves 6 (blue)

*MaryAnn Hennings*

¼ cup dark sesame oil

½ cup vegetable oil

¼ cup rice vinegar

2 tablespoons sweet vermouth

1 tablespoon maple sugar

¼ cup tamari sauce

2 tablespoons chopped fresh ginger

3 garlic cloves, minced

3 to 3½ pounds tuna steaks, about
  1½ inches thick

8 tablespoons unsalted soy margarine

1½ teaspoons green wasabi paste

3 tablespoons chopped fresh cilantro

At least 4 hours before you plan to grill the tuna, in a small bowl, whisk together the oils, vinegar, vermouth, maple sugar, and tamari. Stir in the ginger and garlic. Lay the tuna steaks in a shallow bowl and pour the marinade on top. Cover and marinate in the refrigerator at least 4 hours, turning the fish occasionally.

Meanwhile, prepare the wasabi whip. In a small bowl, beat the margarine and wasabi paste together until creamy. Beat in the cilantro until well blended. Store in a cool place, but let come to room temperature before serving.

Prepare the grill. When hot, remove the tuna steaks from the marinade and grill them a few inches from the heat just until cooked through, 5 to 6 minutes on each side. As the tuna cooks, baste it with some of the marinade to keep it moist. When the tuna is cooked, cut it into serving portions and top each serving with a heaping tablespoon of the wasabi whip.

## Sautéed Asparagus with Shallots

Serves 8 (purple)

2 pounds organic asparagus spears, cleaned
  and trimmed

2 tablespoons soy margarine

3 tablespoons chopped organic shallots

1 tablespoon organic lemon zest

Salt and pepper

Bring a large pan of water to a boil over high heat. Blanch the asparagus for 2 to 3 minutes, or until bright green and just tender. Remove from the water and plunge into ice water; drain and set aside. In a large skillet over medium heat, melt the margarine. Add the shallots and sauté for 3 to 4 minutes, or until the shallots soften. Add the asparagus and lemon zest and sauté until the asparagus is tender. Season to taste with salt and pepper.

## BEVERAGES

- Cucumber water (slices of cucumber in natural spring water—a great refresher)
- Lemon-orange water (slices of lemon and orange in natural spring water—a great cleanser)
- Pineapple-ginger tea (slices of pineapple and ginger in Red Zinger tea—a great energizer)
- Mint tea (a great cure for your ailing stomach)

## HEALTHY HOT TODDY

A great soother.

2 ounces R.W. Knudsen's unsweetened Cider and Spice (or similar all-natural product)

Pour the Cider and Spice into a coffee mug. Add 4 ounces boiling water and garnish with a cinnamon stick (optional).

## THM VIRGIN MARY

There's nothing better for a hangover caused by alcohol (yin) than a Virgin Bloody Mary (very yang). Just don't get cocky and add the hair of the dog.

4 ounces R. W. Knudsen's Very Veggie

1/2 ounce organic natural lemon juice

2 dashes or 1/8 teaspoon Tabasco sauce

Pinch of black pepper

1/4 teaspoon horseradish

Sea salt to taste

Pour all the ingredients over ice in a highball glass. Garnish with a celery stick or lime wedge.

# New Year's Day

## Party Ideas

- 3 A.M. "After Party" party—after everyone celebrates their New Year's Eve, why not have a healthy breakfast to bring everyone back to reality?
- "Morning After" party in the afternoon—to help your friends regroup and recover while they watch the bowl game

Or best of all, start your year with a:

- Spa detox day—you can even find a sponsor/buddy to help you start your year off on the right foot:
  - —Start the party with a yoga class.
  - —Have each guest bring a robe, and give out slippers and a headband as party favors.
  - —Set up a buffet table with different cleansing drinks.
  - —In a quiet room a masseuse/masseur can take each guest in rotation.
  - —In the kitchen set up two pots of boiling water, one with chamomile (to detoxify) and the other with rosemary (to soothe). Depending on your guests' needs, have them place their face over one of the pots, draping a towel over their head to hold in the steam. Then lay out three or four facial concoctions in small sake cups, along with a cup of wooden application sticks.

## Invitations

Calendars start on January 1, so this is the perfect opportunity to use them as invitations:

- Small black day planner, with the first page as the invitation and details of your party on January 1
- Desk calendar with first date circled and information written on first page
- Specialty calendar specific to your guest—i.e., animal lover, Simpsons fanatic, *Sports Illustrated* expert

Or if you really know your crowd:

- An invitation/hangover kit—containing vitamin B, EmergenC, a water bottle, a miso soup packet, an eye mask, and ear plugs.

## Decorations

Fill bowls with flowers, candles, and crystals. Display a clear glass pitcher of cucumber water. Toss around plenty of pillows, play New Age music, and let wind chimes welcome your guests.

## Scents

Use fresh, clean winter scents like:

Wintergreen
Peppermint
Eucalyptus

## BEAUTY RECIPES FOR A SPA PARTY

### Hair

**Hair conditioner**—1 egg yolk, 1 teaspoon baby oil, 1 cup water. Beat the egg, add the oil, and beat again. Mix in the water. Massage into the scalp and hair, then rinse well.

**Hair tonic**—2 egg yolks, 2 teaspoons gin. Beat the eggs until fluffy, add the gin, and beat until foamy. Massage into the scalp. Rinse with warm water.

**Deep hair conditioner**—Mix together ½ avocado and 1 small jar real mayonnaise. Apply to hair and cover with plastic or plastic shower cap. Wait 20 minutes, then rinse well.

### Masks/Scrubs

**Dry skin**—Mix together 1 egg yolk, 1 tablespoon honey, ½ teaspoon olive oil, and 1 tablespoon yogurt. Cleanse the skin thoroughly, apply, wait 5 minutes, and rinse.

**Oily skin**—Mix together 1 egg yolk, 1 tablespoon dry clay (or earth mud, available at health food stores), and ¼ mashed avocado. Add a little witch hazel. Apply. When dry, rinse with warm water.

**Cornmeal/chamomile scrub**—Mix cornmeal and cool chamomile tea into a paste and apply in light circular motions. Rinse with warm water.

**Blackhead treatment**—Mix together equal parts baking soda and water. Rub on gently and rinse with water.

**Almond scrub**—Grind 1 tablespoon almonds into a meal and mix with 1 tablespoon honey and 1egg white. Apply and let set for 15 minutes. Gently wipe with warm cloth.

## ACTIVITIES AND GAMES

New Year's Day is a great time to have a tarot card reading, throw the runes, have your tea leaves read, or see a psychic. Or if you want to be your own psychic, play:

- The Prediction Game: Have each person write out three predictions for the coming year: one for him- or herself, one for someone else in the room, and one for the world. Plan to get together the following year to compare results.
- The Resolution Game: Have each person write out his or her New Year's resolutions. Put them in a bowl, and have each person guess which person belongs to each resolution.
- The Hot Seat: For very close—and willing—friends. Have everyone at the party write a resolution for every other person. Each person takes a turn in the "hot seat," everyone else votes on a resolution for that person, and he or she must follow the winning resolution for a month.

## PRIZES, GIFTS, AND PARTY FAVORS

We all need new things at the beginning of the year, so depending on your crowd, present them with: a gift certificate for a yoga or Pilates class or a massage; a journal; a calendar; new toothbrush and floss; various sized batteries (for fire alarm, remote control, digital scale, and so on) to energize their year; sage to purify their home; or the hangover kit, if you haven't already used it as an invitation, and add an umeboshi plum to really do the job. The Japanese use these salt plums to neutralize and balance the body.

If you are throwing a spa party, give a robe or slippers or a headband; you can even embroider a small workout towel with the date.

## MUSIC

| | | |
|---|---|---|
| *Every Day Is a New Day* | Diana Ross | Album |
| *Brand New Day* | Sting | Album |
| *A New Day Has Come* | Celine Dion | Album |
| *New Day Dawning* | Wynona Judd | Album |
| *January* | George Winston | Album |
| *Something for Everyone* | Baz Luhrman | Album |
| *Everybody Wear Sunscreen* | Baz Luhrman | Album |
| *"New Year's Day"* | U2 | Song |

## MOVIES

| | |
|---|---|
| *New Year's Day* | (1989–R) |
| *2001: A Space Odyssey* | (1968–G) |
| *All That Jazz* | (1979–R) |
| *History of the World Part One* | (1981–R) |

# Toasts

May we all live to be a hundred years, with one extra year to repent.
—ANONYMOUS

A man's health can be judged by which he takes two at a time—pills or stairs.
—JOAN WELSH

Here's a toast to the future,

A sigh for the past;

We can love and remember,

And hope to the last;

And for all the base lies

That the almanacs hold,

While there's love in the heart,

We can never grow old.
—ANONYMOUS

## EXERCISE AND CALORIE CHART

It's best to start your year with a flexible body, a flexible mind, and a flexible spirit. That is why I recommend the following for New Year's Day:

| Activity | Calories Burned/Hour |
|---|---|
| Stretch class | 170 |
| Yoga | 336 |
| Pilates | 378 |
| Walking | 176 |
| Cleaning house | 246 |
| Watching Rose Bowl Parade | 77 |

## ETHNIC TRADITIONS

In many countries, traditional foods are eaten on New Year's Day to bring good luck the rest of the year.

- The Netherlands—hot spiced wine with apple fritters or doughnuts
- Germany—white cabbage, to symbolize silver money
- Switzerland—whipped cream, to symbolize fatness and riches

New Year's Day

- India—newly harvested foods, such as new rice
- Bulgaria—cakes with holes in the center, to represent life's circle
- Armenia—fruit and candles, for food and light

## FOR THE KIDS

New Year's Day is the perfect opportunity to teach your child how to start a new year off in the right way.

- Start a "Slam Book" for your child. Get a notebook or journal or diary. On each day of the year, ask a question, from "What is your favorite color?" to "How do you feel today?" to "What does this day mean to you?" and have your child answer it in his own words. If he can write it himself, great. If you must write the answer for him, do not coax or edit but write exactly what he says, exactly as he says it. You will be surprised years from now when you read his answers and know they were truly his and not yours. I have done this with my children, and I am amazed at how a three-year-old's comments foreshadow those of the eight-year-old he becomes.
- Make a kid's resolution chart. Talk to your children about what they think they can resolve to do every day, and give them a check mark every time they live up to it. At the end of the month, they can get a privilege or points or whatever you like—as long as it's *not* food. Rewarding with food is one of the worst things you can do to your child's natural appetite.

## FOR COUPLES

New Year's Day is a perfect time to take stock of what is important and discard what is holding you back. Therefore, when examining your relationship, it may be beneficial to do the following:

- Make New Year's resolutions that improve not only you but also your relationship:
  - —Listen better to your partner.
  - —Get off the line when your partner calls.
  - —Be more tolerant of your partner's family.
  - —Be more tolerant of your partner's friends.
  - —Be patient with your partner's faults, and remember the good things first.
- Make resolutions for each other, and follow them for one week to see if they will stick.
- Live up to your own resolutions.

# Super Bowl Sunday

Six percent of Americans will call in sick the day after Super Bowl Sunday.
—*Dayton Daily News*

The Super Bowl is the number one home party event of the year, surpassing even New Year's Eve. If you're hosting the party yourself, you can serve a lot of healthy options, like the recipes in this book. They're tasty, healthier versions of standard Super Bowl dishes and are sure to please even the most polluted palates. But what if you attend someone else's party and they serve nothing but junk foods like nachos and Cheese Whiz, burgers and fries, and buffalo wings? Can you enjoy the holiday and stay healthy when your healthiest option is guacamole? The trick is to make a plan beforehand and stick to it. There are several things that work in this situation, but the one I want to focus on most is *food-combining*. (See "Food-Combining," page 11, for more information.)

When you food-combine, your food gets broken down more efficiently, and therefore you can splurge a little more. Before eating, decide whether you're going for a protein meal or a starch meal during the party. Remember that vegetables go with both groups, and fruits go with neither. Let me give you an example. Before putting anything on your plate, take a quick inventory of all the food at the party and mentally divide it into three categories: starches, proteins, and foods you won't eat no matter what—heavy meats, sugar, dairy, and foods loaded with chemicals. Let's say, for example, that the buffet table has turkey, bread, cheeseburgers, chicken wings, shrimp with cocktail sauce, chips and dip, guacamole, salsa, crudités, lettuce salad, pasta salad, creamed spinach, potato salad, popcorn, chocolate and other kinds of candy, and at the bar you see beer, wine, and vodka.

Right off the bat, you're better off nixing the cheeseburgers, cheese dip, creamed spinach, chocolate, and candy, and if you really want to improve your health, I would dump the chicken wings, too—lots of bad fat and usually filled with chemicals. If you decide to go the protein route, you can have the turkey, shrimp cocktail with sauce, and all the crudités dipped in guacamole, salsa, or dressing, as long as you don't overdo the fatty choices.

If you choose to go the starch route, you can have bread, pasta salad, potato salad, chips and salsa, guacamole, and all the crudités you want. I would go easy on all the chips, even though they fit in this category, unless they are Guiltless Gourmet or something comparable that contains no hydrogenated oils. For beverages, water is always the best choice. But if you want alcohol, beer or vodka combine better with starches than proteins because they are made from starches (barley and corn), and always drink water in addition to whatever you are drinking.

Those are the basics of food-combining, but it can get more complicated. For instance, if you've crossed that line and had both starches and proteins at a meal (as most people do), you can add a legume such as beans, peas, peanuts, or even steamed soybeans (edamame) to make a complete protein and connect the two food types. Legumes act as a bridge for your digestive juices. A combination of proteins and starches can be digested more efficiently when a legume is added to the mix. Legumes act as a sort of first-aid kit for some bad food combinations. Try food-combining this Super Bowl Sunday and continue doing it for a while. I have been doing it for twenty-three years now, and I love it. It may change the way you eat at parties—or at every meal, for that matter.

Another digestion trick is to limit your choices to just five items, and one of those choices must be a raw whole food like crudités. Or eat many choices, but limit yourself to smaller portions. Or eat whatever you want (avoiding heavy meats, sugar, dairy, and chemicals, as much as possible), but only after you've done a serious workout earlier in the day. It's all about picking a plan and then sticking with that plan. Since Super Bowl Sunday is such a junk food holiday, you really shouldn't go in with no game plan at all. If you do, you are sure to be on the losing team. Leave that to the Minnesota Vikings. In case you don't know, they're 0–4 in the Super Bowl. I'm sure they never properly food-combine.

## HISTORY, FACTS, AND FOLKLORE

The Super Bowl started after the two football leagues, the original NFL (now NFC) and the newer AFL (now AFC) merged in 1966. When Kansas City Chiefs owner Lamar Hunt formed the American Football League in 1960, many thought the idea of a new conference was so crazy that they referred to it as the "Foolish Club."

As it turns out, the American Football League has had a profound effect on pro football. The merger between the two leagues was announced on June 8, 1966, and that's what led to the first Super Bowl in 1967, in which the Green Bay Packers of the NFL beat the Kansas City Chiefs of the AFL 35–10.

The term Super Bowl was not used until 1969. In fact, tickets and programs from Super Bowls I and II from 1967 and 1968 say *The AFL and NFL World Championship Game.* Lamar Hunt coined the phrase after his kid's popular toy *Superball. Super* because it was the battle of champions, and *bowl* from college championships. After 1969, the name Super Bowl stuck for good.

## RECIPES

"Super Bowl Sunday is the second largest day of food consumption, behind only Thanksgiving."—AMERICAN INSTITUTE OF FOOD DISTRIBUTION

# Roasted Nuts Serves 8 (green)

2 cups mixed organic unsalted nuts
  (almonds, cashews, pecans)
1 tablespoon peanut oil or light olive oil
Sea salt to taste

Preheat the oven to 450°F.
Toss all the ingredients in a medium bowl. Spread out evenly on a cookie sheet and bake until slightly browned, about 10 minutes, stirring occasionally.

# Vegetable Dip Serves 8 (blue/green)

1 organic cucumber, peeled
1 organic scallion, minced
1 tablespoon minced organic fresh dill
  weed
1 cup soy sour cream
Salt and pepper

Slice the cucumber in half lengthwise, scoop out the seeds, and mince the cucumber. In a medium bowl, mix the minced cucumber and scallion with the dill, sour cream, and salt and pepper. Adjust the seasoning to taste. Cover and refrigerate.

## Onion Dip Serves 8 (blue/green)

1 organic scallion, minced

½ cup finely minced organic white onions

¼ cup minced organic parsley

1 cup soy cream cheese

In a medium bowl, mix all the ingredients together. Cover and refrigerate. Serve with fresh vegetables or potato chips.

## Potato Skins with Cheese and Bacon

Serves 6 (yellow with turkey bacon/green with Fakin' Bacon)

4 medium baking potatoes (about 2 pounds)

¾ cup grated soy Cheddar cheese
   (3 ounces)

¼ cup soy sour cream

4 slices cooked, crumbled turkey bacon
   or [¼ cup Fakin' Bacon bacon bits]

1 tablespoon minced fresh organic chives

Preheat the oven to 425°F.
   Bake the potatoes for 1 hour, or until done. Cool slightly. Cut each potato in half lengthwise and scoop out the potato pulp, leaving a ¼-inch-thick shell. Place the potato shells on a baking sheet. Spray the inside of the shells with cooking spray and bake for another 8 to 10 minutes, or until the potatoes are crisp. Add the soy cheese and bake another 5 minutes to melt the cheese. Add a dollop of soy sour cream to each potato, sprinkle with the bacon and chives, and serve.

## Sweet Pea Guacamole

Serves 6 (purple/blue)

1 1-pound bag frozen peas

½ large avocado, peeled, seeded,
   and cut into chunks

1 teaspoon fresh lime juice

¼ cup chopped fresh cilantro leaves
   (optional)

Salt and pepper

Fill a medium saucepan halfway with water and add the peas. Bring to a boil over high heat and simmer for 3 to 5 minutes, or until the peas are soft. Drain and set aside. In a food processor, add the peas and process until smooth. Add the avocado chunks and process until smooth. Add the lime juice, cilantro (if using), and salt and pepper to taste and process a few more seconds until smooth. Chill for 1 to 2 hours and serve with chips.

# A Super Bowl of Chili  Serves 6  (green)

1 teaspoon olive oil

1 Spanish onion, chopped

4 garlic cloves, chopped

1¼ pounds ground lean free-range turkey or
  Gimme Lean soy protein

2 tablespoons chili powder

2 tablespoons dried oregano

1 teaspoon ground cumin

1 cup vegetable broth or stock

1 28-ounce can crushed tomatoes

2 16-ounce cans dark red kidney beans,
  drained and rinsed

1 bay leaf

2 tablespoons Bragg's Liquid Aminos

Salt and pepper

In a large stockpot over medium-low heat, heat the oil. Add the onion and garlic and cook until golden, about 3 to 5 minutes. Add the turkey, chili powder, oregano, and cumin and cook until the turkey meat is white, about 10 minutes. Using a spoon, remove any excess fat from the pan. Add the vegetable broth or stock and simmer for about 1 hour, or until the turkey meat is tender. Add the tomatoes, beans, and bay leaf and cook for 20 to 30 minutes, or until the beans have softened a bit. Add the Bragg's and salt and pepper to taste, remove the bay leaf, and serve.

Fans spend more than $50 million on food during the four days of the Super Bowl weekend, Thursday through Sunday.— *Dayton Daily News*

A San Diego State University professor of telecommunications calculated that a four-hour Super Bowl telecast contains less than 10 minutes of football action. — *Dayton Daily News*

## Safety Lasagna  Serves 6 to 8  (blue/green)

*MICHEL°LE FLANAGAN*

- 1 pound firm tofu
- 1 tablespoon apple cider vinegar
- 2 tablespoons lemon juice
- 1½ tablespoons minced onion
- 1 tablespoon minced chives
- 2 tablespoons chopped dill weed
- ½ teaspoon Spike seasoning
- Olive oil
- 2 pounds frozen spinach, thawed and squeezed dry
- 2 egg whites
- 1 teaspoon crushed red pepper flakes
- 2 pounds prepared polenta, cut into 24 slices
- 3 cups low-fat, sugar-free marinara sauce
- ½ cup grated soy Parmesan cheese (optional)
- ½ cup grated soy mozzarella cheese (optional)
- ½ cup chopped fresh basil

To make the Steda Feta (tofu feta), place half the tofu, the vinegar, lemon juice, onion, chives, dill, and Spike in a blender and process to form a cream. Transfer to a bowl and set aside. Mash the remaining tofu with a fork, then mix it into the herb mixture. Cover and refrigerate until ready to use.

Preheat the oven to 400°F. Coat a 13 × 9-inch baking dish with a tiny bit of olive oil or cooking spray.

In a large mixing bowl, combine the tofu feta, spinach, egg whites, and red pepper flakes. Arrange 12 of the polenta slices in the baking dish. Top with half of the tofu mixture, then cover with half of the marinara sauce. Repeat with the remaining polenta, tofu mixture, and marinara. Cover the pan with aluminum foil and bake for 40 minutes. Uncover, sprinkle with the soy Parmesan and soy mozzarella cheeses (if using), and bake again until the cheese is melted, about 10 minutes. Remove the pan from the oven and sprinkle with the basil. Let stand for 10 minutes before serving.

The average number of people attending a Super Bowl party is seventeen.— Hallmark

Nine of the ten most-watched TV programs of all time are Super Bowls. —NFL Enterprises

An estimated 14,500 tons of chips and 4,000 tons of popcorn are eaten on Super Bowl Sunday.— California Avocado Commission

On Super Bowl Sunday, Americans scarf down eight million pounds of guacamole. —California Avocado Commission

# Carol's Super Bowl Stew   Serves 6   (green)

*CAROL SIEGEL*

¼ cup vegetable oil

3 to 3½ pounds free-range organic chicken breasts, cut into 1-inch cubes

1 large onion, chopped

3 garlic cloves, cut in half

1 tablespoon paprika

1 teaspoon salt

½ teaspoon ground pepper

1 teaspoon dried thyme

1 cup dry white wine

1 28-ounce can roma tomatoes, chopped

1 ounce assorted dried mushrooms

2 whole garlic bulbs

1 1-pound bag frozen organic peas

In a large Dutch oven or 5-quart saucepan over medium-high heat, add the oil and the chicken and cook about 5 to 7 minutes on each side, or until browned. Remove the chicken and set aside on a plate covered with foil. Add the onion and garlic cloves to the oil in the pan and sauté until the onion is translucent, about 5 to 10 minutes. Add the paprika, salt, pepper, and thyme and stir an additional minute. Add the chicken, white wine, tomatoes, and mushrooms, lower the heat, and stir well. Simmer for about 1½ hours, uncovered, to let the flavors come together. Fill a large stockpot halfway with water and bring it to a boil over high heat. Add the garlic bulbs and boil until soft, about 10 to 15 minutes. Drain the bulbs and cool. Push out the soft garlic pulp and stir it into the stew. Fifteen minutes before the stew is done simmering add the frozen peas and stir. Serve over a slice of polenta or a scoop of rice.

Sales of antacid increase 20 percent the day after Super Bowl Sunday.— 7 – E l e v e n

Fans spend an average of $15 on food and drink at the stadium during Super Bowl.
— S e r v i c e   A m e r i c a

## Oven-Fried Chicken  Serves 4  (green)

*MaryAnn Hennings*

- ³/₄ cup soy cream
- 2 organic skinless, boneless chicken breast halves (about 1 pound)
- 2 organic chicken drumsticks, skinned (about ½ pound)
- 2 chicken thighs, skinned (about ½ pound)
- ½ cup whole wheat flour
- 2 teaspoons Spike seasoning
- ½ teaspoon red pepper flakes
- ¼ teaspoon white pepper
- ¼ teaspoon ground cumin

Combine the soy cream and chicken pieces in a large zip-top plastic bag; seal. Marinate in the refrigerator for 1 hour, turning occasionally.

Preheat the oven to 450°F.

Combine the flour, Spike, red pepper flakes, white pepper, and cumin in a second large zip-top plastic bag. Remove the chicken from the first bag, discarding the marinade. Add the chicken, one piece at a time, to the flour mixture, shaking the bag to coat the chicken. Remove the chicken from the bag, shaking off the excess flour. Lightly coat each chicken piece with cooking spray. Return the chicken one piece at a time to the flour mixture, shaking the bag to coat thoroughly. Remove the chicken from the bag, shaking off the excess flour. Place the chicken on a baking sheet lined with parchment paper. Lightly coat the chicken with cooking spray. Bake for 35 minutes, turning after 20 minutes. The chicken is done when the thigh pieces, pricked with a fork at their thickest, yield a clear liquid.

## Sweet Potato Chips  Serves 8  (purple)

- 1 tablespoon extra-virgin olive oil
- 4 sweet potatoes
- Kosher salt
- Freshly ground black pepper

Preheat the oven to 325°F. Oil two baking sheets and put them in the oven for 10 minutes to preheat.

Slice the potatoes on the narrow side lengthwise on a mandoline so they are thin and flexible, about ¹/₁₆ inch thick. Place the slices on the hot sheet pan, making sure they don't touch at all. Sprinkle with salt and pepper. Bake the chips for 10 minutes, then rotate the pans in the oven and bake for another 10 minutes. Flip each chip and then bake for another 5 to 6 minutes, or until golden brown. Remove the chips to paper towels to cool. Repeat with the remaining potato slices. To store the chips, cool completely and place in a plastic zip-top bag. They will stay crisp for several days.

# Baked Garlic Fries Serves 6 (purple/blue)

3 pounds peeled organic baking potatoes, cut into 1/4-inch-thick strips

8 to 9 organic garlic cloves, minced (about 5 teaspoons)

2 tablespoons finely chopped organic parsley

Salt

Preheat the oven to 400°F.

Combine the potatoes, garlic, and parsley in a large zip-top plastic bag, tossing to coat. Arrange the potatoes in a single layer on a baking sheet coated with cooking spray. Bake for 50 minutes, or until the potatoes are tender and golden brown, turning after 20 minutes. Add salt to taste. Serve immediately.

# Touchdown Brownies

Makes 24 brownies (yellow)

3/4 cup (1 1/2 sticks) soy margarine

4 ounces unsweetened baking chocolate

8 ounces grain-sweetened or semisweet baking chocolate

2 cups Sucanat

1 tablespoon vanilla extract

5 large cage-free organic eggs, beaten

1 1/4 cups unbleached flour

1/2 teaspoon salt

Preheat the oven to 350°F. Grease a 13 × 9-inch metal baking pan.

In a 3-quart saucepan over low heat, melt the margarine and chocolate. With a wooden spoon, stir in the Sucanat and vanilla. Beat in the eggs until well blended. In a medium bowl, combine the flour and salt; stir into the chocolate mixture just until blended. Spread the batter evenly in the prepared pan. Bake for 30 minutes, or until a toothpick inserted 1 inch from the edge of the pan comes out clean. Cool completely in the pan on a wire rack. When cool, cut lengthwise into 4 strips, then cut each strip crosswise into 6 pieces.

## BEVERAGES

Beer, beer, and beer! Did I mention beer? Beer is the official beverage of the Super Bowl. Consider renting a keg instead of buying bottles or cans. Kegs add a fun-frat-boy-Animal House-community-spirit to the event. And just for the health of it, place a water cooler next to the keg with a sign saying, FOR A GOOD TIME, PLEASE DRINK EQUAL AMOUNTS OF BOTH. You can do the exact same thing with a tub of beer bottles in ice and a tub of bottled spring water in ice. And don't forget about nonalcoholic beer as an option. You may even want to have a taste test among the better brands to satisfy your guests' urge for that beer taste but without the alcohol. Just a footnote: Beer is considered to be one of the two healthiest alcoholic beverages (sake being the other), for several reasons. Beer and sake are naturally fermented and not distilled, and therefore not as potent as wine and hard liquor. And they are both made from grains rather than fruit, so they combine and metabolize much better with food.

## PARTY IDEAS

The Super Bowl is the top at-home party event of the year, surpassing New Year's Eve.
—Hallmark

- Consider a costume theme: guys in jerseys, girls as cheerleaders. Or have everyone dress in support of his or her team, with pins, jerseys, hats, and so on. Seat everyone based on which team they are rooting for.
- Hire a manicurist and/or pedicurist for the women attending who really don't care about the game. This adds a funny counterbalance to all the testosterone in the room.

## INVITATIONS

- Design invitations to look just like Super Bowl tickets, with all the information for the party on the ticket.
- Cut them in the shape of a football or gridiron.
- Include a line or two for Super Bowl predictions in the RSVP. Give a prize to the prediction that comes closest. Some possibilities: winning team, final score, combined score, point spread, MVP, total interceptions, first team to score, and so on. And make predictions about your guests, too:
  —Guest most likely to do an end zone victory dance.
  —Guest most likely to comment about the cheerleaders' . . . um . . . er . . . pompoms.
  —Guest most likely to comment about a cute tight end.
  —Guest most likely to Monday-morning quarterback . . . during the game.

## DECORATIONS

- Anything and everything that has to do with football works here. Every pro team has a website that allows you to buy team souvenirs, or go to a sporting goods store or souvenir store for posters, banners, T-shirts, and so on. Also consider the towns and colors of the teams involved.
- Have your kids cut out shapes from colored construction paper to tape to the walls: footballs, end zones, referees, banners, or green gridirons.

## SCENTS

The Super Bowl is such a guy event that it's hard to think of scented candles or potpourri. However, the way most of them leave the bathroom, same counterscent might be needed more than ever. You may want to appeal to their sense of humor by providing a scent that's connected to the playing teams. For example, Miami—tropical; Denver—pine, Seattle—coffee.

# T o a s t

The game of life is a lot like football. You have to tackle your problems, block your fears, and score your points when you get the opportunity.
—LEWIS GRIZZARD

## ACTIVITIES AND GAMES

- Draw a typical football pool (you know, the ones that are used in practically every sports bar in the country on Super Bowl Sunday) with one hundred squares, ten rows across and ten rows down. Decide how much per square, then let everyone purchase as many squares as they want, but only after everybody has had a chance to buy one. Randomly choose the numbers for the top row and side row, but only after all the squares have been filled in. Award prizes for each quarter, depending on what the score is for each team at that point. The largest prize should be awarded for the final score.
- Variation for a small group: Write numbers 0 through 9 on folded pieces of paper and place them in a hat. Each participant picks a number. The winning ticket is the final digit of the combined total score. If the score is 28 to 14, the winning ticket is number 2, because the combined total is 42, and the final digit of 42 is 2.
- Hire a masseuse to give everyone a rubdown during the most tense parts of the game.
- Have ballots for everyone to rate the commercials on a scale from 1 to 10. This often leads to some fun disagreements after the game when everyone compares ballots. After all, "Viewers who pay more attention to the commercials than they do to the game . . . 16 percent," according to the *Dayton Daily News*.

And, for the manicure/pedicure party . . . a good game of "Would You Rather." For example, Would you rather . . .

- Date Joey, Ross, or Chandler (or Monica, Rachel, or Phoebe if the guys want to play)?
- Win the lottery or fall in love with your soul mate?
- Have a cat or a dog?
- Remarry your ex or let his second wife move in for two years?
- Completely relive the first moment that you met your mate or go to the Caribbean without him or her?
- Be sixteen for one night or see what your life will be like at sixty?
- Be broke and thin or rich and heavy?
- Feed a hungry nation for a year or put your family members in their dream homes?
- Without science or plastic surgeons, would you rather have longer legs or bigger breasts (or for men, longer length or longer lasting)?

## PRIZES, GIFTS, AND PARTY FAVORS

Fans spend an average of $15 on souvenirs at the stadium.—Facility Merchandising

T-shirts, Nerf footballs, hats, pompoms, megaphones, wristbands, "team" photos of partygoers (possibly in a calendar), pennants, trophies, ace bandages, ice packs, Tiger Balm, Igloo Playmates (as gift basket).

For a manicure party: thong shoes, nail polish, sample perfume, shampoo, conditioner, bath gel, shower caps, Super Bowl chili recipe.

## MUSIC

| | | |
|---|---|---|
| *Chariots of Fire* | Vangelis | Album |
| *Whoomp! (There It Is)* | Tag Team | Album |
| "Another One Bites the Dust" | Queen | Song |
| "We Are the Champions" | Queen | Song |
| *Jerry Maguire* | Various Artists | Soundtrack |
| "Super Bowl Shuffle" | Chicago Bears | Song |

## MOVIES

| | |
|---|---|
| *The Longest Yard* | (1974–R) |
| *Semi-Tough* | (1977–R) |
| *North Dallas Forty* | (1979–R) |
| *The Replacements* | (2001–R) |
| *Brian's Song* | (1971–NR) |
| *Black Sunday* | (1977–R) |
| *Knute Rockne All-American* | (1940–NR) |
| *Jim Thorpe All American* | (1951–NR) |
| *Any Given Sunday* | (2000–R) |
| *Horsefeathers* | (1932–NR) |

For a manicure party:

| | |
|---|---|
| *Main Event* | (1970–PG) |
| *Pat and Mike* | (1952–NR) |
| *Woman of the Year* | (1942–NR) |
| *Heaven Can Wait* | (1977–PG) |
| *Jerry Maguire* | (1996–R) |
| *A League of Their Own* | (1992–PG) |
| *Everybody's All-American* | (1988–R) |

## EXERCISE AND CALORIE CHART

| Activity | Calories Burned/Hour |
|---|---|
| Cheerleading | 422 |
| Half-time tag football game | 563 |

Tell your guests to arrive an hour or two early for the more important event: the touch football game in your backyard or nearby park. It could be guys vs. girls, kids vs. adults, AFC vs. NFC supporters, fire signs vs. water signs, "innie" belly buttons vs. "outies"—whatever you think will work best. If the weather is too cold, you can also do football calisthenics in your living room or basement. I would skip the running-between-the-tires drill; that one's pretty rough on the carpet. Do consider setting up an obstacle course competition in the yard for the kids or as an alternative to the touch football game.

## FOR THE KIDS
- Your children can dress as grandstand vendors with cardboard boxes and a piece of rope. It's always fun to put your kids to work and make them feel like they're involved!
- If your children love to dance, you may want to have them put on their own half-time talent show. They'll jump at the chance to be 'NSYNC or Britney.

## FOR COUPLES
You and your mate each choose a team. Each play or score means you must "do" something to your partner, and you have to keep doing it until some other play or score replaces that action. Here are a few suggestions: first down = back rub, field goal = foot massage, touchdown = (I'll leave that up to you!), and making the extra point means you do it with *honey!* An interception or fumble at any time means you must immediately switch places. If the two of you are still watching TV by the end of the game, you're either married or Packer fans.

# Chinese New Year

I wanted to include Chinese New Year because I've always been fascinated with Chinese culture, and I've been in love with the food since I was six. My dad would go to Lee's Chinese take-out on Diversey Avenue every Sunday and bring home a feast. Over the years, I've eaten in Chinese restaurants hundreds of times. The experience usually leaves me feeling either great or terrible. I finally realized that it has everything to do with how real and fresh the ingredients are and whether or not the food contains MSG. (Of course, none of our recipes here use MSG.)

Another factor is that most Chinese restaurants use a lot of cornstarch, which can leave you feeling heavy and bloated. Other factors common in Chinese food leave you feeling this way as well: too much sodium, sugar, and bad food-combining. The recipes here are lighter, and they contain no sugar, no MSG, more real vegetables, natural spices, and kuzu in place of cornstarch. Chinese food lends itself nicely and naturally to a healthy, clean palate, and Chinese New Year itself is a great celebration. I love the fact that it celebrates our families and can truly be appreciated by all ages and cultures. I'm definitely going to throw a big Chinese New Year party this year. I hope you do, too!

## History, Facts, and Folklore

The thing I like most about Chinese New Year, besides a good reason for gathering friends and family and eating healthy food, is that it's a time to honor ancestors. The Chinese burn incense to call forth their ancestors, who help them leave the past year and ring in the new. I may not be able to eat with my mother and father, but if their presence were invited, it would be nice to assume they accepted. Also, the customs and rituals hit my organization bone. A haircut, a clean house, and debts paid promptly? I'm in! Here's what the Chinese do:

Preparations begin a few days before New Year's Eve. This is the time to cut your hair, buy new clothes, and settle your finances. Tie up loose ends and reconcile grievances. Anything you do right before the New Year determines the tone of the whole year to come. If you're in debt, you'll continue to be so. If you lend money, you will be asked for loans throughout the year. If you cry, you will cry for the year. After you clean your house, all the tools you use—a broom, vacuum, and so on—are put out of sight (a good idea anyway). Last, you decorate your doors with the color red and paper Chinese symbols for happiness, wealth, and longevity.

On their New Year's Eve, the Chinese prepare a great feast with generous portions on a family-size table, which asserts that the year ahead will be bountiful. On the first day of the New Year they welcome the gods of heaven and earth. How? They abstain from meat. Here's my suggestion: abstain from meat and dairy all year long and really welcome the gods. The Chinese believe this will ensure a long and happy life, and I have to add the word *healthy*.

Only after New Year's Day is it okay to sweep the floors of your house again, and when you do, please start at the door, sweep to the center of the room, and carry the dust out the back door. If you push it over your front door threshold, you'll sweep away good fortune for the family.

On the second day, besides the requisite prayers to the ancestors, you have to be nice to dogs. It is considered the birthday of all dogs. Dog lovers get ready, today is the day to indulge . . . Rover.

On the third and fourth day, all sons-in-law show respect for their in-laws. Go ahead. Just do it.

On the fifth day, everyone stays home and waits for the god of wealth to bless their house. Any socializing could bring both parties bad luck, so stay home, because on the sixth day you visit friends and family.

On the seventh day, farmers put out their produce and concoct a special drink made from seven vegetables. This day is also considered the birthday of human beings. Noodles are eaten to promote longevity, and raw fish to promote success.

On days eight through twelve you continue to visit friends and family, make offerings to the gods, and eat together, which brings us to day thirteen, when you cleanse with a simple meal of rice and mustard greens.

With the celebrations coming to an end, on day fourteen you prep for the Lantern Festival, held on the fifteenth and last day of the Chinese New Year's celebrations. Besides celebrating family and reconciling loose ends and grievances, the ideas behind Chinese New Year are happiness, wealth, and longevity. Don't forget, if you have health, the rest come easily. So pull it together, and don't forget to wear red, which the Chinese believe brings high spirits and bright thoughts ahead.

Now do you see why I love this holiday?

## RECIPES
# Spicy Noodle Bowl with Mushrooms and Spinach  Serves 6 (green)

8 cups chicken broth

1 teaspoon peeled and grated fresh ginger

1/2 teaspoon crushed red pepper

6 cups thinly sliced shiitake mushroom caps (about 1/2 pound)

4 ounces somen (wheat noodles)

6 2-ounce skinless, boneless chicken breast halves (1/4 inch thick), poached and sliced thinly

3 cups organic chopped spinach

1 3/4 cups enoki mushrooms (about 3 1/2 ounces)

3 scallions, green parts only, chopped

1/2 teaspoon kosher salt

1/4 cup chopped organic cilantro

In a large Dutch oven, bring the broth, 2 cups water, ginger, and pepper to a simmer. Stir in the shiitake mushrooms and simmer 10 minutes, or until the mushrooms are tender. Stir in the noodles and cook 2 minutes, or until tender. Stir in the chicken, spinach, enoki mushrooms, scallions, and salt; cook 1 minute, or until the spinach wilts. Sprinkle with the cilantro.

## Seared Tuna on a Bed of Asian Noodles

Serves 4    (green)

6½ ounces dry somen noodles

½ cup shelled edamame

1 teaspoon sesame oil

2 tablespoons vegetable oil

2 tablespoons lime juice

1 teaspoon wasabi paste, plus more for
    serving

¼ cup pickled ginger, drained

¼ cup snipped garlic scapes

¼ cup black sesame seeds

12 ounces sashimi-quality tuna

Soy sauce

Place the noodles and edamame in a saucepan of boiling water and cook for 2 minutes, or until the noodles are soft. Drain, cool under running water, and drain again. In a small bowl, combine the sesame oil, vegetable oil, lime juice, and wasabi paste and pour over the noodles and edamame. Add the pickled ginger and garlic scapes and toss to combine. Place the black sesame seeds in a small bowl and press the tuna into the seeds. In a nonstick frying pan over high heat, cook the tuna for 1 minute on each side, or until just seared. Cut into thick slices. To serve, divide the noodles and edamame among the bowls and top with the tuna slices. Serve with soy sauce and wasabi in dipping bowls.

## Chinese-Style Steamed Fish

Serves 2    (purple/blue)

2 6-ounce cod fillets

Salt and pepper

2 tablespoons dry vermouth

1½ teaspoons peeled and minced organic
    ginger

2 small organic garlic cloves, minced

4 teaspoons low-sodium tamari sauce

1½ teaspoons oriental sesame oil

2 tablespoons chopped organic cilantro

Place a small cake rack in a large (12-inch-diameter) skillet; place a 9-inch-diameter glass pie dish on the rack. Put the fish in the dish and sprinkle lightly with salt and pepper. Sprinkle the vermouth, ginger, and garlic in the dish around the fish. Top the fish with the tamari, sesame oil, and 1 tablespoon of the cilantro. Pour enough water into the skillet to reach a depth of 1 inch and bring the water to a boil. Cover the skillet and steam the fish until just opaque in the center, about 10 minutes. Transfer the fish to plates. Top with the juices from the dish and the remaining cilantro.

# Cod in a Soy Pan Sauce Serves 4 (blue)

2 teaspoons sesame oil

1 tablespoon peanut oil

2 large mild red chili peppers, shredded

½ cup low-sodium soy sauce

⅓ cup mirin

2 tablespoons Sucanat

4 ½ pounds cod fillets

In a large frying pan over medium-high heat, heat the oils. Add the peppers and cook for 2 minutes, or until crisp. Add the soy sauce, mirin, and Sucanat; simmer for 1 minute, or until the sauce has slightly thickened. Add the fish to the pan and simmer in the sauce for 3 minutes each side, or until cooked. To serve, place piles of steamed rice on serving plates and top with the fish and pan sauce. Serve with steamed greens or asparagus.

# Honey-Glazed Mahimahi Serves 4 (blue)

3 tablespoons honey

3 tablespoons mirin

1 teaspoon peeled and minced ginger

3 garlic cloves, crushed

4 4-ounce slices mahimahi fillets

1 ½ teaspoons olive oil

¼ teaspoon salt

⅛ teaspoon freshly ground black pepper

In a large bowl, combine the honey, mirin, ginger, and garlic. Add the fish, turning to coat well. Cover and marinate in the refrigerator for 20 minutes, turning the fish once. Remove the fish from the marinade, reserving the marinade.

Heat the oil in a nonstick skillet over medium-high heat. Add the fish and cook 6 minutes, or until golden on one side. Turn the fish, season with the salt and pepper, and cook 3 minutes more, or until the fish flakes easily with a fork. Remove the fillets from the skillet; keep warm.

Add the reserved marinade to the skillet and cook 1 minute over medium-high heat, deglazing the skillet by scraping the particles that cling to the bottom. Spoon the glaze over the fish when serving.

## Gingered Snow Pea Stir-Fry

Serves 2    (blue/green)

- 1 teaspoon sesame oil
- $\frac{1}{2}$ 12.3-ounce package extra-firm tofu, drained and cubed
- 2 garlic cloves, minced
- 3 tablespoons low-sodium soy sauce
- 1 cup vegetable broth
- 1 $\frac{1}{2}$ tablespoons arrowroot
- 1 cup sliced organic carrots (about 2)
- 1 teaspoon peeled and minced ginger
- $\frac{1}{2}$ pound organic snow peas, trimmed

Heat the oil in a wok or large nonstick skillet over medium-high heat until hot. Add the tofu and garlic and stir-fry 7 minutes, or until the garlic starts to brown. Add 1 tablespoon of the soy sauce; stir-fry 2 minutes, or until the tofu is browned. Remove from the pan; set aside. In a small bowl, combine the remaining 2 tablespoons soy sauce, vegetable broth, and arrowroot. Stir until smooth and set aside. Add the carrots and ginger to the pan and stir-fry 5 minutes. Add the broth mixture and snow peas and stir-fry 2 more minutes. Return the tofu mixture to the pan. Cook until well heated, stirring gently. Serve over brown rice or soba noodles.

## Braised Baby Bok Choy  Serves 2    (blue)

- 1 cup vegetable broth
- 3 tablespoons soy margarine
- $\frac{3}{4}$ pound organic baby bok choy, trimmed
- $\frac{1}{2}$ teaspoon Asian sesame oil
- Pepper

Bring the broth and soy margarine to a simmer in a large, deep, heavy skillet. Arrange the bok choy evenly in the skillet and simmer, covered, until tender, about 5 minutes. Transfer the bok choy with tongs to a serving dish, cover, and keep warm. Boil the broth until reduced to about $\frac{1}{4}$ cup, then stir in the sesame oil and pepper to taste. Pour the broth over the bok choy and serve.

# Sautéed Asparagus and Snap Peas

Serves 8    (blue)

*BETH EVIN HEFFNER*

2 pounds asparagus spears

1½ pounds sugar snap peas

1 tablespoon olive oil

1 tablespoon sesame oil

Kosher salt

Freshly ground black pepper

Red pepper flakes (optional)

3 tablespoons sesame seeds, both black and
    white, if available

Cut off the tough ends of the asparagus and slice the stalks diagonally into 2-inch pieces. Snap off the stem ends of the snap peas and pull the string down the length of the vegetable.

In a large sauté pan over medium-high heat, warm the olive oil and sesame oil and add the asparagus and snap peas. Add salt, pepper, and red pepper flakes, if desired, to taste. Sauté about 10 minutes, or until crisp-tender, tossing occasionally. Sprinkle with the sesame seeds and serve hot.

# Sautéed Mustard Greens with Garlic

Serves 6    (purple)

2 large garlic cloves, minced

½ teaspoon sea salt

¼ cup light sesame oil

1½ pounds organic mustard greens, stems
    and center ribs discarded and leaves
    halved (2 bunches)

Soy sauce

With a mortar and pestle, mash the garlic to a paste with the salt. In a 5-quart pot over medium heat, heat the oil and sauté the garlic paste until fragrant, about 2 to 3 minutes. Add half the greens and toss with tongs to coat with the oil. Add the rest of the greens as they wilt. Add ½ cup water and cook 5 minutes, covered, stirring occasionally. Continue to cook, uncovered, until the greens are just tender and most of the liquid is evaporated, about 5 minutes. Season to taste with soy sauce.

## Almond Cookies   Makes 2 dozen   (yellow)

1 cup whole almonds

1 cup whole wheat pastry flour

1 cup unbleached all-purpose flour

¼ teaspoon fine sea salt

⅛ teaspoon baking soda

½ cup pure maple syrup

½ cup soy margarine, melted

1 teaspoon vanilla extract

½ teaspoon almond extract

½ cup sliced almonds

Preheat the oven to 350°F. Spread the whole almonds on an ungreased baking sheet and toast in the oven for 8 minutes. In a food processor fitted with a metal blade, combine the toasted almonds, flour, salt, and baking soda and grind to a fine meal. In a medium bowl, whisk together the maple syrup, soy margarine, vanilla, and almond extract. Add the almond mixture and sliced almonds and mix well with a wooden spoon. Moisten your hands and form the dough into walnut-sized balls.

Lightly grease 2 baking sheets. Place the dough balls 3 inches apart on the sheets and gently flatten each ball into a 2-inch round. Bake for 15 to 18 minutes, rotating the baking sheets halfway through for even baking, until cookies are golden brown. Let cool for 1 minute on cookie sheet, then cool completely on wire rack.

### BEVERAGES

Green tea, plum spritzers, Tsing-Tao beer.

### INVITATIONS

- Red cards and envelopes with Chinese characters stamped on them in black or gold, a gold coin in each envelope
- Invitations sent inside Chinese food take-out boxes

### DECORATIONS

Everything on your table should symbolize:

- Sweetness in the New Year—bowls of oranges, incense placed in orange halves drizzled with honey, bowls of rice and plum candy
- Prosperity in the New Year—gold coins, bowls of goldfish on each table, bowls of water with floating votives and exotic red flowers, or red envelopes symbolizing the gifts to come.

Place noisemakers at each table setting and paper lanterns around the room.

### SCENTS

Green tea

Red plum

Sandalwood

Patchouli

Sesame

# Toasts

*To have attained to the human form is a source of joy.... What an incomparable bliss it is to undergo these countless transitions.*
—CHANG TZU, THIRD CENTURY B.C.

Happy New Year, and to those changes—welcome!
May there be a generation of children of the children of your children.

Ginger
Fennel

## ACTIVITIES AND GAMES

- Play Chinese Checkers.
- Cook together. Chinese food lends itself to community preparation. Get everyone to slice and dice while listening to some of the music listed below.
- Match celebrities and/or your guests to their Chinese Zodiac signs. Have fun matching up the best combinations.

## PRIZES, GIFTS, AND PARTY FAVORS

Chinese cooking and feng-shui books, Chinese silk pajamas, gold coin earrings, soup bowls and spoons, chopsticks, sparklers, masks, puppets, slippers, Chinese handcuffs, fortune cookies, green tea, brooms, Chinese checkers set, Chinese take-out box as gift basket, fans, origami, astrological charts, wood incense burners, a goldfish in a bowl and a sack of supplies for its care, red scarves, pots of honey sealed with a red ribbon and gold emblem, abacus, red envelopes with a gold coin. You may also want to visit your local Chinatown for inspiration and ideas.

## MUSIC

In addition to traditional Spring Festival music or recordings of Chinese poetry or flute music:

| | | |
|---|---|---|
| *Miss Saigon* | Original Broadway Cast | Soundtrack |
| *Flower Drum Song* | Original Broadway Cast | Soundtrack |
| *China* | Vangelis | Album |
| *Great Wall of China* | Tangerine Dream | Album |
| *Chinese Work Songs* | Little Feat | Album |

## MOVIES

| | |
|---|---|
| *Flower Drum Song* | (1961—NR) |
| *The World of Susie Wong* | (1960—R) |
| *The Last Emperor* | (1987—PG-13) |

| | |
|---|---|
| *Joy Luck Club* | (1993—R) |
| *Crouching Tiger, Hidden Dragon* | (2001—PG-13) |
| *Big Trouble in Little China* | (1986—PG13) |
| *Shanghai Surprise* | (1986—PG-13) |
| *With Six You Get Eggroll* | (1968—G) |
| *Rush Hour* | (1998—PG-13) |
| *Rush Hour 2* | (2001—PG-13) |
| *Enter the Dragon* | (1973—R) |
| *Red Square* | (2001—R) |

## EXERCISE AND CALORIE CHART

| Activity | Calories Burned/Hour |
|---|---|
| Tai chi | 288 |
| Yoga | 384 |
| Chinese jump rope | 493 |

## FOR THE KIDS

- All children receive a red envelope from their parents on New Year's morning that contains a little money and something sweet.
- Teach your children how to use chopsticks.
- Make a Chinese dragon. Check out the website www.family.go.com for instructions.

## FOR COUPLES

Create your own fortune cookies by writing on little pieces of paper things you're hoping will be in your future together, such as a weekend getaway, dinner at a favorite restaurant, a fun field trip, or even a trip somewhere exotic. Fold the pieces of paper, put them into a bowl, and each choose one. Open it up and immediately buy tickets, make a deposit or reservation, or do whatever else you need to do to put the wheels in motion to fulfill your fortune together.

Or, write on several pieces of paper all the things you would like to do for each other (such as foot massage, back rub, or other things—use your imagination!). Take turns opening the pieces of paper and fulfilling each other's wishes.

# Valentine's Day

February 14 is the second most celebrated day in the United States, after December 25.—The Romantic

It's a good thing we associate the color red with Valentine's Day because red also means stop—and stopping is what I want you to do this Valentine's Day. Don't worry, I'm not talking about stopping in the middle of a hot and heavy passionate moment with your sweetie. I would never want to stop that kind of fun. Besides, that burns some serious calories! No, I'm talking about stopping something else. Valentine's Day means chocolate, and chocolate usually means sugar and dairy—double trouble! If you're going to indulge in naughty treats like sugar-filled, dairy-laden chocolate on Valentine's Day, make sure that you stop immediately when the holiday is over.

It is too common to wake up on February 15 with a stomach that's been up all night gurgling from fermentation caused by excess sugar and dairy. It's the perfect environment for bad digestion, constipation, pimples, and making cheap wine. And it leaves you feeling lethargic, stressed, and (believe it or not) wanting more sugar! This is the beginning of what I call the "sugar treadmill." If you had the willpower to say, "Okay I'm going to pig out this one day and then stop," that would be fine. But you can't stop, can you? You just have to keep that huge box (the I-love-you-*so*-much size) of Godiva chocolates around for a couple of days until every single piece is gone. And right after you've finished it, you're out searching for another box. Only this time you're not just searching for an innocent little treat. This time it's the buzz . . . the fix . . . the *addiction*! This time it's not Godiva at all, it's a cheap Whitman's Sampler box concealed in a brown paper bag tucked into the inside pocket of a dirty trench coat. How pathetic! Don't deny it. You're on the sugar treadmill. And it's all because of one big box of chocolates your sweetheart gave you knowing damn well it would eventually make you fat enough to fit perfectly under his thumb.

This year, try something different. Tell him you want sexy lingerie and if he plays his cards right, you just might model it for him . . . in heels! And if you really must have your candy, try substituting the legal sweets we suggest in this book. They won't make you sick, hyper, or craving more. And no matter what kind of sweets you choose to overeat (legal or illegal), decide in advance that at midnight you are going to stop and that first thing in the morning, all the junk goes right in the garbage. Start the next day with a sugar-detox breakfast—lots of grapes (or other watery fruit) and a tall glass of fresh water. They both help clean the sugar out of your system. Throw in a wet whole food at lunchtime to really get yourself back on track. Most important, though, is to start your day with fruit because it will to help you digest all that chocolate, which is very concentrated and constipating. Sludge like that takes a long time to pass through your digestive tract. Hydrate your system enough to keep everything moving, and get back to balanced eating right away to avoid the sugar and spicy food treadmill. Balanced meals keep you from craving extremes, and the sooner you return, the easier it is to adjust. Anything too salty or too spicy induces extreme cravings as well. In short, for Valentine's Day (or any holiday, for that matter), think good, clean, simple food as much as possible. Set a timer to *stop,* and then stick with your plan.

We often talk about self-sabotage during the on-line classes I teach at Marilu.com. I always say, "If you're going to go through a period of indulgence, that's fine. Enjoy it, and do it with gusto. But then set a timer and say to yourself, 'When that timer goes off, I'm going to stop.' And really make yourself stop."

There is one last point I want to stress here, and that is *awareness.* As painful as it is, you should always be conscious of and accountable for what you are consuming by writing everything down. It is amazing how seeing it in black and white can make you stop. If you write "chateaubriand, potatoes au gratin, three candy bars, and six Godiva chocolates," and actually see the decadence written down on paper, it makes a deeper impression on your psyche, and you'll be more likely to do something about it.

If you want to simplify this, just write down the sweets you eat. I know that many of you have a big thing for sweets, especially chocolate. But hang in there. Just as Nancy Reagan suggested saying no to drugs, I believe you can say *stop* to chocolates on Valentine's Day.

Or why not be your own valentine today? February is Heart Healthy Month. So along with (or maybe instead of) all the hearts and flowers and chocolates and kissy sweetheart stuff, do something nice for your heart. Make an appointment with your doctor for a stress test and/or cholesterol and blood pressure check. Or get out and do some cardiovascular exercises. If you're not sure what to do, check the chart in the exercise section for ideas. This is the perfect day to start a love affair with your heart.

## HISTORY, FACTS, AND FOLKLORE

In ancient Rome, February 14 was the day to honor Juno, goddess of women and marriage. This was also the night before the Feast of Lupercalia, a spring festival. On the eve of the festival, girls' names were put in a jar, and each boy reached in and chose a partner for the duration of the festival. These pairings often led to marriage and children, so the reasons for doing it went beyond momentary carnal pleasures.

When Claudius II was emperor, he ordered all the Roman military not to marry, fearing it would deter them from being committed to battle. However, a Christian priest named Valentine took it upon himself to secretly marry those couples in love and looking to make it legal before the soldier had to leave. Valentine was arrested, and whether by coincidence or cruel intention he was put to death on February 14. When Valentine was canonized as a saint, the holiday became Saint Valentine's Day in honor of the priest.

I always find it odd that we set aside only one day a year for love. Most of us are conceived in love, sense it immediately upon arrival, and, with our first crush, have experienced almost every aspect of love there is. There's parental love, sibling love (and that natural rivalry). We become boy-crazy, then fall seriously in love. Then, out in the world, we look for something we love to do, so that we can find more love and someone who loves us. We love them back, and in that love we create something to love. We conceive and begin the entire cycle again when a child is born and senses immediately upon arrival that he is loved, and so on.

I guess we'd go crazy if we celebrated love more than one day a year, so let's make sure that day is worth it.

## HENNER HOLIDAY TRADITIONS AND STORIES

I've always loved Valentine's Day because I've always been a little boy-crazy. I remember one particular Valentine's Day when I was eight years old. I arrived at school with my little bag of cards from Woolworth's. You know—the pack of thirty for sixty-nine cents. My mother was politically correct long before it was fashionable; she made sure we gave cards to every kid in the class to avoid hurting anyone's feelings. When the cards were handed out, it was important to get a pile that was large enough to show I was popular, and most important, to get a special one from . . .

*Tommy Donovan.* Well, my pile was respectable enough, but the card from Tommy looked just like the ones he gave out to all the other kids—until I opened it and compared. To other kids he signed it *from Tommy Donovan,* but on mine it said *from Tommy D.* Shortening Donovan to simply D must have meant true love.

## RECIPES
# Warm Wild Mushroom Salad

Serves 6    (blue)

*MaryAnn Hennings*

6 cups torn organic mixed greens

3 tablespoons olive oil

3 tablespoons walnut oil

1 pound fresh organic wild mushrooms (chanterelles, cepes, shiitakes), tough stems discarded, sliced about $1/4$ inch thick

2 tablespoons white wine vinegar

1 teaspoon Dijon-style mustard

Salt

Freshly ground black pepper

$3/4$ cup chopped toasted almonds

Arrange the greens on six plates. In a sauté pan or skillet, combine the oils and warm over medium heat. Add the mushrooms and sauté until just tender, 3 to 4 minutes. Remove from the heat and cool for about 1 minute. Stir in the vinegar and mustard and season to taste with salt and pepper. Spoon the mushrooms over the greens, toss on the nuts, and serve.

# Honey-Baked Chicken Serves 6    (blue)

$1^{1}/_{2}$ to 2 pounds chicken on the bone, cut up

$1/2$ cup (1 stick) soy margarine, melted

$1/2$ cup honey

$1/4$ cup Dijon-style mustard

1 teaspoon salt

1 teaspoon curry powder (optional)

Preheat the oven to 350°F.
Place the chicken pieces in a shallow baking pan, skin-side up. In a small bowl, combine the soy margarine, honey, mustard, salt, and curry powder. Pour the mixture over the chicken and bake for about $1^{1}/_{4}$ hours, basting every 15 minutes, until the chicken is tender and nicely browned.

# Red Endive Salad Serves 4 (blue)

¼ tablespoon white wine vinegar

Salt

1 tablespoon honey

1 small organic shallot, minced

¾ cup olive oil

2 heads organic Belgian endive,
  preferably red

6 ounces organic frisée, torn into bite-size
  pieces (4 cups)

⅓ cup thinly sliced organic red onion

½ cup chopped toasted walnuts

Pepper

1½ ounces organic baby red oak-leaf
  or green-leaf lettuce (2 cups)

To make the dressing, in a small bowl, whisk together the vinegar, ½ teaspoon salt, honey, and shallot. Add the oil in a slow stream, whisking until emulsified.

To make the salad, reserve 8 endive leaves. Coarsely chop the remaining endive. In a large bowl, toss the chopped endive, frisée, onion, walnuts, and lettuce, and enough dressing to coat. Season the salad with salt and pepper to taste. Divide the reserved endive leaves among four plates, and place the tossed salad in between each of the 2 endive leaves.

# Salmon in Orange-Ginger Cream Sauce

Serves 4 (yellow)

*MARY BETH BORKOWSKI*

¾ cup Vegenaise

¾ cup Whole Soy plain yogurt

1 teaspoon freshly grated ginger

2 tablespoons freshly grated orange zest

2 tablespoons orange juice

1 tablespoon bottled capers

1 teaspoon pink peppercorns

1 bay leaf

4 6- to 8-ounce salmon fillets

Preheat the oven to 350°F.

In a medium bowl, whisk together the Vegenaise, yogurt, ginger, orange zest, orange juice, and capers. Refrigerate until ready to serve.

In a small saucepan over medium heat, boil 1½ cups water. Add the peppercorns and bay leaf and simmer for 3 minutes. Place the salmon fillets in a 9 × 11-inch baking dish and pour the water over the fillets. Poach for 20 to 30 minutes, or until the fish is flaky. Serve with the chilled cream sauce.

## Pasta with Smoked Salmon and White Beans Serves 4 (green)

2 tablespoons Dijon-style mustard

1/4 cup red wine vinegar

1/4 cup fresh organic lemon juice

6 tablespoons olive oil

2 tablespoons soy sour cream (optional)

2 cups dried bow tie pasta

1 1/2 cups sliced organic asparagus spears (about 12 ounces)

1 15-ounce can organic Great Northern beans, drained well

1 4-ounce pakcage smoked salmon, cut into 1/2-inch-wide strips

1 1/4 cups grape or cherry tomatoes

To make the vinaigrette, in a small bowl, blend the mustard, vinegar, and lemon juice. Slowly add the oil and soy sour cream; set aside.

In a large saucepan of boiling water, cook the pasta 10 minutes. Add the asparagus and drained beans and cook 4 to 5 minutes more, or until the asparagus is tender. Drain the pasta mixture, rinse with cold water, and drain well again. Combine the pasta mixture, salmon, and tomatoes in a large bowl. Toss with the vinaigrette.

## Roasted Beets and Carrots

Serves 6 (purple)

6 small beets trimmed, with 1 inch of stems attached (2 1/2 pounds with greens)

2 pounds carrots, peeled and cut diagonally into 3/4-inch-thick slices

2 tablespoons olive oil

Salt and pepper

Preheat the oven to 425°F.

Wrap the beets tightly in foil, making two packages, and roast in the middle of the oven until tender, about 1 1/4 hours. In a shallow baking pan, toss the carrots with the oil and salt and pepper to taste. Roast the carrots in the middle of the oven until tender, about 20 minutes. While the carrots are roasting, unwrap the beets and when just cool enough to handle, slip off the skins and remove the stems. Cut each beet into 6 wedges. Add the beets to the carrots, tossing to combine, and roast until the beets are hot and the carrots are very tender, about 15 minutes more.

# Roasted Cherry Tomatoes

Serves 8    (purple)

*BETH EVIN HEFFNER*

2 pints organic cherry tomatoes

2 pints organic yellow teardrop tomatoes

2 tablespoons olive oil

Kosher salt

Pepper

10 basil leaves, cut into chiffonade

2 tablespoons red wine vinegar

Preheat the oven to 400°F.

In a large bowl, toss the tomatoes lightly with the olive oil. Spread them in one layer on a baking sheet and sprinkle generously with kosher salt and pepper. Roast for 15 to 20 minutes, until the tomatoes are soft. Transfer the tomatoes to a serving platter and sprinkle with the basil leaves, salt, and red wine vinegar. Serve hot or at room temperature.

# Peas with Celery Root   Serves 8    (blue)

*Celery root, a popular fall vegetable, tastes like a cross between celery and parsley.*

1½ pounds celery root (celeriac), peeled and cut into ½-inch pieces

4 tablespoons (½ stick) soy margarine

1 shallot, chopped

1 16-ounce package frozen organic petit peas, thawed

1 teaspoon celery salt

Salt and pepper

In a large pot of boiling salted water, boil the celery root until just tender, about 5 minutes; drain. Melt the margarine in a large, heavy pot over medium heat. Add the shallot and sauté until just tender, about 3 minutes. Add the celery root, peas, and celery salt and sauté until the vegetables are heated through and steaming, about 8 minutes. Season to taste with salt and pepper.

Today, over one billion Valentine cards are sent in the United States—second in number only to Christmas cards.—Did you know.com

The wholesale value of domestically produced roses in 2000 was $69 million. Roses generated the highest receipts of any type of cut flower category, followed by lilies at $59 million.

Twenty-nine pounds per capita consumption of candy by Americans in 2000; it is believed a large portion is consumed around Valentine's Day.—U.S. Census Bureau

Valentine's Day

## Cupid's Chocolate Cake  s e r v e s   9   ( y e l l o w )

8 ounces soy margarine, softened

1 cup Sucanat

6 large organic eggs

1½ cups unbleached white flour

½ teaspoon baking powder

¾ cup cocoa powder

9 ounces grain-sweetened chocolate chips

¾ cup soy cream

Preheat the oven to 350°F and grease and flour an 8-inch-square cake pan.

In a large bowl with an electric mixer, beat the margarine and Sucanat until creamy. Add the eggs one at a time, beating well. Sift the flour, baking powder, and cocoa powder over the margarine mixture and stir until combined. Pour into the prepared cake pan and bake 40 minutes, or until a toothpick inserted into the center comes out clean. Cool on a rack, chill in the refrigerator for 30 minutes, and cut into squares.

To make the glaze, in a small saucepan over low heat, melt the chocolate chips in the soy cream, stirring until smooth. Cool to room temperature. Pour the glaze over the cake and refrigerate to set.

## Stuffed Oranges  s e r v e s   1 2   ( y e l l o w )

*M A R Y   B E T H   B O R K O W S K I*

6 large oranges

1 pint orange sorbet, softened

1 pint vanilla soy dream, softened

Raspberry Sauce (recipe follows)

Cut a half dollar–sized slice from the top of each orange. Using a grapefruit knife and spoon, scoop out the inside of each orange, leaving a shell. Push 3 tablespoons of sorbet into the bottom of each orange. Arrange in a flat baking dish and freeze for half an hour. Remove from the freezer and push 3 tablespoons of vanilla soy dream into each orange. Spoon the raspberry sauce over the soy dream to cover and freeze another half hour. Repeat with another layer of orange sorbet, vanilla soy dream, and raspberry sauce. Freeze until ready to serve. Just before serving, slice through from top to bottom, using a large, nonserrated knife. They will fall open to form their own cups and show the ingredient layers.

### RASPBERRY SAUCE

1 10-ounce bag frozen raspberries, thawed

2 tablespoons evaporated cane juice crystals

2 tablespoons Grand Marnier (optional)

In a large bowl, roughly mash the berries, using a hand-held potato masher. Stir in the cane juice crystals and Grand Marnier, if using. Heat over low heat, stirring occasionally, for 3 to 5 minutes, until the crystals dissolve. Refrigerate until ready to use.

# Chocolate Lovers' Hazelnut Macaroons

Makes 2½ dozen cookies    (yellow)

1 cup hazelnuts

1 cup Sucanat

¼ cup unsweetened cocoa

2 ounces unsweetened chocolate chips

⅛ teaspoon salt

2 large organic egg whites

1 teaspoon vanilla extract

Preheat the oven to 350°F. Place the hazelnuts in a 9 × 13-inch metal baking pan and bake 15 minutes, or until golden brown. Cool. Line 2 large cookie sheets with foil. Place the hazelnuts in a clean dish towel and rub them back and forth to remove the skins. In a food processor with a metal blade, process the hazelnuts, Sucanat, cocoa, chocolate chips, and salt until the nuts and chocolate are finely ground. Add the egg whites and vanilla and process until blended. On a prepared cookie sheet, drop the dough by rounded teaspoons, using another spoon to release batter and leaving 2 inches between the macaroons. Bake 10 minutes, rotating sheets between upper and lower racks halfway through baking, or until the tops feel firm when pressed lightly. Cool on the cookie sheets on wire racks.

# Chocolate Mousse    Serves 8    (yellow)

¾ cup semisweet grain-sweetened
    chocolate chips

1 12.3-ounce package reduced-fat, extra-firm
    organic silken tofu (such as Mori-Nu)

¼ teaspoon salt

3 large organic egg whites

½ cup Sucanat

Place the chocolate chips in a small glass bowl and microwave on high 1½ minutes, or until almost melted, stirring after 1 minute. Place the chocolate and tofu in a food processor or blender and process 2 minutes, or until smooth. In a medium bowl, beat the salt and egg whites with a mixer on high speed until stiff peaks form. In a small saucepan, combine the Sucanat and ¼ cup water and bring to a boil over medium heat. Cook, without stirring, until a candy thermometer registers 238°F. Pour the hot sugar syrup in a thin stream over the egg whites, beating at high speed. Gently stir ¼ of the meringue into the tofu mixture, then gently fold in the remaining meringue. Spoon ½ cup of the mousse into each of 8 6-ounce custard cups. Cover and chill at least 4 hours.

## BEVERAGES

Anything with cranberry, strawberry, or cherry, of course. There are plenty of healthy, all-natural brands available. For grown-up tastes, with or without the alcohol, try these. (All recipes make 1 serving.)

## THM COSMOPOLITAN

2½ ounces organic fruit juice–sweetened lemonade (I recommend R. W. Knudsen's or Santa Cruz lemonade)

1½ ounces vodka (optional)

1 teaspoon unsweetened natural cranberry juice

1 orange wedge (¼ orange) or 1 tablespoon orange juice

Combine the lemonade, vodka, if using, and cranberry juice. Squeeze in the orange juice. Shake with ice, strain into a martini glass, and serve.

## DREAMSICLE

3 ounces strawberry purée

1½ ounces Vanilla Silk

1½ ounces vodka (optional)

Pour the strawberry purée, Vanilla Silk, and vodka, if using, over ice. Shake, pour into a highball glass, and serve.

## TOOTSIE ROLL

1 ounce Silk Soymilk Creamer

1 ounce orange juice (no pulp)

1 ounce Kahlúa (optional)

Sparkling mineral water

Combine the creamer, orange juice, and Kahlúa if using, over ice. Shake, pour into a rocks glass, and top off with sparkling mineral water.

## Pear Bellini

2 ounces pear juice or nectar
  (I recommend Ceres brand)
1/4 ounce natural unsweetened cranberry
  juice
4 ounces champagne

Combine the pear juice and cranberry juice.
Slowly pour in the champagne. Serve in a wine or champagne glass.

## Nonalcoholic Pear Bellini

2 ounces sparkling mineral water, like
  Pellegrino or Perrier
2 ounces pear juice or nectar
  (I recommend Ceres brand)
2 ounces Martinelli's Sparkling Cider

Combine the mineral water and pear juice. Add the cider. Serve in a wine or champagne glass.

## THM Pinklúa and Cream

*Warning: not lo-cal!*

2 ounces Silk Coffee Soylatte
2 ounces Silk Vanilla Creamer or soy milk
1 tablespoon fresh strawberry purée
1 1/2 ounces vodka (optional)
Grated nutmeg or ground cinnamon
  (optional)

Combine the coffee soylatte, vanilla soy milk, strawberry purée, and vodka, if using. Shake or stir, pour into a rocks glass, and serve. Sprinkle with nutmeg or cinnamon, if using.

## PARTY IDEAS

- *Couples Party*—Avoid the restaurant shuffle. There's nothing worse than trying to be cozy in a restaurant while the two of you are jammed up against another couple also trying to be cozy and romantic. Instead of jamming yourself up with strange couples, get jammed up with couples you know. Invite three to five couples over for dinner. One of my best Valentine's Days ever was celebrated with four other couples. We talked about everything from morning rituals to sleeping habits to the unusual signals each person used to initiate sex. It was a blast! And I think we all better appreciated our own mates by the end.
- *Singles Party*—Throw a party for all your unattached friends and celebrate your singleness. (What kind of party would Carrie from *Sex and the City* throw?)
- *Party for Two*—Celebrate a romantic evening in the privacy and comfort of your own home. Be adventurous. Pick a room you don't ordinarily use for eating. I always love to spread a blanket on the living room floor and have a picnic with candles, a fire in the fireplace, and beautiful music. Changing environments always leads to some interesting adventures.

## INVITATIONS

- *Couples Party*—Send invitations that you might send out for a children's party—or perhaps write invitations on those multipack children's valentines.
- *Singles Party*—Cut out hearts from colored paper. Rip them or cut them decoratively in half. Send one person half a heart, and another half to a person who you think might hit it off with them, whether romantically or as friends. Explain on the invitation that when they arrive they have to find their other half. If there is an uneven number of people, cut a heart in three parts.
- *Party for Two*—Plan a scavenger hunt for your loved one. Place notes around the house that slowly reveal the time and place of the dinner.

## DECORATIONS

- Use heart string lights, red candles, red heart confetti, roses.
- Replace the regular light bulbs in your house with red or pink ones.
- Cover the doormat with rose petals, and carve white princess pumpkins with heart shapes, using them as votives to line the steps or flank the doors.
- Make a Heart Tree—Any trees in the yard can be decorated with construction paper hearts in red and pink hung on clear string. Or drape several garlands of these hearts around the house.

## SCENTS

Chocolate
Rose
Merlot
Strawberries and champagne
Candy hearts
Aromatherapy scents if it is a private evening for two

# Toasts

Never go to bed angry. Stay up and fight.
— PHYLLIS DILLER

This is the miracle that happened every time to those who really love; the more they give, the more they possess.
— RILKE

Here's to love, the only fire against which there is no insurance!

Here's to the sweets that are out of sight
And not on our lawful diet,
To the stolen day and pilfered night,
To each and every dear delight,
Including the kiss on the quiet.

May we have those in our arms whom we love in our hearts.

Here's to the one and only one,
And may that one be he
Who loves but one and only one
And may that one be me.

Drink to the man who keeps his head though he loses his heart

May we kiss whom we please and please whom we kiss.

I have known many,
Liked a few,
Loved one,
Here's to you!

She: Just for today, I won't care where this is going.
He: Just for today, I'll say I love you first.

## ACTIVITIES AND GAMES

### Couples Party

- Play The Newlywed Game—Have each couple come to the party with a question. Or as host, make all the questions up yourself. The couple who wins gets a massage kit, soy margarine, and a copy of *Last Tango in Paris*.
- Blindfold the wives and have each of them feel the hands of the men at the party. See if they can pick out their husband's hand. Blindfold the men and see if they can do any better.
- Each person hides an item of clothing that belongs to him or her in a certain area in the house. All the men have to look for their wives' items at the same time. The women do the same after the men find all their items.

### Singles Party

- The Dating Game—Match up bachelor contestants with three bachelorettes each, or each women with three bachelors. Have the other guests make up the questions.
- Personal Ad Game—Each person comes to the party having written his or her own ad. Put all the ads in a pile to be read aloud. Have everyone guess the author and match them with their date for the evening based on their ads.
- Hide Valentine-appropriate items, such as roses or cut-out hearts, in two different rooms. The guys look for an object in one room while the women look in another. When everyone

has found an object, for example, the guy who found a rose is matched with the woman who found a rose. (No switching allowed!)

- Collect several clever one-page cartoons with captions, such as those found in the *Saturday Evening Post* or *Playboy*. When guests arrive, give each girl a cartoon without its caption and every guy a caption without its cartoon. During the party, guests are to find their matching cartoon half. This usually leads to some odd matches and funny conversation.
- Pretend you're back in eighth grade and play spin the bottle; slap, kiss, hug; or choo-choo.

## Party for Two

- Strip Poker, Strip Hearts, or even Strip Yahtzee, and for you eggheads—Strip Scrabble.
- Play the 9½ *Weeks* refrigerator game as Kim Basinger and Mickey Rourke. Make sure you taste only THM-approved foods—no sugar, no dairy, no chemicals—but keep the blindfold. And try to use *organic* strawberries with your nondairy whipped cream.
- If you're really brave, ask personal questions about each other and give rewards for the correct answers. For example, the woman asks the man her shoe size or her favorite color, and if he answers correctly, she takes off an article of clothing.

## PRIZES, GIFTS, AND PARTY FAVORS

Underwear, stuffed animals, love potions, candles, poetry books, *True Romance* comic books, massage oils, romance novels, blindfolds, little black books, sex slave coupons, apology coupons, coupons to see "whatever movie you want."

## MUSIC

You could fill an entire book with music selections that get you in the mood. My personal favorites are Frank Sinatra, Barry White, and, if truth be told, I tried to conceive both of my children to Van Morrison. So anything by those three artists is a good place to start.

| | | |
|---|---|---|
| "You Are So Beautiful" | Joe Cocker | Song |
| *I'm Your Baby Tonight* | Whitney Houston | Album |
| XO | Elliot Smith | Album |
| *I Never Loved a Man the Way I Love You* | Aretha Franklin | Album |
| *Where the Heart Is* | Various | Soundtrack |
| (anything by) | Heart | Band |
| *Only Trust Your Heart* | Diana Krall | Album |
| *Amplified Heart* | Anything but the Girl | Album |
| "Loved" | Merrick | Song |
| *I Can Hear the Heart Beating as One* | Yo La Tengo | Album |

| | | |
|---|---|---|
| *Heart & Soul* | Vonda Shepard | Album |
| *One from the Heart* | Tom Waits | Album |
| *Heart Like a Wheel* | Linda Ronstadt | Album |
| *Song from the Heart* | Nat King Cole | Album |
| *Seasons of the Heart* | John Denver | Album |
| *Warm Your Heart* | Aaron Neville | Album |
| *State of the Heart* | Mary Chapin Carpenter | Album |
| *Transmissions from the Satellite Heart* | The Flaming Lips | Album |
| *Heart & Soul* | Elvis | Album |
| *Heart in Motion* | Amy Grant | Album |
| *The Heart of a Woman* | Etta James | Album |
| *The Wild Heart* | Stevie Nicks | Album |
| *My Cherie Amour* | Stevie Wonder | Album |
| *Harden My Heart* | Quarterflash | Album |
| *Matters of the Heart* | Tracy Chapman | Album |
| *You Belong to My Heart* | Engelbert Humperdinck | Album |
| *Groove Is in the Heart* | Deee Lite | Album |
| *Heart's Horizon* | Al Jarreau | Album |
| *Untamed Heart* | Various | Soundtrack |
| *Sgt. Pepper's Lonely Hearts Club Band* | Beatles | Album |

The human heart creates enough pressure when it pumps out to the body to squirt blood 30 feet. Consider how much blood it moves in a lifetime!

Humans and dolphins are the only species that have sex for pleasure.

Some lions mate over fifty times a day.

40 percent of women have hurled footwear at a man.

The average sexual experience lasts about thirty-nine minutes.—s q u a r e w h e e l s . c o m

Valentine's Day

## MOVIES

### For Couples

| | |
|---|---|
| *Two for the Road* | (1967–NR) |
| *An Affair to Remember* | (1957–NR) |
| *Sleepless in Seattle* | (1993–PG) |
| *Romeo and Juliet* | (1936, 1954, 1966, 1968–PG; 1996–PG-13) |
| *Pretty Woman* | (1990–R) |
| *Somewhere in Time* | (1980–PG) |
| *Bridges of Madison County* | (1995–PG13) |
| *Four Weddings and a Funeral* | (1994–R) |
| *Bridget Jones' Diary* | (2001–R) |
| *Thomas Crown Affair* | (1968–NR; 2001–R) |
| *Shakespeare in Love* | (1998–R) |
| *Love in the Afternoon* | (1957–NR) |
| *9½ Weeks* | (1989–R) |

### For Singles

| | |
|---|---|
| *My Best Friend's Wedding* | (1997–PG-13) |
| *Casablanca* | (1942–NR) |
| *Shampoo* | (1975–R) |
| *Unmarried Woman* | (1978–R) |
| *Fatal Attraction* | (1987–R) |

## Exercise and Calorie Chart

| Activity | Calories Burned/Hour |
|---|---|
| Aerobic class | 422 |
| Running | 363 |
| Dancing | 320 |
| Dirty dancing | 640 |
| Sex | 258 |
| Great sex | 516 |
| Proposing | 302 |
| Seeing an old boyfriend while looking good | 192 |
| Seeing an old boyfriend while looking bad | 292 |
| Waiting for a first date | 182 |
| Waiting for a blind date | 232 |
| Stolen kisses in a broom closet | 202 |
| Stolen kisses in a broom closet while your date is knocking on the door | 404 |
| Fighting with your soon-to-be ex | 346 |
| Makeup sex | 516 |

## Celebrity Holiday Stories

| Celebrity | Event |
|---|---|
| Sharon Stone | Married Phil Bronstein on 2-14-98 |
| Prince | Married Mayte Garcia on 2-14-96; marriage annulled 1998; recommitted their love on 2-14-2000; broke up 2000 |
| Christian Slater | Married Ryan Haddon on 2-14-2000 |
| Elle Macpherson | Gave birth to baby boy on 2-14-98 in New York City |
| Noah Wylie | Proposed to Tracy Warbin on 2-14-1999 |

Valentine's Day

Women feel more comfortable undressing in front of men than they do undressing in front of other women. Women are too judgmental, whereas men are just grateful.
—ROBERT DE NIRO

See, the problem is that God gives men a brain and a penis, and only enough blood to run one at a time.
—ROBIN WILLIAMS

Women might be able to fake orgasms. But men can fake whole relationships.
—SHARON STONE

## FOR THE KIDS

For an invitation to a children's party, send a plain white T-shirt with a red heart safety-pinned to it that says, "Please come to a Valentine's Party (date, time, and so on). Bring this T-shirt to decorate."

Throw a craft party for children at which they can assemble and decorate their own:
- Paper kites
- Paper fans
- Beaded necklaces, bracelets, and so on
- Candles
- Soap
- Handmade books
- Rag dolls
- T-shirts with Valentine's theme

Be sure to check that all materials are machine washable and child safe. You may want to buy extra T-shirts or provide some of your old shirts to be used as children's smocks. It has been my experience that children will eat far less candy if they are involved in an activity that interests them and sparks their interest and imagination.

You may also want to take advantage of the fact that February is American Heart Month and teach your children about their heart. My son Joey surprised me one day by making a fist and telling me that he'd learned in school that his fist is the size of his heart. It's a lesson he will never forget. Children are great sponges for information, and what a great opportunity to introduce your children to the value of cardiovascular exercise and information about a healthy heart.

# Academy Awards

I have two words for you today: *star food.*

Tonight, for the Academy Awards, I want you to think like a star, feel like a star, and, most important of all, *eat* like a star.

When I first began working on *Taxi*, I knew it was going to be different from any other professional acting job I had ever done. It was the first time I was costarring as a regular on a major sitcom, and the buzz was that *Taxi* was going to be a big hit. It was time to really take my career seriously. On the first day of rehearsal, I went up to the craft service table to get a snack. The craft service table is a snack table for the cast and crew and has all the stuff you usually see at a bad teen party: potato chips, M&Ms, brownies, soft drinks, cheese, and crackers.

One of the older crew guys, Jack Mann, saw me eyeballing the table and said, "You don't really want to eat this junk, do you?" I laughed and said, "Well, maybe just a little something to tide me over until dinner." And he said, "No, you can't. This is what the crew eats. Look at these guys around here. Look how out of shape they are. You wanna look like this crew? This isn't star food. This is crew food! I love these guys, but let's be honest; most of them look like John Madden. Is that the kind of body you want? You know, you're in a sitcom now, young lady. You've got an obligation to watch that figure. You've got to eat star food now!"

Well, I never forgot Jack's great advice. Since then, I've always looked at that stuff as junk food that makes everybody who eat it look . . . well . . . um . . . less than stellar.

So for tonight's Oscar party, reach for the star food. Imagine that you're going to be filmed tomorrow. How would you eat tonight? Nobody wants to look puffy and bloated on camera. The camera never lies. Skip the chips, dips, candy, and cheese.

You are what you eat. And tonight, you're a star!

## HISTORY, FACTS, AND FOLKLORE

Once upon a time there were no E-channel, *People* magazine, *In Style,* and access shows that revealed everything from a celebrity's bathroom to his or her shoe collection. If you wanted to see what Elizabeth Taylor was like when she was Elizabeth Taylor the movie star (the jewels, the dress, the walk), you had to watch the Academy Awards. And it happened only once a year.

Once a year! Now that's a holiday. That's what made young girls in the Midwest willing to do "bus and truck" tours and Samsonite commercials and live in New York studios the size of dimes.

Who doesn't like movies? The Academy Awards is about flourishing in an art that entertains the world, people reveling in the results of creative efforts, drive, and tenacity. Now that takes stamina and energy and—you know what's coming next—*health!* So plan your party and make it healthy.

## HENNER HOLIDAY TRADITIONS AND STORIES

I grew up in a very theatrical, artsy kind of family. My mother ran a dancing school in our remodeled garage and a beauty shop out of our kitchen, while my uncle taught art classes in his upstairs apartment. Both of them were obsessed with old movies. She loved Lana Turner, and he loved Betty Grable. They argued over who was sexier with the same intensity that countries argue over border disputes. Movies were so important to my mother that she would actually encourage us to take naps after school so we could stay up to watch the Late Show. She felt as if she was on a first name basis with most of the stars, so I went into show business thinking that movie stars were our friends. Academy Awards night was obviously big in our house. We were up-to-date on all the nominees and always had a lot of friends over to watch. We didn't have shows like *Entertainment Tonight* back then, and many of the big movie stars would not be seen on *The Tonight Show* or game shows, so Oscar night was a rare opportunity to see many of the stars be themselves.

I've been practicing my own acceptance speech in my head since I was four, especially during

Oscar parties. I used to look around the room and think about whom I would thank first, and depending on which brother or sister I was fighting with, who was going to be left out.

I've carried the Oscar party tradition into adulthood and have friends over almost every year. (I'm still practicing my speech, so be nice to me if you want to be mentioned.) My parties are always great fun. I give out ballots, usually ten dollar to play—winner take all. If you want to be a guaranteed winner, do as my brother Lorin does and research all the other award shows and critics' lists.

In 1992, the year *Silence of the Lambs* won, I went to a memorable star-studded Academy Awards party in New York, hosted by Michael Fuchs of HBO. Judith Regan brought me as her guest, and I won the pool. Sonia Braga collected my ballot. The moment she told me I had the winning ballot was the moment I met her for the first time. It was surreal, because I've always been a enormous fan of hers, and there she was, excited because she was correcting the winning ballot. I was also excited because I usually don't win pools, and the twenty-dollar-per-person pot was huge at $1,760. I gave the money to my sister Christal's charity, the Scholarship Builder Fund, a program for inner city kids that she managed in New York. If you feel awkward about having a pool at your party, decide ahead of time that the winner will donate the money to charity.

I've been to the Academy Awards ceremony twice, once in 1978 with John Travolta, who was nominated for *Saturday Night Fever,* and once in 1980 with Frederic Forrest, who was nominated for *The Rose.* It was really exciting both times, of course. But the first time I went, in 1978 with Johnny, it surprised me. I spent the day as most people do, getting ready for the big night, bursting with anticipation, too excited to relax or eat. When we finally got there, everyone was so excited, it felt like a bunch of kids playing dress-up for the evening. In fact, I was surprised to find that it had such a neighborhood-production, church-basement feel to it. Every time there was an embarrassing moment or a glitch, Johnny and I joked with each other, "I hope the PTA likes our show!" You realize that behind the scenes, behind all the glamour, it's just people putting on an assembly. That was the feeling. Watching it on television, I never saw the miscues, the professional seat fillers, or how tipsy and nervous the nominees really are.

Anyway, there is nothing like the Academy Awards. It is the most popular awards show on the planet, with over a billion viewers every year, and it is the perfect excuse for a great party!

## RECIPES

For your party you can make the star recipes in this chapter, or if you would like your party to favor a nominated movie, here are some suggestions that might spark your imagination.

- Hollywood in general: Champagne, caviar, spa cuisine
- *Silence of the Lambs:* Chianti with fava beans
- *Gosford Park:* Pheasant and red wine
- *Titanic:* Caviar, champagne, and English tea
- *Forrest Gump:* Shrimp gumbo
- *Gandhi:* Everyone has to fast and wear a loincloth (only kidding).
- *Tess:* Strawberries and nondairy whipped cream.
- *The Apartment:* Spaghetti strained through a tennis racquet.
- *Shakespeare in Love:* Turkey drumsticks to be eaten by hand, Henry VIII style.

## Salmon Dip  Serves 8  (yellow)

1 organic scallion, minced

½ cup minced smoked salmon

2 tablespoons minced organic parsley

1 cup soy sour cream

In a small bowl, mix all the ingredients well. Refrigerate for 2 to 3 hours and serve with baked whole wheat pita chips.

## Roasted Red Pepper and Hummus–Stuffed Cucumber

Serves 4  (blue)

1 large red bell pepper

2 teaspoons salt

2 cucumbers, peeled

1 15-ounce can chickpeas, rinsed

1 tablespoon olive oil

¼ cup fresh lemon juice

Toast the pepper on the stovetop over an open flame, turning with tongs until the pepper is completely blackened. Put the pepper into a paper bag with ½ teaspoon of the salt and close the bag airtight. The result should look like a blackened, shriveled pepper. Cut off the ends of the cucumbers. Cut each cucumber lengthwise, then into 6 half circles. Use a melon baller or spoon to gently scoop out seeds from each cucumber piece. In a food processor or blender, make the hummus by combining the chickpeas, oil, 1 tablespoon water, lemon juice, and the remaining 1½ teaspoons salt. Purée, adding more water if needed for creaminess. Remove the pepper from the bag and scrape off the black outer layer under cold running water. Cut the pepper open and remove the seeds and stem. Chop the pepper and add it to the hummus mixture. Purée until smooth. Spoon the mixture into the hollowed-out part of each cucumber round.

The first television broadcast of the Oscars took place in 1953—and was shown throughout the United States and Canada. Telecasting in color begun in 1966, and since 1969 the Oscars have been telecast throughout the world. By the mid-1990s the show was telecast in more than a hundred countries.

In 1970 George C. Scott refused the Oscar for his performance in *Patton*, and in 1972 Marlon Brando refused the Oscar for his role in *The Godfather*. They weren't the first, though. In 1935 a writer named Dudley Nichols refused to accept the Oscar for his movie *The Informer* because the Writers Guild was on strike against the movie studios at the time.

# Crab Canapes Serves 10 (green)

MARY BETH BORKOWSKI

8 slices white spelt bread

1 cup crabmeat

2/3 cup Vegenaise

2/3 cup grated soy Parmesan cheese

4 scallions, diced into small pieces

Paprika

Preheat the oven to 400°F.

Remove the crusts from the bread and slice into 4 pieces on the diagonal, to form triangles. Lay the bread triangles on a baking sheet and toast for 4 to 5 minutes, taking care not to allow them to get too brown. Lower the heat to 375°F.

In a medium bowl, blend the crabmeat, Vegenaise, soy Parmesan, and scallions. Top the toast triangles with the crab mixture and sprinkle lightly with paprika. Bake for 10 minutes, or until golden on top.

# Scallion Puffs with Bacon

Serves 10 (yellow)

MARY BETH BORKOWSKI

1/4 cup (1/2 stick) Earth Balance margarine

Salt

1/2 cup flour

2 large cage-free eggs

3 tablespoons minced scallions

4 slices soy bacon, cooked and crumbled

1 cup shredded soy cheese, Cheddar style
  (optional)

Pepper

Preheat the oven to 425°F.

In a small saucepan over medium heat, bring 1/2 cup water and the margarine to a boil. Stir in a pinch of salt. Add the flour all at once. Beat the ingredients with a wooden spoon until the mixture pulls away from the pan and forms a ball. Remove the pan from the heat and add the eggs; beat well. Stir in the scallions, bacon, and cheese, if using. Add salt and pepper to taste.

Drop by rounded teaspoons on a lightly greased baking sheet about 2 inches apart. Bake in the oven for 20 minutes, or until golden brown.

The Hustons are the only family to have produced three generations of Oscar winners: Walter Huston was named Best Supporting Actor in 1948 for his role in *The Treasure of the Sierra Madre*, John Huston was awarded Best Director/Adapted Screenplay for the same movie, and Anjelica Huston received an Oscar for Best Supporting Actress in *Prizzi's Honor*, 1985.

## Spicy Vodka Tomatoes  Serves 10  (green)

*MARY BETH BORKOWSKI*

- 1 pint cherry tomatoes, washed, stems removed
- 2 cups good-quality vodka
- 1 jalapeño pepper, sliced
- 1 cup coarse-ground sea salt

Pierce each tomato 4 to 5 times with a toothpick. Place the tomatoes in a straight-sided bowl and add the vodka over the top to cover. Add 4 or 5 jalapeño slices. Cover the bowl and refrigerate 8 hours or overnight.

When ready to serve, lay the tomatoes in a shallow bowl and pour enough vodka to come about halfway up the side of the tomatoes. Place the salt in a small bowl for dipping the tomatoes. (A small dip is all it takes.)

## Potato Caviar Cups  Serves 10  (green)

*MARY BETH BORKOWSKI*

- 1 slice lavash bread
- 1 to 1½ cups light oil for frying
- 2 medium potatoes, peeled and cubed
- 2 teaspoons Earth Balance margarine
- 2 teaspoons homemade, nondairy yogurt cheese (recipe follows)
- Salt
- 2 teaspoons caviar

Using a round 2-inch cookie cutter, cut circles in the lavash bread. In a medium frying pan over medium-high heat, add the oil and bread and cook until light brown on both sides, about 5 minutes. Do not allow the bread to get too brown.

Place the toast circles in nonstick mini-muffin tins, pressing in with your knuckle or the back of a wooden spoon to form small cups. Refrigerate in an airtight container until set, about an hour. These may be made up to a day in advance.

In a small saucepan of boiling water, cook the potatoes until soft, about 25 minutes. Drain and mash with the margarine, cheese, and salt to taste. This can be made a day in advance and stored, covered, in the refrigerator.

Before assembling the ingredients, bring the cups to room temperature and heat the potato mixture just until slightly warm. Fill each toast cup with a teaspoon of the potato mixture and top with ⅛ teaspoon caviar.

# Coconut Chicken Serves 10 (yellow)

*MARY BETH BORKOWSKI*

2 cups nondairy pancake mix

2 tablespoons garlic powder

1 to 2 cups unflavored seltzer water

3 whole skinless, boneless chicken breasts,
  cut into 1 1/2-inch chunks

4 cups unsweetened shredded coconut

Canola oil for frying

In a shallow baking dish, mix the pancake mix with the garlic powder and add the seltzer a bit at a time to make a thick batter. Dip the chicken pieces in the batter, then roll them in the coconut.

In a large frying pan, add 1/8 inch of oil and heat on medium-high heat. When the oil is hot, fry the chicken in batches, browning both sides, about 5 to 7 minutes. Drain on paper towels.

# Moroccan Grilled Salmon Serves 4 (green)

1 cup chopped fresh organic parsley

1 cup chopped fresh organic cilantro

3 organic garlic cloves, minced

1 tablespoon chopped almonds

3/4 teaspoon salt

2 teaspoons sweet paprika

1 teaspoon black pepper

3/4 teaspoon ground cumin

Pinch of hot pepper flakes

3 tablespoons fresh organic lemon juice

1/3 cup vegetable broth

1 1/2 tablespoons extra-virgin olive oil

4 1/2 pounds salmon fillets

In a food processor, finely chop the parsley, cilantro, and garlic. Add the almonds, salt, paprika, pepper, cumin, hot pepper flakes, lemon juice, vegetable broth, and olive oil and grind to a coarse purée, running the machine in short bursts. Taste, adding salt and pepper if needed.

Run your fingers over the pieces of fish, feeling for bones and removing any you may find with a tweezers. Pour a third of the sauce over the bottom of a baking dish just large enough to hold the salmon. Arrange the salmon pieces on top. Spoon another third of the sauce over the fish and marinate in the refrigerator for 1 to 4 hours, covered. (The longer you marinate, the richer the flavor.)

Preheat the grill to high. Oil the grill grate. Grill the fish 4 to 6 minutes per side, turning with a spatula until it reaches the preferred doneness. Transfer the fish to plates or a platter and spoon the remaining sauce over it.

## Linguine with Garlic and Red Pepper

Serves 6    (purple)

Salt

1 pound dried linguine noodles

3 or 4 tablespoons olive oil

1/4 to 1/2 teaspoon dried crushed red pepper
   flakes

3 garlic cloves, sliced

1/2 cup chopped fresh organic parsley

1/2 teaspoon black pepper

In a large pot over high heat, add 6 quarts of water and bring to a boil. Add a teaspoon of salt and the linguine. Cook for 11 minutes, until al dente. Drain and set aside.

In a large nonstick skillet over medium-high heat, add the oil and red pepper flakes; cook 2 minutes. Add the garlic and sauté until the garlic is lightly browned, about 30 seconds. Remove from the heat. Stir in the pasta, parsley, salt to taste, and pepper. Combine the sauce with the linguine and serve immediately.

## Coconut Macaroons

Makes 3 1/2 dozen    (yellow)

3 cups flaked sweetened coconut

4 large cage-free organic egg whites

3/4 cup Sucanat

1 teaspoon vanilla extract

1/4 teaspoon salt

1/8 teaspoon almond extract

Preheat the oven to 325°F. Line 2 large cookie sheets with cooking parchment. In a large bowl, combine the coconut, egg whites, Sucanat, vanilla, salt, and almond extract. Scoop the dough into rounded teaspoons and drop onto the cookie sheets, keeping 1 inch between the cookies. Bake 25 minutes, or until set and lightly golden, rotating sheets between the upper and lower racks halfway through baking. Cool 1 or 2 minutes on the cookie sheets. With a spatula, transfer the cookies to a wire cooling rack to cool completely.

# Truffle Cookies  Serves 6  (yellow)

4 ounces unsweetened chocolate, chopped

6 tablespoons (¾ stick) soy margarine, cut into small pieces

2 cups semisweet grain-sweetened chocolate chips

½ cup unbleached flour

2 tablespoons unsweetened cocoa powder (not Dutch process)

¼ teaspoon baking powder

½ teaspoon salt

1 cup Sucanat

3 large cage-free organic eggs

1½ teaspoons vanilla extract

Melt the chocolate, margarine, and 1 cup of the chocolate chips in a 1-quart heavy saucepan over low heat, stirring occasionally. Cool. In a large bowl, stir together the flour, cocoa, baking powder, and salt. In another bowl, beat together the Sucanat, eggs, and vanilla with an electric mixer until pale and frothy, about 2 minutes. On low speed, mix in the melted chocolate mixture and then the flour mixture until well combined. Stir in the remaining cup of chocolate chips. Chill, covered, until firm, about 2 hours.

Preheat the oven to 350°F.

With a dampened hand, roll heaping teaspoons of dough into 1-inch balls and arrange 2 inches apart on ungreased baking sheets. Bake in batches in the middle of the oven until puffed and set, about 10 minutes. The cookies will be soft in the center. Transfer to racks to cool.

Only two married couples have won Oscars for acting roles: Laurence Olivier (*Hamlet*, 1948) and Vivian Leigh (*A Streetcar Named Desire*, 1951); and Joanne Woodward (*The Three Faces of Eve*, 1957) and Paul Newman (*The Color of Money*, 1986). The only sisters to have won Oscars are Joan Fontaine (*Suspicion*, 1941) and Olivia de Havilland (*To Each His Own*, 1946, and *The Heiress*, 1949).

Each year, about 800 movies are released annually in India, about twice the output of Hollywood.—D i d y o u k n o w . c o m

That first year, 1929, fifteen statuettes were awarded, all of them to men except for Janet Gaynor.

## BEVERAGES

Champagne, *dahling!* Or anything bubbly, like carbonated apple juice, but definitely served in stemware.

## PARTY IDEAS

The key to planning an Academy Awards party is to base your party choices on the main movies involved, usually the five Best Picture nominees. Since the nominations come out only six weeks before the awards, you will have to wait until then to plan your menu, decorations, activities, games, ballot, and almost everything else. However, the Hollywood theme in general works for every year, so for some of the categories I will give you suggestions that work no matter what films are nominated. Plus, I'll give examples from past years that fit perfectly to help you plan using the films you'll have to work with.

## INVITATIONS

- Send a video of your kids or you walking down the red carpet or giving acceptance speeches with information about the party given at the end of the speech.
- Along with the invitation, send a ballot to be filled out and brought to the party. Sending the ballot ahead of time will give your guest time to fill it out.

## DECORATIONS

Movie posters, Hollywood signs, Walk of Fame place mats with each person's name, director's chairs, clapboards, popcorn cups, movie stubs, posters, or anything that reflects the themes of current nominees. For example:

- *Gladiator*—any ancient Roman art-architecture-Coliseum-Ben Hur-type stuff.
- *Shakespeare in Love*—anything ye wishes as long as 'tis "olde" and hast that look of yore. At least that's what methinks.
- *Forrest Gump*—Smile buttons, American flags, Vietnam War symbols.
- *Braveheart*—Scottish plaids, medieval castles, posters of Scotland. Have the kids greet guests dressed and painted like William Wallace.

## SCENTS

Roses
Scented candles
Greasepaint

## ACTIVITIES AND GAMES

- Have an Academy Awards pool. To make ballots, start with a complete list of all the nominees, which you can get online or from *Variety* or the *Hollywood Reporter* following the release of the nominees in mid-February. Decide if your pool will include *all* the categories or just the top awards. I highly recommend including all the categories (or as many as possible). That way your guests will stay interested throughout the night and not be bored during the minor categories. Type up the ballot, leaving a space for guests to mark their choices. The ballot with the most correct choices wins. Some trade magazines like *Entertainment Weekly* and *Movieline* print a ballot for you. All you need to do is make copies and give one to each guest. Or better yet, as I mentioned, mail them with the invitation.

- Buy disposable cameras and have your kids act as paparazzi as guests arrive.
- Have someone film your guests' walk-ins and show them after the awards or during the commercials. You can even have one of your children interview your guests à la Joan Rivers and get that on film.
- Have one of your guests pretape an interview (à la Barbara Walters) with three of your other guests, or have your kids interview each other before or during the awards.
- Star Search—Have each guest choose a movie star and pick three of their movies. Find the ratings for those movies in a movie book (e.g., by Leonard Maltin or Roger Ebert). The highest cumulative rating wins.
- Divide your guests into teams. Lay out the fixings for pizza-making. Have each team design a pizza based on a movie. The winning team for most imaginative pizza gets a Wolfgang Puck (caterer for Academy Awards Governors Ball) cookbook.

## PRIZES, GIFTS, AND PARTY FAVORS

*AFI Book of Greatest Movies,* movie books by famous directors, movie posters, disposable cameras, Hollywood Walk of Fame place mats, Glam nail polish, sun glasses, Hollywood memorabilia.

## MUSIC

Along with Academy Award collections or soundtracks from Oscar winners:

| | | |
|---|---|---|
| *Fame and Fortune* | Bad Company | Album |
| *Paradise Theater* | Styx | Album |
| "Magic Carpet Ride" | Steppenwolf | Song |
| *Roll Out the Red Carpet* | Buck Owens | Album |
| *Superstar Car Wash* | Goo Goo Dolls | Album |
| "Superstar" | Carpenters | Song |
| *Fame* | Various | Soundtrack |
| "Fame" | David Bowie | Song |

Academy Awards

| | | |
|---|---|---|
| "Fashion" | David Bowie | Song |
| *Fashion Nugget* | Cake | Album |
| *Songs from an American Movie* | Everclear | Album |
| *The Movie Song Album* | Tony Bennett | Album |

## Movies

| | |
|---|---|
| *The Oscar* | (1966–NR) |
| *The Player* | (1992–R) |
| *All About Eve* | (1950–NR) |
| *Plaza Suite* | (1971–PG) |

Or any great Oscar-winning movie, such as these Best Picture winners:

| | | |
|---|---|---|
| 1927–28 | *Wings* | NR |
| 1928–29 | *Broadway Melody* | NR |
| 1929–30 | *All Quiet on the Western Front* | NR |
| 1930–31 | *Cimarron* | NR |
| 1931–32 | *Grand Hotel* | NR |
| 1932–33 | *Cavalcade* | NR |
| 1934 | *It Happened One Night* | NR |
| 1935 | *Mutiny on the Bounty* | NR |
| 1936 | *The Great Ziegfeld* | NR |
| 1937 | *The Life of Emile Zola* | NR |
| 1938 | *You Can't Take It With You* | NR |
| 1939 | *Gone With the Wind* | NR |
| 1940 | *Rebecca* | NR |
| 1941 | *How Green Was My Valley* | NR |
| 1942 | *Mrs. Miniver* | NR |
| 1943 | *Casablanca* | NR |
| 1944 | *Going My Way* | NR |
| 1945 | *The Lost Weekend* | NR |

| 1946 | The Best Years of Our Lives | NR |
|------|------|------|
| 1947 | Gentlemen's Agreement | NR |
| 1948 | Hamlet | NR |
| 1949 | All the King's Men | NR |
| 1950 | All About Eve | NR |
| 1951 | An American in Paris | NR |
| 1952 | The Greatest Show on Earth | NR |
| 1953 | From Here to Eternity | NR |
| 1954 | On the Waterfront | NR |
| 1955 | Marty | NR |
| 1956 | Around the World in 80 Days | NR |
| 1957 | The Bridge on the River Kwai | NR |
| 1958 | Gigi | NR |
| 1959 | Ben-Hur | NR |
| 1960 | The Apartment | NR |
| 1961 | West Side Story | NR |
| 1962 | Lawrence of Arabia | NR |
| 1963 | Tom Jones | NR |
| 1964 | My Fair Lady | NR |
| 1965 | The Sound of Music | NR |
| 1966 | A Man for All Seasons | NR |
| 1967 | In the Heat of the Night | NR |
| 1968 | Oliver! | G |
| 1969 | Midnight Cowboy | R |
| 1970 | Patton | PG |
| 1971 | The French Connection | R |
| 1972 | The Godfather | R |
| 1973 | The Sting | PG |

# Academy Awards

| Year | Film | Rating |
|---|---|---|
| 1974 | The Godfather Part II | R |
| 1975 | One Flew Over the Cuckoo's Nest | R |
| 1976 | Rocky | PG |
| 1977 | Annie Hall | PG |
| 1978 | The Deer Hunter | R |
| 1979 | Kramer vs. Kramer | PG |
| 1980 | Ordinary People | R |
| 1981 | Chariots of Fire | PG |
| 1982 | Gandhi | PG |
| 1983 | Terms of Endearment | PG |
| 1984 | Amadeus | PG |
| 1985 | Out of Africa | PG |
| 1986 | Platoon | R |
| 1987 | The Last Emperor | PG-13 |
| 1988 | Rain Man | R |
| 1989 | Driving Miss Daisy | PG |
| 1990 | Dances with Wolves | PG-13 |
| 1991 | The Silence of the Lambs | R |
| 1992 | Unforgiven | R |
| 1993 | Schindler's List | R |
| 1994 | Forrest Gump | PG-13 |
| 1995 | Braveheart | R |
| 1996 | The English Patient | R |
| 1997 | Titanic | PG-13 |
| 1998 | Shakespeare in Love | R |
| 1999 | American Beauty | R |
| 2000 | Gladiator | R |
| 2001 | A Beautiful Mind | PG-13 |

## EXERCISE AND CALORIE CHART

Rent or buy your favorite celebrity exercise video to kick-start your day. Consider Jane Fonda if you want an actual Oscar winner (twice, in fact!), or if you want someone who's been there twice—*Dancerobics* by me.

| Activity | Calories Burned/Hour |
|---|---|
| Lifting weights the same weight as Oscar (8.5 pounds) | 211 |
| Walking the red carpet | 176 |
| Running from the paparazzi | 323 |
| Sprinting to the podium | 354 |

## FOR THE KIDS

One year as I was organizing an Academy Awards party and calling friends to invite, I kept saying Oscar party this and Oscar party that. A couple of days before the party, my son Joey, who was four at the time, asked me, "When is the Grouch party?" I said, "What are you talking about? What Grouch party?" And then I realized that he thought it was an Oscar the Grouch party, as on *Sesame Street.* So now we call it the Grouch Party in my house.

The Academy Awards have always been held on a school night, so most kids will be in bed before the end. Actually, most adults are in bed before the end—even on the West Coast! But keep the following in mind to get the kids involved: buy or make a zoetrope wheel so that your children can create their own short animated films. This will keep kids of all ages (and grownups) busy for hours making their own one-second cartoons. The DaMert Company makes an animation kit for kids (between $10 and $20) that includes a small zoetrope. You can find them at educational arts and crafts stores. You can make your own zoetrope if you're patient and skilled at that sort of thing; there's even a website dedicated to making your own: www. digitalstudio.ucr.edu.

## FOR COUPLES

Act out a juicy scene from one of the nominated films. For example, during the year *Titanic* ruled, you could have taken turns sketching each other in the buff. Or surprise each other by privately dressing up as Hollywood sex symbols. Try to pick someone who's very different from you to add to the surprise. Or how about playing Powerful Hollywood Mogul meets Demure, Innocent Ingenue, and have fun watching the awards from the casting couch.

If you don't feel that daring, then go head-to-head in an Oscar pool. The loser has to treat the winner to dinner.

# Mardi Gras

**M**ardi Gras is that final blowout before Lent, so please tread carefully; otherwise it's going to take you forty days to recover. It's really a shame that people tend to go on a binge before starting a healthy program. It's as if their main purpose for starting that program is to have carte blanche to binge the night before. They then have to spend the first few days, sometimes weeks, recovering from that binge—and wondering how they got so many beads! Bingeing like that is terribly taxing on both the cardiovascular and digestive system. Don't do this on Mardi Gras! You don't have to! It is so easy to make healthier versions of traditional Cajun-style dishes and enjoy Mardi Gras without moaning in bed the morning after. Let's be honest, New Orleans cooking is not known for being light and healthy, but those Cajun flavors can be easily achieved by applying a few tricks. Try one of the dishes in this book, like seafood gumbo, and you'll know exactly what I mean.

So go easy this year, and you will enjoy Mardi Gras more than ever. Eat light, drink light, and skip the cameo on *Girls Gone Wild.*

## HISTORY, FACTS, AND FOLKLORE

When the French settled in New Orleans, they brought the Mardi Gras holiday with them. It literally translates as "Fat Tuesday" and is normally celebrated with extreme decadence on the night before Ash Wednesday, the first day of the Lenten season. After Ash Wednesday the discipline begins, as people give something up for Lent such as sugar, alcohol, smoking, and so on.

About two weeks before Mardi Gras, the season begins with nightly parades and weekend festivals, or what they call Carnival. All the traditions are in full swing: balls are organized, trinkets are thrown from floats, favors are given away, costumes are displayed and put on parade, and spectators line the streets to watch. Everything in moderation, including it seems, moderation.

The official colors for Mardi Gras are purple, green, and gold. These colors were chosen by the King of Carnival in 1872, purple to represent justice, green to stand for faith, and gold to stand for power. (Sounds a lot like my rainbow theory!)

Speaking of my rainbow theory . . . before you settle in for purple mode, boot camp, or a THM Lenten regime, go to New Orleans, or better yet, make your own Mardi Gras at home.

## HENNER HOLIDAY TRADITIONS AND STORIES

Even as a child, I loved the concept of Lent. The whole idea of giving up something for the forty days before Easter really appealed to my sense of discipline, organization, and perseverance. Each year I would try to give up something that I was obsessed with, just to see if I could do it. Usually it was candy because of my enormous sweet tooth. I would struggle through the forty days not eating one bite, but come Easter morning—look out! I would devour anything and everything sweet in sight, including my little brother Lorin's cheeks. But occasionally, instead of giving something up, only to go back to it Easter morning, I would think of something to give up (I hoped) forever.

This happened when I was thirteen. I was a notorious nail-biter. I chewed those ten little guys down to the quick until there was nothing left except swollen, puffy stumps. My fingers would bleed and hurt like hell, but I didn't care. I kept chewing in spite of the pain, blood, and shredded skin. My mother hated this habit so much that she tried everything to get me to stop, including buying pepper-flavored nail polish. This did nothing but reinforce my love for spicy food. But being thirteen and in the eighth grade made me rethink this whole nail-biting thing. I was a teenager at last, and girly things like pretty nails were becoming important to me. So I gave up biting my nails for Lent.

Oh, my gosh! To this day, I don't think *anything* (except maybe giving up dairy products) has ever been so difficult. But I did it. I soldiered on and made it all the way to Easter without so much as a nibble. Imagine my surprise when I discovered that I had good nails. So good, in fact, that years later, during my young-actress-in-New-York days, I worked as a hand model in many commercials.

See that? You never know where giving up your unhealthy habits will lead.

## RECIPES
# Seafood Gumbo  Serves 6  (green)

*JAN DAVIS*

1 pound okra, sliced

¼ cup plus 2 tablespoons soy margarine, melted

¼ cup unbleached white flour

1 bunch green onions, sliced

½ cup chopped celery

2 garlic cloves, chopped

1 16-ounce can chopped tomatoes, undrained

1 bay leaf

1 tablespoon chopped fresh parsley

1 fresh thyme sprig

1½ teaspoons salt

½ to 1 teaspoon crushed red pepper flakes

1 pound fresh shrimp, peeled and deveined

1 pound fresh crabmeat

In a large skillet over medium-high heat, sauté the okra in 2 tablespoons of the soy margarine until the okra is lightly browned, about 7 to 10 minutes. Set aside. Combine the remaining ¼ cup margarine and the flour in a large iron skillet. Make a roux by cooking it over medium heat, stirring constantly, until the roux is the color of chocolate, about 20 to 25 minutes. Stir in the green onions, celery, and garlic and cook until the vegetables are tender, about 12 minutes.

In a large Dutch oven, combine the roux, okra, tomatoes, bay leaf, parsley, thyme, salt, red pepper, and 2 quarts water. Bring the mixture to a boil over high heat. Reduce the heat and simmer, uncovered, for 2 hours, stirring occasionally, or until it thickens.

Add the shrimp and crabmeat and simmer 10 minutes more. Remove the bay leaf and serve.

## Okra with a Kick  Serves 4  (purple/blue)

½ teaspoon ground cumin

½ teaspoon ground coriander

1 teaspoon turmeric

1 teaspoon mustard seeds

Small pinch of dried red pepper flakes

1 medium organic Spanish onion, finely chopped

1¾ cups fresh organic okra, cut into thirds on the diagonal

In a large nonstick skillet over medium-high heat, combine the cumin, coriander, turmeric, mustard seeds, and pepper flakes and cook, stirring with a wooden spoon, until the mustard seeds pop, about 2 minutes. Heat a wok or a large nonstick skillet over medium heat. Add the onion and cook for 2 minutes, until the onion is soft and translucent. Turn the heat to high and add the okra. Cook, stirring occasionally, until the okra gives slightly when pressed with a spoon, about 2 minutes.

## Mustard Greens with a Kick

Serves 4  (purple)

2½ tablespoons extra-virgin olive oil

1 onion, roughly chopped (about 1 cup)

3 cloves garlic, chopped

1 organic red jalapeño pepper, seeded and finely chopped, or ½ teaspoon hot red pepper flakes

1½ teaspoon cumin seeds

1 large bunch of organic mustard greens (about 2 pounds), chopped into bite-size pieces

3 tablespoons Braggs Liquid Aminos

Coarse sea salt

Freshly milled black pepper

In a large pot over medium heat, warm the oil. Add the onion and sauté about 5 minutes, or until softened. Add the garlic, jalapeño, and cumin and sauté 3 minutes more, or until the garlic is golden. Add the mustard greens and raise the heat to medium-high. Stir until the greens wilt, about 7 minutes. Reduce the heat to low and simmer, covered, for 25 to 30 minutes, or until the greens are tender. Season with the Braggs, add salt and pepper to taste. Serve hot or at room temperature.

# Spicy Chard and Collard Greens

Serves 6    (green)

1 pound fresh collard greens, washed and
coarsely chopped

1 cup vegetable broth

1 large red onion, cut in half

½ teaspoon crushed red pepper

1 bunch chard, washed and coarsely chopped

Salt

Pepper

Tabasco or other hot sauce

In a large stockpot over medium-high heat, add the collard greens, vegetable broth, onion, and red pepper and cover with water. Bring to a boil, lower the heat to medium, and simmer about 2 hours, or until the greens are tender. Add the chard and simmer 7 to 10 minutes, or until wilted. Remove the onion and season with salt, pepper, and hot sauce to taste.

Throws are inexpensive trinkets tossed from floats by costumed and masked Krewe members. Among the more popular items are krewe emblemed doubloons, plastic cups, and pearl, gold, or purple necklaces.

A King Cake is an oval, sugared pastry that contains a plastic doll hidden inside. The person who finds the doll is crowned "king" and buys the next cake or throws the next party.

The season of merriment begins annually on January 6, the Twelfth Night (feast of the Epiphany), and ends at midnight on Fat Tuesday.

—Home and Away

# Emeril's Pasta Salad with Garden Vegetables, Oven-Roasted Tomatoes, and Herbed Vinaigrette

Serves 6 (purple/blue)

*EMERIL LAGASSE*

1 pint red grape tomatoes

1 tablespoon extra-virgin olive oil

1/4 teaspoon salt

1/8 teaspoon freshly ground black pepper

1 pound farfalle (bow tie pasta)

1 small zucchini, trimmed, cut in half lengthwise, and thinly sliced

1 small yellow squash, trimmed, cut in half lengthwise, and thinly sliced

1 small red onion, cut in half and thinly sliced

1/2 cup diced red bell pepper

Herbed Vinaigrette (see recipe below)

Preheat the oven to 400°F.

Place the tomatoes on a baking sheet. Toss with the olive oil, salt, and pepper to lightly coat. Roast until the tomatoes are tender and starting to split, 10 to 15 minutes. Remove from the oven and let cool.

Bring a large pot of salted water to a boil. Add the pasta and cook, stirring occasionally to keep it from sticking, until tender but firm to the bite. Drain in a colander and rinse under cold running water. Drain well. Transfer to a large bowl and toss with the roasted tomatoes and the remaining ingredients. Toss with enough dressing to lightly coat. Adjust the seasoning to taste, adding more dressing if desired.

## HERBED VINAIGRETTE Makes about 1 1/4 cups (blue)

1/4 cup chopped fresh basil

2 tablespoons chopped fresh parsley

2 tablespoons white wine vinegar

2 teaspoons fresh lemon juice

1 teaspoon minced garlic

1/2 teaspoon salt

1/4 teaspoon freshly ground black pepper

1/4 cup olive oil or vegetable oil

1/4 cup extra-virgin olive oil

In a medium bowl, combine the herbs, vinegar, lemon juice, garlic, salt, and pepper and whisk to blend. Slowly add the oils in a steady stream, whisking constantly until the mixture thickens. Use immediately, or cover and refrigerate until ready to use.

# Emeril's Gumbo L'Herbes

Serves 8 to 10   (yellow with chicken/
green without)

*EMERIL LAGASSE*

1½ pounds chicken or smoked turkey
  (optional)

1 teaspoon salt

½ teaspoon cayenne

5 bay leaves

8½ cups water

4 pounds assorted greens, such as collards,
  mustard, turnip, spinach, chard, and kale,
  trimmed, washed, and dried

2 tablespoons vegetable oil

2 cups chopped yellow onions

1 cup chopped bell peppers

1 cup chopped celery

½ teaspoon dried thyme

½ teaspoon dried oregano

½ teaspoon dried basil

¼ cup chopped fresh parsley leaves

4 tablespoons soy margarine (optional)

Steamed white rice (optional
  accompaniment)

Filé powder

Put the chicken, if using, with the salt, cayenne, and bay leaves in a large, deep pot and add the water. Bring to a boil over medium-high heat and cook for 30 minutes. With a slotted spoon, remove the chicken and when cool enough to handle, chop it. Set aside.

Reduce the heat to medium and add the greens, a handful at a time, and blanch until wilted. Drain, reserving the liquid. Coarsely chop the greens and set aside.

In the same pot, heat the oil over medium heat and add the onions, bell peppers, and celery. Cook, stirring often, until the vegetables are wilted and golden, about 10 minutes. Add the chicken, greens, reserved liquid, thyme, oregano, basil, and parsley. Bring to a gentle boil and simmer for 1½ hours. Remove the bay leaves. (If not using meat, add 4 tablespoons soy margarine to the pot just before removing from the heat.)

Serve in deep soup bowls over rice, if desired, with filé powder passed at the table for guests to thicken the gumbo to their personal taste.

Moon Pies became the official food of Mardi Gras in Mobile, Alabama. Pies became objects to throw at carnival, when mystic societies were ordered to find something soft and aerodynamic to replace the Cracker Jack boxes that had been used previously.

# Blackened Sea Bass  Serves 4  (purple)

2 teaspoons paprika

1½ teaspoons cayenne

1 teaspoon salt

1 teaspoon onion powder

1 teaspoon black pepper

½ teaspoon dried thyme

½ teaspoon dried oregano

½ teaspoon white pepper

½ teaspoon cumin

4 4 to 6 ounce sea bass fillets,
  boned and skin removed

2 tablespoons olive oil

2 teaspoons soy margarine

4 lemon wedges (optional)

Preheat the oven to 400°F. In a large plastic bag, combine the paprika, cayenne, salt, onion powder, black pepper, thyme, oregano, white pepper, and cumin and shake until well blended. Brush each fillet lightly on both sides with olive oil and toss in the bag of spices until well coated. Heat a large cast-iron skillet on high heat for 3 to 5 minutes (you can't get it too hot). When the skillet begins to smoke, add the fillets and cook 2 to 3 minutes on each side, or until the outside is blackened. Remove from the heat and top each fillet with ½ teaspoon margarine. Place the skillet in the oven and cook for 5 minutes, or until the fish flakes apart gently with a fork.

# Red Beans and Rice Serves 6 to 8 (green)

*THIS RECIPE IS BEST IF YOU SOAK THE BEANS OVERNIGHT*

1 onion, finely chopped

2 tablespoons olive oil

1 pound spicy chicken sausage, cut into 1-inch pieces

1 red bell pepper, seeded and chopped

3 cloves garlic, chopped

2 cups dried red kidney beans, soaked overnight

3½ cups vegetable broth

3 cups water

1 bay leaf

2 cups uncooked rice, rinsed

Salt

Pepper

Tabasco

In a large skillet over medium heat, sauté the onion in the olive oil until translucent, about 5 minutes. Add the chicken sausage, bell pepper, and garlic and sauté about 7 to 10 minutes, or until the chicken sausage is no longer pink.

In a large stockpot over medium-high heat, add the drained beans, broth, water, and bay leaf and bring to a boil. Add the sausage mixture, cover, reduce the heat to medium-low, and simmer 45 to 60 minutes, or until the beans are soft. Add the rice and ½ cup water (or more if needed; there should be enough liquid to be absorbed by the rice). Cover and simmer until the rice is cooked, about 25 minutes. Season with salt, pepper, and Tabasco.

# Crabmeat Salad with Celery, Peppers, and Cayenne Serves 4 (blue/green)

JONATHAN WAXMAN, WASHINGTON PARK RESTAURANT

1 head baby romaine, washed and cut into
   long strips

1 pound Louisiana jumbo lump crabmeat

1 stalk celery, diced

1 red bell pepper, diced

1 green bell pepper, diced

1 poblano pepper, diced

Pinch cayenne

Juice of ½ orange

Juice of 1 lime

¼ cup sake

1 teaspoon fresh thyme leaves

¼ cup olive oil

Chill the romaine in a bowl of ice water for 10 minutes. Drain and dry the romaine, then place it on a platter and chill in the refrigerator.

In a large bowl, toss the crabmeat, celery, and peppers. In a small bowl, whisk together the cayenne, orange juice, lime juice, sake, and thyme. Whisk in the olive oil. Add the dressing to the crabmeat mixture and toss. Place the crabmeat salad over the chilled romaine and serve.

# Baked Oysters with Wilted Chard and Black Truffle  Serves 2    (green)

*Jonathan Waxman, Washington Park Restaurant*

1 scallion, chopped

1 garlic clove, chopped

1 bunch red chard, washed and chopped into small pieces

2 tablespoons olive oil

1 black truffle, washed and diced

Salt

Freshly ground black pepper

12 oysters on the half shell

In a large sauté pan over medium heat, sauté the garlic, scallion, and chard in the olive oil for 5 minutes. Add 1 cup water, lower the heat, and simmer for 10 minutes. Add the truffle and cook for 5 minutes. Season with salt and pepper to taste.

Place the oysters on a baking sheet and top each oyster with a spoonful of the truffle mixture. Broil the oysters for 5 to 8 minutes and serve hot.

## BEVERAGES

## HEALTHY HURRICANE

2 ounces orange juice (without pulp)

2 ounces organic fruit-juice sweetened lemonade (I recommend R.W. Knudsen's or Santa Cruz lemonade)

2 ounces natural fruit punch or natural passion fruit juice

3 ounces light and/or dark rum (optional)

Pour all the ingredients over ice in a pint-size or hurricane glass. Shake or blend and garnish with an orange slice.

## THM Ramos Fizz

2 ounces organic fruit-juice sweetened
   lemonade

2 ounces orange juice

2 ounces gin (optional)

2 ounces Silk Soy Creamer or regular soy milk

½ cup cracked ice

Sparkling mineral water

Pour all the ingredients into a collins glass, shake or stir, and top with sparkling mineral water. Garnish with an orange slice.

## Mimosa

3 ounces orange juice

4 ounces champagne

Pour the orange juice into a wine or champagne glass, then add the champagne.

## Non-alcoholic Mimosa

2 ounces sparkling mineral water, such as
   Pellegrino or Perrier

2 ounces orange juice

2 ounces Martinelli's Sparkling Cider

Pour the mineral water and orange juice into a wine or champagne glass, then add the cider.

## Party Ideas

- Invite your friends for a Mardi Gras party—a last wild fling before Lent. Do it New Orleans style using the recipes in this book. Don't tell them they're eating healthy food until they wake up the next day surprised at how much better they feel than usual.

## Invitations

- Send a mask with feathers to be decorated and worn to the party.
- Include a coloring book with three pencils: purple, gold and green, the official Mardi Gras colors.
- Confetti is always festive, but it's better to warn your invitees before they open the envelope. Many a computer keyboard has been ruined because of errant confetti-filled party invitation opening.

# Toasts

The floats are floating and
The hurricanes are blowing
May we toast to Lent before we all get spent.

I vow to give up . . . [say what you plan to give up or do for Lent].
—ELIZABETH CARNEY

Let's have wine and women, mirth and laughter, sermons and soda water the day after.
—LORD BYRON

## DECORATIONS

Masks, colored lights, banners, flags, beads, and pirate-themed decorations in green, gold, and purple.

## SCENTS

Mint
Seaside
Jasmine
Magnolia
Honeysuckle

## ACTIVITIES AND GAMES

- Throw a best craft and costume contest, complete with face painting, decorating masks, stringing beads, and making minifloats out of shoeboxes.
- Organize a treasure hunt all over your house and/or neighborhood. Use a pirate theme, complete with maps, gold coins, and buried treasure.
- Design a Jeopardy board that includes New Orleans jazz and trivia.
- Have your guests write out suggestions of things to give up for Lent. Place all suggestions in a pile and have each guest pick one. Invite the same crowd for an Easter brunch and compare notes.

## PRIZES, GIFTS, AND PARTY FAVORS

Beads; masks; coins; *Let's Go New Orleans* travel book; packets of dried red beans and rice; hot sauces; cajun spices; Ann Rice books; CDs burned from your favorite jazz and Zydeco artists; voodoo dolls of meat, sugar, and dairy.

## MUSIC

Anything by Buckwheat Zydeco, Professor Longhair, the Neville Brothers, the Radiators, Wayne Toups and the Zydecajuns, Al Hirt, the Meters.

| | | |
|---|---|---|
| *Tattoo You* | Rolling Stones | Album |
| *Goin' Back to New Orleans* | Dr. John | Album |
| *Down on Bourbon Street* | Terry Lightfoot | Album |
| *The Soft Parade* | The Doors | Album |
| "Pageant" | Merrick | Song |

## MOVIES

| | |
|---|---|
| *The Big Easy* | (1987–R) |
| *Angel Heart* | (1987–R) |
| *Ash Wednesday* | (1973–R) |
| *Mardi Gras* | (1958–NR) |

## EXERCISE AND CALORIE CHART

Whatever you usually do, you may want to "kick it up a notch," as Emeril would say, because you'll need it with this cuisine.

| Activity | Calories Burned/Hour |
|---|---|
| Watching a parade | 176 |
| Throwing beads | 211 |

## ETHNIC TRADITIONS

Lent is a solemn time of reflection for Christians everywhere. So the Tuesday before Lent or Mardi Gras (also known as Shrove Tuesday) begins a time of merrymaking not only in this country but for many people around the world. In Brazil, the wildest of all Mardi Gras festivals, known as Carnavale, goes on for days before and features parades, costumes, and music. In England, some towns have contests in which women run a race while flipping a pancake at least three times.

## FOR THE KIDS

Mardi Gras is a wonderful, whimsical holiday that inspires all sorts of creativity that has nothing to do with debauchery. Your children can string beads, make floats from shoeboxes, or design masks using jewels, beads feathers, glitter, sequins, or even beans, dried pasta, dried fruits, and vegetables.

## FOR COUPLES

The guy starts out with metallic-colored necklaces, while the girl starts out with neon- or pastel-colored necklaces. The colors don't really matter, as long as his beads look different from hers. Throughout the day, she must do something fun and/or naughty to earn one of his necklaces, and he must do the same to earn one of hers. By the end of the day, all the necklaces should end up on the opposite neck from whence they came.

# Saint Patrick's Day

Top o' the mornin' to ya! And a fine healthy one it's going to be at that. What kind of healthy plans do you have today? How about eating green for Saint Patrick's Day? Green fruits and green vegetables, that is. Consider focusing your meals today on lots of whole green foods. Here are some suggestions to work with:

- Breakfast: honeydew melon, grapes, pears, apples, kiwi
- Lunch and dinner: spinach, soybeans, avocado, cucumbers, green beans, lettuce, green

peppers, peas, cabbage, kale, dandelion greens, broccoli, brussels sprouts, zucchini, olives, green tomatoes

Another way to make this day healthier is to go easy on the beer. Try this at your Saint Patrick's Day party: provide equal amounts of nonalcoholic and regular beer, and encourage people to alternate between the two. Instead of having two beers, they're really having only one. You can make the beer green by adding a few drops of liquid chlorophyll, available at health food stores.

Don't assume that you must serve corned beef and cabbage on Saint Patrick's Day. The Irish in Ireland eat as much fish as they do beef. That's not really surprising, considering that Ireland is completely surrounded by the ocean and has lots of rivers and lakes teeming with salmon, trout, and other fish. Cod, mackerel, swordfish, prawns, oysters, and scallops are commonly found in restaurants throughout Ireland, so serving fish on Saint Patrick's Day is just as traditional as corned beef.

One last thought: avoid heavy combinations like corned beef, cabbage, and potatoes. They're very taxing on the digestive system and arteries. Instead, try some of the recipes from this book. They're lighter, much healthier, and just as traditional as corned beef. Oi tink Pahtty en Moike eat 'em ahl da toime!

## HISTORY, FACTS, AND FOLKLORE

Saint Patrick, originally named Maewyn, was born in the late fourth century in Wales. When he was a teenager, he was abducted and sold into slavery by Irish marauders. He found God during his six years of captivity in Ireland. After escaping, he studied in a monastery for twelve years under the bishop of Auxerre in Gaul.

He eventually decided that his calling was to return to Ireland and convert the pagans to Christianity. Even though Saint Patrick was arrested several times, he was very successful during his thirty years as a missionary and set up many schools and churches. He ultimately died in County Down on March 17, A.D. 461. The date has been set aside to honor Saint Patrick ever since.

There is a lot of folklore associated with Saint Patrick's Day, but not much of it has actually been authenticated. The two most popular stories are that Saint Patrick raised people from the dead and that he gave a sermon from a hilltop that drove all the snakes from Ireland (actually, snakes were never found in Ireland in the first place). Most believe this myth was created as a metaphor for his conversion of the pagans. Though originally a Catholic holy day, Saint Patrick's Day has become more secular over the years.

The shamrock has always been associated with Saint Patrick's Day. This idea originated from an Irish tale in which Patrick used the three-leafed shamrock to explain the Trinity—how the Father, the Son, and the Holy Spirit could all exist as separate elements of the same entity. His followers adopted the custom of wearing a shamrock on his day.

Saint Patrick's Day was first celebrated in the United States on March 17, 1737, in Boston.

# Cream of Asparagus Soup Serves 4 (green)

3 cups organic asparagus spears, cut into
  ½-inch slices (about 1 pound)

2 cups vegetable broth

¾ teaspoon minced fresh organic thyme

1 bay leaf

1 garlic clove, crushed

1 tablespoon whole wheat flour

2 cups low-fat organic soy milk

Dash of grated nutmeg

1 teaspoon olive oil

Salt

Pepper

In a large saucepan over medium-high heat, combine the asparagus, broth, ½ teaspoon of the thyme, the bay leaf, and garlic. Bring to a boil. Reduce the heat, cover, and simmer 10 minutes, or until soft. Discard the bay leaf. Place the asparagus mixture in a blender and purée until smooth. Place the flour in a medium saucepan and gradually whisk in the soy milk. Add the puréed asparagus and grated nutmeg and stir to combine. Bring to a boil over medium-high heat. Reduce the heat and simmer 5 minutes, stirring constantly. Remove from the heat and stir in the remaining ¼ teaspoon thyme, the oil, and ¾ teaspoon salt. Season to taste with more salt and pepper.

# Henri's Home-Style Split Pea Soup

Serves 6 (green)

1 cup chopped onions

2 cups sliced organic carrots

1 cup chopped organic celery

2 garlic cloves, minced

6 cups organic chicken broth

2 cups dried split peas

1 small organic sweet potato, peeled and
  diced

½ teaspoon salt

½ teaspoon black pepper

2 bay leaves

In a large soup pot over medium-high heat, combine the onions, carrots, celery, garlic, and 1 cup broth. Simmer 3 to 5 minutes, until the onions are translucent. Add the split peas, sweet potato, the remaining 5 cups broth, the salt, pepper, and bay leaves. Bring the soup to a boil over medium-high heat. Reduce the heat to low and let simmer for 1 hour, or until the peas are tender. Mash the soup with a potato masher and put it through a food mill or strainer, or serve it country style, with all the vegetables intact.

## New Potato and Green Bean Salad

Serves 8 (blue)

*BETH EVIN HEFFNER*

- ¼ cup balsamic vinegar
- 2 tablespoons Dijon-style mustard
- 2 tablespoons fresh organic lemon juice
- 1 garlic clove, minced
- Vegan Worcestershire sauce
- ½ cup extra-virgin olive oil
- Salt and pepper
- 1½ pounds organic red potatoes, skinned
- 12 ounces organic green beans
- 1 small organic red onion, finely chopped
- ¼ cup chopped fresh organic basil

To make the dressing, whisk the vinegar, mustard, lemon juice, garlic, and Worcestershire sauce to taste in a medium bowl. Gradually whisk in the oil. Season to taste with salt and pepper.

To prepare the salad, in a steamer over simmering water, steam the potatoes until tender. Cool and cut into quarters. Cook the green beans in a large pot of boiling water until crisp-tender, about 5 minutes. Drain and transfer the beans to a bowl of ice water to cool. Cut the beans in half. Combine the green beans, potatoes, onion, and basil in a large bowl. Add the dressing to coat and season to taste with salt and pepper.

## Sautéed Broccoli with Garlic

Serves 4 (purple)

- 2 teaspoons coarse sea salt
- 1 large organic head broccoli (about 1½ pounds), stem peeled and sliced ½-inch-thick and florets separated
- 2 tablespoons extra-virgin olive oil
- 5 organic garlic cloves, peeled and sliced
- Pinch of hot red pepper flakes (optional)
- 2 teaspoons Bragg's Liquid Aminos

In a large pot over high heat, bring 3 quarts water to a boil. Add the salt. Add the broccoli and cook, uncovered, for 2 to 3 minutes, or until crisp-tender. Drain and immediately plunge the broccoli into a bowl of ice water. Drain and set aside. In a wide, heavy saucepan over medium heat, warm the oil. Add the garlic and sauté for 1 minute, or until pale gold. Do not let the garlic brown. Stir in the red pepper flakes, cooked broccoli, and Bragg's. Cover and cook for 3 to 4 minutes, or until broccoli is tender.

# Pasta, Pesto, and Peas Serves 12 (green)

1½ pounds dried bow tie pasta

1 tablespoon olive oil

1½ cups homemade pesto

1 10-ounce package frozen chopped spinach, thawed and squeezed dry

1¼ cups Vegenaise

½ cup grated soy Parmesan cheese

1½ cups frozen organic peas, thawed

⅓ cup toasted pine nuts

¾ teaspoon kosher salt

¾ teaspoon freshly ground black pepper

Cook the bow tie pasta in a large pot of boiling salted water for 10 to 12 minutes, until al dente. Drain and toss into a bowl with the olive oil. Cool to room temperature.

In the bowl of a food processor fitted with a steel blade, purée the pesto and spinach until almost smooth. Add the Vegenaise and continue to purée until blended. Add the pesto mixture to the cooled pasta, and then add the soy Parmesan, peas, pine nuts, salt, and pepper. Mix well, season to taste, and serve at room temperature.

33.1 million: the number of U.S. residents who in 2000 said they had Irish ancestry. This number was almost nine times the population of Ireland itself (3.8 million).
—U.S. Census Bureau

A leprechaun is no more than 24 inches tall, dresses in bright colors, is usually skilled as a shoemaker, and if surprised, might lead you to his pot o' gold. Your best chance of seeing one will come if you visit one too many pubs. (Ted Kennedy sees 'em all the time.)

The potato did not originate in Ireland. The lowly spud was actually brought to the Emerald Isle in the seventeenth century from America by Sir Walter Raleigh, who had a large estate at Youghal [pronounced "Yawl"] in County Cork.

Saint Patrick's Day

## Lucky Irish Stew Serves 6 (blue)

1 teaspoon olive oil

2$\frac{1}{2}$ medium yellow onions, sliced

$\frac{1}{4}$ cup unbleached flour

1$\frac{1}{2}$ cups diced potatoes

2 cups thickly sliced mushrooms

1$\frac{1}{2}$ cups carrots, sliced into rounds

$\frac{1}{2}$ cup peeled and diced turnips

1 cup diced celery

1 cup Great Northern beans

$\frac{1}{2}$ cup chopped fresh parsley

3 tablespoons soy sauce

1 tablespoon Bragg's Liquid Aminos

2 vegetarian or soy bouillon cubes

1 bay leaf

2 teaspoons yeast extract

1 teaspoon Sucanat

$\frac{1}{4}$ teaspoon dried thyme

$\frac{1}{4}$ teaspoon dried rosemary

$\frac{1}{4}$ teaspoon dried marjoram

Salt and pepper

I n a large, lightly oiled, heavy pot over medium heat, sauté the onions until they turn translucent, about 2 minutes. Add the flour and blend thoroughly. Add 4 cups water and the remaining ingredients, mix well, and bring to a boil. Cover, turn the heat to low, and simmer for about 30 minutes, or until the vegetables are done. Remove the bay leaf and add salt and pepper to taste.

# Honey Oat Bread   Serves 10   (blue/green)

1³/₄ cups warm water (105°F. to 110°F.)

1 tablespoon dry yeast

³/₄ cup quick-cooking oats, plus more for

    sprinkling

¹/₃ cup organic honey

3 tablespoons vegetable oil

2¹/₂ teaspoons salt

5 cups unbleached flour

1 large cage-free egg, beaten

In a large bowl, mix ¹/₄ cup of the warm water and the yeast. Let stand 10 minutes to dissolve the yeast. Stir in the remaining 1¹/₂ cups water, oats, honey, oil, and salt. Stir in enough flour to form a soft dough, up to 5 cups. Coat another large bowl with oil. Transfer the dough to the oiled bowl and turn to coat. Cover with plastic wrap, then a kitchen towel and let rise at room temperature until doubled in volume, about 1 hour.

Oil two 8¹/₂ × 4¹/₂ × 2¹/₂-inch loaf pans. Punch down the dough and shape it into 2 loaves. Place 1 loaf in each pan. Cover and let rise in a warm draft-free area until almost doubled in volume, about 20 minutes.

Preheat the oven to 350°F.

Brush the tops of the loaves with the beaten egg and sprinkle with additional oats. Bake until brown on top and a tester inserted into the center comes out clean, about 40 minutes. Cool completely. (The bread can be prepared up to 1 day ahead. Store airtight at room temperature.)

# Irish Tea Bread   Serves 10   (yellow)

1¹/₂ cups brewed decaffeinated black tea,

    cold

¹/₂ cup organic golden raisins

¹/₂ cup organic dark raisins

¹/₄ cup dried currants

2 eggs, lightly beaten

¹/₂ cup packed maple sugar

¹/₄ cup (¹/₂ stick) soy margarine, melted

1¹/₂ cups unbleached flour

1 teaspoon baking powder

Place the tea, raisins, and currants in a medium bowl. Cover and soak at least 3 hours or overnight. Drain the tea from the fruit and reserve the fruit and ¹/₂ cup of the tea.

Preheat the oven to 350°F. Grease and flour an 8-inch round pan.

In a large bowl, beat the eggs and sugar until fluffy. Add the margarine and reserved ¹/₂ cup tea and mix well. Sift together the flour and baking powder and beat into the mixture until just combined. Stir in the fruit until evenly distributed throughout. Pour the batter into the prepared pan. Bake for 40 minutes, or until a wooden pick inserted into the bread comes out clean. Cool the bread in the pan for 5 minutes, then turn out onto a wire rack to cool completely, or serve warm. Serve cut into wedges.

## BEVERAGES

- Guinness, of course.
- THM Green Beer. You can make green beer using your favorite lager and nonalcoholic beer without using artificial food coloring. A few drops of liquid chlorophyll does the job, and it's actually good for you. Get it at health food stores.
- 40 Shades of Green: Wheat Grass Shooter

## THM IRISH COFFEE

1½ ounces Jameson's (or Bushmill's) Irish whiskey (optional)

1 teaspoon organic honey

6 ounces cold-pressed decaffeinated coffee

Splash of Silk Soymilk Creamer

Combine all ingredients and serve in an Irish coffee mug or regular coffee mug.

## THM MICHAEL COLLINS

4 ounces organic fruit juice–sweetened lemonade (I recommend R.W. Knudsen's or Santa Cruz)

1½ ounces Jameson's (or Bushmill's) Irish whiskey (optional)

Sparkling mineral water

Combine the lemonade and whiskey, if using, over ice. Shake or blend and pour into a collins glass, top with sparkling mineral water, and garnish with an orange slice and a fresh cherry (not maraschino).

# Toasts

May the sound of happy music and the lilt of Irish laughter fill your heart with gladness that stays forever after.

Here's to the land of the shamrock so green,
Here's to each lad and his darling Colleen,
Here's to the ones we love dearest and most,
And may God bless old Ireland!—that's an Irishman's toast.

Saint Patrick was a gentleman
Who thro' strategy and stealth
Drove all the snakes from Ireland,
Here's a bumper to his health.
But not too many bumpers,
Lest we lose ourselves, and then
Forget the good Saint Patrick,
And see the snakes again.

May the grass grow long on the road to hell for the want of use.

As you slide down the banisters of life, may the splinters never point the wrong way.

May you live as long as you want, and never want as long as you live.

May the best day of your past be the worst day of your future.

May you be in heaven half an hour before the devil knows you're dead.

May the wind at your back always be your own.
May those who love us, love us,
And for those who don't love us,
May God turn their hearts.
And if he cannot turn their hearts,
May he turn their ankles,
So we may know them by their limping.

May the road rise up to meet you,
May the wind be always at your back,
May the sun shine warm upon your face,
And the rains fall soft upon your fields,
And until we meet again,
May God hold you in the palm of His hand.

# Saint Patrick's Day

## INVITATIONS

- If you're artistic, try making the invitations in the style of the Book of Kells, a gorgeous illuminated manuscript created in Ireland in the early ninth century. Make the first letter take up nearly the whole page, and decorate it elaborately. Try to find a copy of the Book of Kells to use as an example.
- Write as a limerick on a paper shamrock:

We want you to come to a party
The food will be healthy and hearty
We'll toast to good luck
We might even . . . dance
Wear green, and don't ya be tardy!

- On the invitations, give everyone Irish names like O'Henner, O'Lieberman, McDanza, O'DeVito, and so on.

## DECORATIONS

Shamrocks, leprechauns, harps, Irish flags, Guinness mugs, travel posters for Ireland, hurlies.

## SCENTS

Shamrock/clover
Sea breeze
Rain
Ocean
Irish cream
Irish coffee
Fresh-baked bread
Irish toffee

## ACTIVITIES AND GAMES

- Organize a hurling game using whiffle balls and whiffle bats. (It would be too difficult to get real hurlies and far too dangerous, especially for Yanks.) Use football uprights instead of goals, and play the game using similar rules to soccer. You can touch the ball with your hand, but only to toss it up to hit it with the bat.
- How about "legal" gambling! In the same way that people hire a bartender for their parties, consider hiring a blackjack or craps dealer and let your guests have the luck o' the Irish. Give each party guest forty chips when they arrive, but instead of playing for money, they play for gifts. Perhaps the person with the most chips at the end of the night wins the grand prize.
- Play Mr. Potato Head (possibly blindfolded), but use a real potato instead.
- Play Hot Potato, and the loser gets to be the subject of a limerick.

## PRIZES, GIFTS, AND PARTY FAVORS

Many cities have Irish stores full of fun souvenirs. They typically carry Guinness bar towels and coasters, claddagh rings, Irish coffee mugs, Murphy's and Guinness pint glasses, green glycerin soap, family names and crests laminated on place mats, stickers saying "Let's go Ireland," Himself/Herself buttons and T-shirts, linens, yarn, lottery tickets, Waterford crystal, Avoca wool, and books by James Joyce, Oscar Wilde, and Samuel Beckett, to name a few.

## MUSIC

| | | |
|---|---|---|
| *Riverdance* | Bill Whelan | Soundtrack |
| *Otherworld* | Lunasa | Album |
| *Dance of the Celts* | Narada Collection Series | Album |
| *The Book of Secrets* | Loreena McKennitt | Album |
| (anything by) | The Chieftains | Band |
| (anything by) | The Corrs | Band |
| (anything by) | The Cardigans | Band |
| *Lord of the Dance* | Ronan Hardiman | Soundtrack |
| (anything by) | U2 | Band |
| *The Bells of Dublin* | The Chieftains | Album |
| (anything by) | Sinead O'Conner | Artist |
| (anything by) | Green Day | Band |
| (anything by) | Al Green | Band |
| *Out of Bad Luck* | Al Garrett | Album |
| *Luck Be a Lady* | Mel Torme | Album |
| *Pot Luck* | Elvis Presley | Album |
| *Gaelic Heart* | Michael Atkinson | Album |
| *Breathe* | Young Dubliners | Album |
| *Luck of the Draw* | Bonnie Raitt | Album |

## MOVIES

| | |
|---|---|
| *The Wrong Man* | (1957–NR) |
| *Darby O'Gill and the Little People* | (1959–NR) |
| *Waking Ned Devine* | (1998–G) |
| *The Commitments* | (1991–R) |
| *Riverdance* | (1996–G) |
| *Michael Collins* | (1996–R) |
| *Matchmaker* | (1997–R) |
| *Brigadoon* | (1954–NR) |
| *Angela's Ashes* | (2000–R) |
| *Going My Way* | (1944–NR) |
| *Luck of the Irish* | (2001–PG) |
| *Odd Man Out* | (1947–NR) |
| *Ryan's Daughter* | (1976–PG) |
| *Shake Hands with the Devil* | (1959–NR) |
| *Dancing at Lughnasa* | (1998–PG) |
| *Finian's Rainbow* | (1968–G) |
| *The Informer* | (1935–NR) |
| *Secret of Roan Irish* | (1994–PG) |
| *Leprechaun* | (1993–R) |
| *Far and Away* | (1992–PG) |
| *State of Grace* | (1990–R) |
| *The Devil's Own* | (1997–R) |

## EXERCISE AND CALORIE CHART

Everyone knows that Irish dancing is beautiful and exciting. It is also wonderful exercise, and learning the basics is easier that you think. If you can do the pony (you know, the popular dance from the 1960s), you should be able to handle most of the basic steps. For a party activity, teach your guests one or two simple Irish dance combinations. There are several Celtic dance instructional videos available; try a local Irish store or the Internet (activevideos.com or angelfire.com, for example). Collin Dunne from *Riverdance* made a pretty good video. Your guests will love this unique activity, and they'll burn up the extra calories from dinner.

| Activity | Calories Burned/Hour |
|---|---|
| Irish dancing | 493 |
| Irish dancing like Michael Flatley | 824 (and four T-shirts) |
| Kissing the Blarney stone | 135 |
| Chasing a leprechaun | 456 |
| Catching a leprechaun | Never worry about calories again |

## FOR THE KIDS

Here's a great opportunity to get your kids to eat their fruits and veggies. Tell them that if they conquer the rainbow on Saint Patrick's Day, they will get a pot of gold. The pot of gold could be a toy, a bag of pennies, or even little toys wrapped in gold paper—whatever you like. To conquer the rainbow, the kids must eat a fruit or vegetable from each color of the rainbow. Make sure you stock up ahead of time with lots of colorful choices. Here are some suggestions:

- Red—apples, cherries, beets, strawberries
- Orange—oranges, carrots, yams, sweet potatoes, peaches
- Yellow—bananas, yellow squash, corn, golden delicious apples
- Green—spinach, green beans, broccoli, cucumbers, peas, kiwi, honeydew
- Blue—blueberries
- Purple—eggplant, grapes, prunes, plums

- Get lots of green construction paper, glue, scissors, and crayons, and have the kids make decorations for the grown-up party.
- Ask the kids what three wishes they would want granted if they caught a leprechaun.

## FOR COUPLES

- Get edible, nontoxic body paints and doodle shamrocks on each other's lucky charms. You'll be magically delicious!
- Wearing something green, according to Irish tradition, protects you from getting pinched. Don't worry. It does nothing to protect you from getting "lucky"!

# Passover

The Jewish people take pride in being survivors. In ancient times, there was no refrigeration and little sanitation, and kosher eating began as a dietary standard to ensure survival. It was based on cleanliness and what they believed to be the healthiest diet at the time. Times have changed, but the basic idea hasn't—a kosher diet aims for health and high standards. Keep that in mind as you celebrate this wonderful holiday about freedom, health, and survival.

## HISTORY, FACTS, AND FOLKLORE

Passover celebrates the Israelites' escape to freedom from their Egyptian oppressors during the reign of the Pharaoh Ramses II more than 3,000 years ago in 1134 B.C. (Some historians believe it happened in 1476 B.C., during the reign of Thutmose III.) Each aspect of the Passover celebration today symbolizes that historic journey. It is a time for families to celebrate, observe specific religious rituals, and share lavish symbolic meals called Seders. The *Haggadah,* the narrative of Exodus, is read during the Seder to retell the story of Passover.

## The Story of Passover

When the Israelites were enslaved by the Egyptians under Pharaoh, Moses, a common Jewish shepherd, went to the Pharaoh (following orders from God) and demanded, "Let my people go!"

Moses' plea was ignored even after Moses warned Pharaoh of the punishments God would inflict on the people of Egypt if the Jews were not set free. God then sent a series of terrible plagues (ten to be exact) on the Egyptians.

1) Nile waters turn into blood
2) Frogs
3) Lice
4) Flies
5) Livestock disease
6) Boils
7) Hailstorm
8) Locusts
9) Darkness
10) Slaying of the firstborn

The Pharaoh agreed to free the Israelites during each plague, but changed his mind as soon as the plague stopped.

It was from the tenth and final plague that Passover (or *Pesach* in Hebrew) got its name. God intended to kill the firstborn of every family of man and beast in Egypt. To protect themselves, Moses told the Israelites to mark their homes with lamb's blood so that God would know they were Jews and *pass over* their homes.

The slaying of the firstborn finally convinced Pharaoh to free his Jewish slaves. The Jews, now free, left in such a hurry there wasn't enough time to bake their bread. The dough later baked into hard crackers in the hot desert. This is why matzoh is the only bread eaten during Passover.

Pharaoh once again changed his mind and sent his Egyptian army after the Jews in the desert, heading toward the Red Sea. When the Jews reached the sea, they were trapped—until a miracle occurred!

The Red Sea parted, and the Israelites simply walked across to the other side. After all of the Israelites were safely on the other side of the sea, the waves of the Red Sea closed again, and the Pharaoh's army drowned. It was very dramatic. (Rent the movie!)

It is this compelling historical event that Passover celebrates, especially during Seder, a very symbolic Passover meal.

## The Seder

The Seder takes place on the first two nights of Passover (the first night only for Reformed Jews). Led by the head of the family, the Seder is a way for participants to relive the Exodus as a personal spiritual event and, by doing so, feel their ancestors' pain, exaltation, and pride. It is also a great thought-provoking experience for the children in the family. The youngest child traditionally reads and/or answers the four big questions (see For the Kids), which are meant to summarize and illustrate the uniqueness of the Passover holiday compared to other days of the year.

Throughout the meal, four glasses of wine are served to represent the four stages of exodus: freedom, deliverance, redemption, and release. Then a fifth and final glass is poured to invite the prophet Elijah. The final phase of the Seder is when the children find the broken Afikomen (matzoh), and everyone eats a piece.

Here are the seven main symbolic foods eaten during Passover:

1) Matzah (or matzoh): Unleavened bread symbolizes the Jews' hasty exit.
2) Charoseth (or haroset): A mixture of crushed nuts, apples, cinnamon, and honey, symbolizing the mortar the Jewish slaves used in construction for the Pharaoh in Egypt.
3) Egg: A hard-boiled egg is used to symbolize life and rebirth.
4) Saltwater: The egg is dipped in saltwater, which symbolizes both the tears of oppression and the joy in freedom.
5) Maror: Horseradish symbolizes the hardships of slavery.
6) Karpas: A mixture of boiled potatoes or radishes and parsley, which is dipped in salt water and symbolizes the undernourishment of the Jewish slaves, along with the new spring season.
7) Z'roah: A shank bone, which symbolizes the Paschal lamb and refers to God's kindness and guidance from slavery in Egypt.

Passover is observed for eight days (seven for Reformed Jews) and always begins at sundown on the fourteenth day of the Hebrew month of Nisan (or Nissan). The actual starting date changes every year, in the Julian calendar but always winds up in March or April. In 2003, Passover will begin at sundown on Wednesday, April 16.

**RECIPES**
# Morning Scrambled Matzo Brei

Serves 4     (blue/green)

- 5 pieces matzo
- 2 eggs and 6 egg whites
- 1 tablespoon vanilla extract
- 1 teaspoon ground cinnamon
- 1 teaspoon Sucanat
- Salt and freshly ground black pepper
- 1½ tablespoons soy margarine
- 2 tablespoons finely chopped onion (optional)
- Honey (optional)

Run each sheet of matzo under warm running water for about 10 seconds per side until moist. Shake off the excess water and break the matzo into pieces into a large mixing bowl. In another bowl, mix the eggs, egg whites, vanilla, cinnamon, Sucanat, and salt and pepper to taste. Add the matzo to the egg mixture and mix. In a nonstick frying pan over medium heat, heat the margarine and the onion, if using, and sauté for about 30 seconds, or until the onion is translucent. Add the matzo mixture to the pan and scramble until cooked through, another 2 to 3 minutes. Transfer to plates and serve with honey, if desired.

# White Horseradish Purée

Serves 12     (purple)

- 1 pound fresh organic horseradish root (enough to make 2 cups grated)
- ⅔ cup white vinegar
- 3 tablespoons mirin
- 1 teaspoon Sucanat
- 1 teaspoon salt, or to taste

Peel the horseradish with a paring knife and cut into ½-inch slices. In a food processor fitted with a metal blade, finely chop the horseradish. Work in the vinegar, mirin, Sucanat, and salt to taste; process into a creamy purée. Store the horseradish purée in a glass jar in the refrigerator. Try to serve it the same day or within a week. Place a piece of plastic wrap under the lid of the jar to seal tightly.

# Gefilte Fish   Serves 6   (green)

4½ pounds fresh skinless, boneless freshwater fish, such as pike, whitefish, or trout, bones, heads, and skin reserved

1 medium organic potato, peeled and grated

1 medium organic Spanish onion, finely chopped

1 tablespoon minced fresh organic ginger

2 tablespoons canola oil

1 tablespoon Sucanat

1½ teaspoons salt

1 teaspoon freshly ground black pepper

1 cage-free egg plus 1 egg white

3 large organic carrots, peeled and cut into ¼-inch slices

3 organic celery stalks, cut into ¼-inch slices

1 large organic Spanish onion, thinly sliced

Organic lettuce leaves for serving

White Horseradish Purée (see recipe page 138)

Wash the fish and blot it dry. Cut each piece of fish into ½-inch cubes, feeling for bones and removing any you find. Place the fish in a food processor, filling the processor bowl not more than a quarter full. Add some grated potato, chopped onion, and ginger. Finely chop the fish by running the processor in short bursts. Do not over-grind. The mixture should resemble ground beef. Transfer to a large bowl. Continue with the rest of the fish, potato, onion, and ginger. Add to the fish mixture the oil, Sucanat, salt, pepper, egg, and egg white and mix well with a wooden spoon.

Line the bottom of a large pot with the fish skins, bones, and heads. Arrange half the sliced carrots, celery, and onion on top. Wet your hands with cold water and form oval balls of the fish mixture; each should be about 3½ inches long and 2 inches wide. Gently lay the fish balls on the sliced vegetables. Arrange the remaining sliced carrots, celery, and onions on top. Add water to cover by 4 inches and salt and pepper to taste and gradually bring to a boil. Reduce the heat to low and gently simmer the gefilte fish until firm and cooked through, about 1 hour. Remove the pan from the heat.

Using a slotted spoon, transfer the fish balls and carrots to a platter and cool to room temperature. Strain some of the cooking liquid on top and discard the rest. Refrigerate the gefilte fish until it is cold; the cooking liquid will gel. Serve on a lettuce leaf with the horseradish purée.

## Matzo Ball Soup   Serves 8   (purple)

4 cage-free organic eggs, separated

2 tablespoons vegetable oil

1½ teaspoons salt, or to taste

½ teaspoon freshly ground black pepper,
   plus additional as needed

¼ teaspoon garlic powder

3 teaspoons finely chopped organic parsley

1 cup matzo meal

2 tablespoons club soda

10 cups NO-chicken broth

In a large bowl, beat the egg yolks with a fork until light-colored and thick. Add the oil, salt, pepper, garlic powder, parsley, and matzo meal and blend; slowly add the club soda. In another large bowl, beat the egg whites until stiff but not too dry; fold into the matzo meal mixture. Refrigerate the batter for about 1 hour, or until it is thick enough to form balls. (If it's too thick, add more club soda.) Boil 1 quart and 2 cups of water with 2 cups NO-chicken broth to make about 2 quarts. Wet your hands and form 1½-inch balls between the palms of your hands. Drop the balls carefully into the pot and cook for 25 minutes, or until cooked in the center. When done, transfer the matzo balls with a slotted spoon and add to the prepared NO-chicken soup. Cook for another 15 to 20 minutes.

## Moroccan Haroset   Serves 10   (yellow)

1 pound dates, pitted and chopped

1½ cups sweet red Passover wine

1½ teaspoons ground cinnamon

¾ teaspoon ground cloves

1 cup coarsely chopped walnuts

In a medium saucepan over medium-low heat, simmer the dates, wine, cinnamon, and cloves, stirring occasionally, until you have a soft paste. Put the mixture through the food processor for a smoother texture. Cool and then stir in the walnuts.

# Dinah's Chicken Soup

Serves 12  (blue/green)

*DINAH WOLKCOFF & BETH EVIN HEFFNER*
*This is best made a day ahead.*

1 4- to 5-pound organic free-range chicken, cleaned

2 large organic carrots, cut into chunks

4 organic celery stalks, cut into chunks

1 onion, peeled

1 bunch organic parsley, chopped

1 organic sweet potato, peeled

2 garlic cloves, chopped

2 peppercorns

1 bay leaf

Salt

2 chicken bouillon cubes

2 vegetable bouillon cubes

5 fresh organic dill weed sprigs

In a large stockpot, place the chicken and cover with 3 quarts cold water. Add the carrots, celery, onion, parsley, sweet potato, garlic, peppercorns, bay leaf, salt to taste, and bouillon cubes. Simmer for 2 to 3 hours. Strain the soup, reserving the carrots, and cool. Refrigerate until the fat rises (overnight is best) and can be separated from the stock. Skim off the fat and bring the stock to a boil, adding the dill. Serve the soup with matzo balls (see page 140) and carrots.

# Zatar Sea Bass  Serves 4  (blue)

*Zatar is a blend of spices from the Mediterranean.*

4 6-ounce sea bass fillets, washed and blotted dry

3 tablespoons zatar spice

1½ tablespoons extra-virgin olive oil, plus more for the grill

1½ tablespoons fresh organic lemon juice

Coarse sea salt and freshly ground black pepper

Lemon wedges for serving

Rub the fish on both sides with the zatar. Place in a medium baking dish and drizzle with the olive oil and lemon juice. Season on both sides with salt and pepper and marinate about 30 minutes in the refrigerator. Heat the grill to high and oil the grill grate. Grill the fish until cooked, 4 to 6 minutes per side, turning with a spatula. Transfer the fish to plates or a platter. Serve with lemon wedges for squeezing over the fish.

# Passover Chicken with Olives

Serves 2     (blue)

- 4 large organic free-range chicken thighs
- 2 garlic cloves, crushed
- 2 teaspoons ground cumin
- 2 teaspoons paprika
- Salt and freshly ground black pepper
- 4 tablespoons olive oil
- 1 organic Spanish onion, finely chopped
- 1 teaspoon saffron threads
- Juice of 1 large organic lemon
- 1 cup organic chicken stock
- 1 large organic lemon, sliced
- 3/4 cup pitted green olives
- 1 cup organic cilantro, chopped
- 1/2 cup organic parsley, chopped

Put the chicken thighs in a baking dish. In a small bowl, mix the garlic, cumin, paprika, salt to taste, and plenty of black pepper. Blend with 2 tablespoons of the olive oil, then spoon the mixture over the chicken and stir well. Cover and marinate for up to 4 hours.

In a small, shallow, heavy pot over medium heat, add the remaining 2 tablespoons oil and the chicken and brown evenly about 10 minutes. Remove with a slotted spoon and drain on paper towels. Add the onion to the pan and fry, stirring occasionally, until soft and golden. Add the saffron and stir for 1 minute, then return the chicken to the pan. Pour in the lemon juice and stock. Add the sliced lemon and simmer. Add the olives, cilantro, and parsley and cover. Adjust the heat so that the liquid gives an occasional bubble. Continue cooking for 15 to 20 minutes, or until the chicken is tender.

The Last Supper was actually a Passover Seder.

# Passover Carrot Ring  Serves 8  (yellow)

3 tablespoons potato starch

½ cup sweet Jewish wine, such as
Manischewitz

¼ cup (½ stick) soy margarine

½ cup matzo meal

1 pound carrots, peeled and grated

¼ cup raisins (optional)

½ cup Sucanat

1 teaspoon ground cinnamon

1 teaspoon ground ginger

Juice and zest of 1 lemon (optional)

1 cage-free organic egg

½ teaspoon salt

Preheat the oven to 350°F.

In a small bowl, dissolve the potato starch in the wine (it takes a bit of mixing). In a large bowl, cream together the margarine and matzo meal. Add the rest of the ingredients and mix well. Pour into a well-greased ring mold or casserole dish and bake for 1 hour, or until firm and golden on top.

# Passover Zucchini Kugel  Serves 6  (green)

2 pounds organic zucchini

Salt

1 tablespoon olive oil

1 large organic Spanish onion, finely chopped

1 garlic clove, minced

1 cage-free organic egg plus 4 egg whites

2 tablespoons chopped fresh organic parsley

2 tablespoons chopped fresh organic mint
leaves or ½ teaspoon dried

½ cup matzo meal

Freshly ground black pepper

Preheat the oven to 375°F.

Trim the zucchini and cut on the diagonal into ¼-inch-thick slices. In a large pot over high heat, bring 2 quarts of salted water to a boil. Boil the zucchini until tender, about 2 minutes. Drain the zucchini in a colander, rinse under old water, and drain again. Blot dry with paper towels. Place the zucchini slices in a mixing bowl; set aside.

In a large nonstick skillet over medium heat, heat the oil; add the onion and garlic and cook over medium heat until soft but not brown, about 4 minutes. Add the onion mixture to the zucchini. Stir the eggs, egg whites, and herbs into the zucchini mixture. Stir in the matzo meal and salt and pepper to taste. Transfer the mixture to an 8 × 8-inch baking dish, lightly greased with cooking spray. Bake until the kugel is set and the top is golden brown, about 45 minutes. Cut into squares for serving.

## Traditional Potato Kugel Serves 8 (green)

3 tablespoons olive oil

1 large organic Spanish onion, finely chopped (about 2 cups)

2 garlic cloves, finely chopped

3 pounds Yukon Gold potatoes, peeled

3 tablespoons finely chopped organic flat-leaf parsley

1/2 cup matzo meal

1 tablespoon sweet paprika

1 teaspoon baking powder

1 egg and 4 egg whites

2 teaspoons salt

1 teaspoon freshly ground black pepper

Preheat the oven to 350°F.

In a large nonstick skillet over medium heat, heat 1½ tablespoons of the oil. Add the onion and garlic and sauté until the onion is lightly browned, 5 to 8 minutes. Coarsely grate the potatoes into a strainer and press out as much liquid as possible. Transfer the potatoes to a large mixing bowl and stir in the sautéed onion, parsley, matzo meal, paprika, and baking powder. Add the egg and egg whites and mix well. Add the salt and pepper; the kugel should be highly seasoned. Spoon the kugel mixture into a 7 × 12-inch ovenproof baking dish, lightly sprayed with cooking spray, and drizzle the top with the remaining 1½ tablespoons olive oil. Bake the kugel until the top is lightly browned and the filling is cooked through, about 30 to 40 minutes. (Test with a metal skewer for doneness.) Cut the kugel into rectangles or squares for serving.

## Baked Asparagus with Toasted Walnuts

Serves 8 (blue)

2 to 3 pounds asparagus spears, peeled, bottoms cut off

Salt and freshly ground black pepper

1 tablespoon soy margarine, cut into small pieces

4 tablespoons finely chopped walnuts

WALNUT TOPPING

3 tablespoons walnut oil

1 tablespoon white wine vinegar

Salt and freshly ground black pepper

Preheat the oven to 300°F.

Place the asparagus in a greased or sprayed 9 × 13-inch glass baking dish. Sprinkle lightly with salt and pepper and dot with the margarine. Cover the dish with foil and bake for 20 to 30 minutes, or until tender but still crisp.

Toast the chopped walnuts in a 350°F. oven until golden, about 10 minutes.

To make the topping, in a small bowl, whisk together the oil, vinegar, and salt and pepper to taste.

Before serving, spoon the topping over the asparagus and sprinkle with the toasted walnuts.

# Ashkenazi Haroset Serves 10 (yellow)

*BETH EVIN HEFFNER*

2 medium to large organic Granny Smith
   apples, peeled, cored, and finely chopped

½ cup chopped walnuts

1 teaspoon ground cinnamon

3 tablespoons sweet red wine (like
   Manischewitz), or more to taste

1½ tablespoons honey, or more to taste

In a large bowl, mix all of the ingredients, adding more wine and honey to taste.

# Passover "Puffs" Serves 12 (yellow)

⅓ cup canola oil

1 teaspoon Sucanat

1 scant teaspoon salt

1½ to 2 cups matzo meal

1 cage-free egg plus 8 egg whites

Preheat the oven to 375°F.

In a medium saucepan, combine 1 cup water, the oil, Sucanat, and salt and bring to a boil over medium-high heat. Remove the mixture from the pan and transfer to a large mixing bowl. Stir in the matzo meal. Stir in the egg, then the whites, 2 at a time, beating until the mixture is smooth before adding more whites. Using two spoons, form the dough into 2-inch balls. Arrange the balls on a lightly greased baking sheet, keeping 3 inches between each. Using a fork dipped in water, smooth the tops of the rolls. Bake the rolls until puffed and golden brown, about 40 to 50 minutes.

## BEVERAGES

Kosher wines for Passover from Israel or France.

## INVITATIONS

Make a tape of all the songs you plan to sing together at the Seder, and supply the lyrics. This way your guests can familiarize themselves with the songs ahead of time so you won't be the only one singing.

## SCENTS

Lilac
Lily of the valley
Hyacinth
Tulips
Daffodils

# Toasts

Blessed art Thou oh Lord our God, King of the universe, who created the fruit of the vine.
— **TRADITIONAL**

May your home be warmed by the love of family and friends.

Here's a joke you could use in a toast:

A Jewish man took his Passover lunch to eat outside in the park. He sat down on a bench and began eating. A little while later a blind man came by and sat down next to him. Feeling neighborly, the Jewish man passed a sheet of matzoh to the blind man. The blind man ran his fingers over the matzoh for a minute or two, looked puzzled, and finally exclaimed, "Who wrote this crap?"
— **LAUGHOUTLOUD.COM**

## MUSIC

### There's No Seder Like Our Seder

*(sung to the tune of "There's No Business Like Show Business")*

There's no Seder like our Seder,
There's no Seder I know.
Everything about it is *halachic*,
Nothing that the Torah won't allow.
Listen how we read the whole Haggadah,
It's all in Hebrew,
'Cause we know how.

There's no Seder like our Seder,
We tell a tale that is swell:
Moses took the people out into the heat,
They baked the matzoh
While on their feet,
Now isn't that a story
That just can't be beat?
Let's go on with the show!

### A Few of My Favorite Things

*(sung to the tune of "My Favorite Things")*

Cleaning and cooking and so many dishes,
Out with the *hametz*, no pasta, no knishes,
Fish that's gefilted, horseradish that stings,
These are a few of our Passover things.

Matzoh and *karpas* and chopped up *haroset,*
Shankbones and kiddush and Yiddish neuroses,
Tante who kvetches and uncle who sings,
These are a few of our Passover things.

*Motzi* and *maror* and trouble with Pharoahs,
Famines and locusts and slaves with wheelbarrows,
Matzoh balls floating and eggshells that cling,
These are a few of our Passover things.

When the plagues strike,
When the lice bite,
When we're feeling sad,
We simply remember our Passover things,
And then we don't feel so bad.

### Take Us Out of Egypt
*(sung to the tune of "Take Me Out to the Ball Game")*
Take us out of Egypt,
Free us from slavery,
Bake us some matzoh in a haste,
Don't worry 'bout flavor—
Give no thought to taste.
Oh it's rush, rush, rush to the Red Sea,
If we don't cross it's a shame,
For it's ten plagues
Down and you're out
At the Pessah history game.

## MOVIES

| | |
|---|---|
| *The Ten Commandments* | (1923–NR; 1956–NR) |
| *Exodus* | (1960–NR) |
| *Fiddler on the Roof* | (1971–G) |
| *Come Blow Your Horn* | (1963–NR) |
| *Apprenticeship of Duddy Kravitz* | (1974–PG) |
| *Gentlemen's Agreement* | (1947–NR) |
| *The Diary of Anne Frank* | (1959–NR) |

| | |
|---|---|
| *Avalon* | (1990–PG) |
| *The Chosen* | (1981–PG) |
| *Marathon Man* | (1976–R) |
| *A Stranger Among Us* | (1992–PG-13) |
| *The Producers* | (1967–NR) |

Anything by Woody Allen or Mel Brooks

## EXERCISE AND CALORIE CHART

| Activity | Calories Burned/Hour |
|---|---|
| Searching for Afikoman | 156 |

## FOR THE KIDS

Many elements in the seder are meant to teach children and spark their curiosity. Have them use paints, crayons, and construction paper to make place mats that represent scenes from Passover. Buy sheets of laminating plastic to cover the place mats when they're done. Here are some suggestions.

- Scenes that answer the four questions:
  1) On all other nights we eat all kinds of breads and crackers. *Why do we eat only matzoh on Passover?*

     Matzoh reminds us that when the Jews left the slavery of Egypt they had no time to bake their bread. They took the raw dough on their journey, and it baked in the hot desert sun into hard crackers called matzoh.
  2) On all other nights we eat many kinds of vegetables and herbs. *Why do we eat bitter herbs at our Seder?*

     Bitter herbs (*maror*) remind us of the bitter and cruel way the Pharaoh treated the Jewish people when they were slaves in Egypt.
  3) On all other nights we don't usually dip one food into another. At our Seder, we dip the parsley in salt water and the bitter herbs in *haroset. Why do we dip our foods twice tonight?*

     We dip bitter herbs into *haroset* to remind us how hard the Jewish slaves worked in Egypt. The chopped apples and nuts look like the clay used to make the bricks to build the Pharaoh's buildings.

     We dip parsley into saltwater. The parsley reminds us that spring is here and new life will grow. The saltwater reminds us of the tears of the Jewish slaves.
  4) On all other nights we eat sitting up straight. *Why do we lean on a pillow tonight?*

     We lean on a pillow to be comfortable and to remind us that once we were slaves, but now we are free.
- Scenes depicting the ten plagues (see list on page 136).

# Easter

Make this Easter the start of a healthier tradition—lighter food and easier digestion. Throw a healthy brunch and make it your big meal of the day. If you must cook dinner, instead of the usual baked ham or lamb, how about a tasty grilled fish like salmon, snapper, or halibut? There are great vegetables available at this time of the year, too, so try to incorporate many of them with that fish. And how about eating earlier than usual? An earlier dinner will give your body more time to digest before bedtime. In general, make the Easter less about food and more about the fun, traditional activities like coloring eggs, an egg hunt, and going to church. And most of all, stay away from the candy! Especially those pink and yellow sugar-coated marshmallow things. You know what I'm talking about. They're either bunnies or baby chicks or some other cute thing, and they're on sale everywhere, especially the ninety-nine-cent store! Think of those tacky little marshmallows sludging their way through your twenty-seven feet of intestinal tract. Those poor chicks! Your poor *intestines!*

Try some of the healthy sweet substitutes that have been mentioned throughout this book, and check out my advice about sweets in the Valentine's Day section.

## HISTORY, FACTS, AND FOLKLORE

Easter is one of those "movable" holidays. It occurs on the first Sunday after the first full moon after the vernal equinox, somewhere between March 22 and April 25. It closes the forty-six-day period of Lent, signifying a rebirth and springtime fertility. The nuns wouldn't like to hear this, but Easter was originally a pagan festival. The Saxons celebrated springtime with a raucous festival honoring Eastre, the goddess of springtime and offspring. It was only diplomatic and determined second-century missionaries who infiltrated the pagan rituals with more Christian-minded ideals. Since the Eastre festival coincided with the celebration of the resurrection of Christ, eventually Eastre became Easter, the Christian holiday that it is today. Now about that Easter bunny and the eggs . . .

The goddess Eastre was symbolized by the rabbit, and the Germans brought the idea to America as a symbol. Sometime after the Civil War the Americans latched onto the iconography of the rabbit, or as we say, the Easter bunny. The symbol of the egg is as old as the Christianized holiday. Giving, exchanging, and hunting eggs are long-standing customs that symbolize fertility and rebirth. Change your habits, clean your body, heighten your palate, and you too could have the proverbial egg—your health.

## HENNER HOLIDAY TRADITIONS AND STORIES

I always loved Easter as a kid because it was close to my birthday, April 6. I was actually born on Palm Sunday, and I've celebrated my birthday on Easter three times in my life so far. In Chicago, Easter also meant it was starting to get warm outside. It was the beginning of that spring fever feeling, in late March or early April, when the air would start smelling different and give you that clean, healthy feeling. You would shed your winter coat and your winter sensibility and feel alive again.

Sunday mass was always wonderful and dramatic during the Easter season. All the statues were covered with dark purple cloth throughout Lent, and when they were removed on Easter morning, the church was beautifully reborn, with lilies, tulips, and candles.

But Easter and the change of season had a much deeper meaning to me—getting a new outfit! Because most Catholic school kids wear uniforms, we rarely got to wear anything different, so clothes were very important to us. Going shopping, getting dressed up, and going to mass in a new spring outfit was a very big deal. I can remember every Easter Sunday outfit I wore since I was five. And because it doubled as my birthday ensemble, I always felt particularly cost-efficient. (Easter was as good a time as any to be shallow—and thrifty!) And it was about that time, often during our shopping field trip, that we would get the one item that pretty much defined what a Henner Easter was all about: our nine-inch-high, 100 percent solid milk chocolate bunnies from the Jewel Supermarket!

I'm sorry—or I should say *glad*—to say, I was never a chocolate person. But I really got into the chocolate bunny thing during Easter because it became an "event." We were each given (or rather, we each adopted) our very own personal chocolate bunny. There was enough chocolate in just one rabbit to keep Fat Albert content until Labor Day, but each of us expected to polish a whole one off over the short Easter weekend.

Of course, you'd always eat the ears first. And then you'd wrap it in tinfoil and hide it in the freezer. Unfortunately, everyone else also started with the ears, wrapped it in tinfoil, and hid it in the freezer. By day three or four, there was no way you knew for sure which was yours and which was your brother's chocolate rabbit. So you would carefully compare teeth marks hoping to find some distinguishing characteristics. Luckily my brother Tommy had some gnarly chipped teeth left over from a one-handed cartwheel that went bad when he was seven, so his bunny was as distinctive as a size thirteen Bruno Magli shoeprint. Back then we didn't need shows like CSI. We had plenty of forensic science happening right in our freezer. And whether it held remnants of carpet fibers or cat hairs, every bunny told a story. Eventually, when our bunnies got to that Monty Python Holy Grail stump stage, we would give up, and the remaining chunks of bunny body parts would sit there until we needed the freezer space for Thanksgiving. I don't think any one of us ever actually finished a whole bunny.

Coloring eggs was a big tradition, too. Our uncle (the eccentric artist who lived upstairs) was in charge, so we couldn't just make an assortment of solid pastel-colored eggs with an occasional multicolored swirl, like other families. *Absolutely not.* He had us making stained glass recreations from the western facade of Chartes Cathedral or panel #17 (Genesis) from the Sistine Chapel. My uncle thought he was Peter Fabergé or something. He had a perfectionist obsession with anything artistic, so it was like growing up with a temperamental child prodigy, a temperamental *middle-aged* child prodigy. One year my mother wrote her name on an egg and got the spacing all wrong. My uncle reprimanded her for writing *Loret* instead of *Loretta*. I don't think she joined any of his OCD egg-coloring workshops again. I never really had that artistic gene myself, so I did a lot of the setting up (the hot water, vinegar, and so on) and cleanup afterward. I never want to be left out of anything, so I get involved where I'm needed most. You know me: plan B.

## RECIPES
# Deviled Eggs Serves 8 (blue)

4 cage-free organic eggs, hard-boiled,
   cooled, and peeled

2 tablespoons Vegenaise

1 teaspoon Dijon-style mustard

1/8 teaspoon cayenne, or to taste

Salt

1/8 teaspoon paprika

1/4 teaspoon minced organic parsley

Cut the eggs in half lengthwise and remove the yolks. Mash the yolks in a bowl with the Vegenaise, mustard, cayenne, and salt to taste. Spoon the filling into the egg whites. Garnish the tops of the eggs with the paprika and parsley.

# Overnight Baked French Toast

Serves 10 to 12 (green)

SUSAN ROMITO

1½ loaves Italian or French bread, cut into
   1-inch slices

2 organic eggs and 8 organic egg whites or 6
   organic eggs

3 cups vanilla soy milk

1/3 cup Sucanat

1/4 teaspoon ground cinnamon

1 teaspoon dried grated orange zest or 2
   teaspoons grated fresh orange zest

1/4 teaspoon grated nutmeg

4 tablespoons (½ stick) Earth Balance
   margarine, melted

1 teaspoon vanilla extract

Warm maple syrup for serving

Lightly oil a 13 × 18-inch pan and cover the bottom with a single layer of bread slices—do not overlap.

In a large bowl, mix the remaining ingredients and evenly pour the mixture over the bread. Cover with foil and refrigerate at least 2 hours or overnight. Preheat the oven to 350°F. Bake, uncovered, for 50 or 60 minutes, until lightly browned. Watch it near the end; it browns very quickly. Serve with warm maple syrup.

# Morning Muffins Makes 12 muffins (green)

*MARY BETH BORKOWSKI*

2 cups organic flour

1 cup evaporated cane juice crystals

2 teaspoons baking powder

¼ teaspoon salt

2 tablespoons (¼ stick) Earth Balance margarine, melted

1 cage-free organic egg

1 cup vanilla soy milk

2 teaspoons vanilla extract

Preheat the oven to 400°F. and spray a 12-cup muffin tin with canola oil.

In a large bowl, stir together the dry ingredients. In a medium bowl, combine the margarine, egg, and soy milk. Beat with a fork until blended, then stir in the vanilla. Pour the liquid ingredients all at once into the dry ingredients and mix just until blended. Do not overmix or the muffins will be tough. Pour the batter into the prepared muffin tins. Bake for 15 to 20 minutes, or until the tops are slightly golden.

# Greek Country Salad Serves 8 (purple/blue)

1 tablespoon white wine vinegar

Salt

1 teaspoon honey

⅓ cup extra-virgin olive oil

½ pound organic escarole, chopped (4 cups)

¼ pound organic tender young mustard greens, trimmed and finely chopped (2 cups)

½ pound organic dandelion greens, tough stems discarded, leaves cut crosswise into ¼-inch slices (2 cups)

2 ounces organic baby spinach (2 cups)

1 cup organic watercress sprigs, trimmed

¼ cup chopped organic Italian parsley

¼ cup thinly sliced organic red onion

Pepper

In a large salad bowl, whisk together the vinegar, ½ teaspoon salt, and the honey. Add the oil in a slow stream, whisking until blended. Add the salad ingredients to the dressing and toss to coat. Season to taste with salt and pepper.

# Grilled Salmon Sandwiches

Serves 6    (yellow)

3 teaspoons olive oil

6 6-ounce pieces fresh salmon fillets, skin on

Kosher salt

Freshly ground black pepper

1 cup Vegenaise

¼ cup soy sour cream

10 large organic basil leaves

¾ cup fresh organic dill weed

1½ teaspoons organic scallion, white and
   green parts only, chopped

3 teaspoons capers, drained

6 whole grain rolls

6 organic red leaf lettuce leaves

For the salmon, prepare a charcoal grill and brush the grilling rack with 1 teaspoon of oil. Rub the outside of the salmon with the remaining 2 teaspoons of oil and salt and pepper to taste. Grill the fish for 5 minutes on each side, or until it is almost cooked through. Remove to a plate and allow it to rest for 15 minutes. Remove any remaining skin.

For the sauce, place the Vegenaise, soy sour cream, basil, dill, scallions, ¼ teaspoon salt, and ¼ teaspoon pepper in the bowl of a food processor fitted with a steel blade. Process until combined. Add the capers and pulse two or three times.

To assemble, slice the rolls in half crosswise. Spread 1 tablespoon of the sauce on each cut side. Place some red leaf lettuce or basil on the bottom half, then a piece of salmon. Place the top of the roll over the salmon and serve.

# Hummus  Serves 8    (blue)

2 cups canned organic chickpeas, drained

½ cup tahini

¼ cup sesame oil

1 garlic clove, peeled and pressed, or more to
   taste

Salt and freshly ground black pepper

1 tablespoon ground cumin, or more to taste,
   plus a sprinkling for garnish

Juice of 1 lemon, or more to taste

½ teaspoon salt

1 teaspoon olive oil, plus more for drizzling

Place everything except the olive oil in the container of a food processor and process; add water as needed to make a smooth purée. Taste and add more garlic, salt, lemon juice, salt, pepper, and cumin as needed. Serve, drizzled with a little olive oil and sprinkled with a bit of cumin.

# Tabbouleh   Serves 4   (purple)

1 cup bulgur wheat

1¼ cups boiling water

1 garlic clove, pressed or finely chopped

2 tablespoons olive oil

2 tablespoons red wine vinegar

2 teaspoons tamari sauce

½ medium red onion, chopped

1 bunch fresh organic parsley, finely chopped
  (about 1 cup)

1 small bunch fresh organic mint leaves,
  finely chopped (about ½ cup)

2 organic cucumbers, peeled and diced

1 pint organic cherry tomatoes, cut in
  eighths

Salt and pepper

Combine the bulgur wheat and the boiling water in a medium mixing bowl and let sit for about 15 minutes, or until the water has been absorbed. Add the remaining ingredients and stir gently to combine. Refrigerate for at least 2 hours to let the flavors blend. Add salt and pepper to taste.

# Streusel Sour Cream Coffee Cakes

Makes 18     (yellow)

- 1 cup fruit juice cane sugar
- 2½ cups flour
- ½ teaspoon salt
- ¾ cup packed maple sugar
- 1 cup (2 sticks) soy margarine, cut into ½-inch cubes
- 1 teaspoon ground cinnamon
- 1½ cups chopped toasted pecans (6 ounces)
- 1 cup soy sour cream
- 1 large organic egg
- 1 large organic egg yolk
- 1 teaspoon vanilla extract
- 1 teaspoon baking soda

Preheat the oven to 350°F. Using cooking spray, thoroughly spray two muffin tins, each with 12 ½-cup muffin cups.

In a large bowl, blend the sugar, flour, salt, and ½ cup of the maple sugar. With your fingertips or a pastry blender, blend in ¾ cup (1½ sticks) of the soy margarine until the mixture resembles a coarse meal with some pea-size butter lumps.

To make the streusel topping, transfer ¾ cup of the mixture to a medium bowl. With your fingertips or a pastry blender, blend in the cinnamon, the remaining ¼ cup (½ stick) soy margarine, and the remaining ¼ cup maple sugar until crumbly. Stir in the pecans, then chill for 15 minutes.

In a medium bowl, whisk together the soy sour cream, egg, egg yolk, vanilla, and baking soda. Stir the sour cream mixture into the remaining flour mixture until just combined. The batter will be stiff. Divide the batter among 18 of the muffin cups. Sprinkle each with streusel topping, pressing it lightly into the batter. Bake the coffee cakes in the middle of the oven until golden brown and a toothpick inserted in the center comes out clean, 20 to 25 minutes. Cool the cakes in the pans on racks for 30 minutes. Loosen the cakes with a sharp knife, and then carefully remove the cakes from the pans.

## Beverages

- Easter Shake—Make pink, purple and yellow shakes with soy ice cream, crushed ice, and strawberries, blueberries, and bananas. Garnish with a little carob bunny on the top.
- Bunny Juice—Fresh squeezed carrot juice for the Easter bunny in you. Add fresh parsley leaves or a celery stalk for garnish.
- Springtime for Spritzers—Mix your favorite fruit with sparkling mineral water and garnish with a fresh lily.

## Easter Eggnog

*(warning: not lo-cal)*

4 ounces Silk Vanilla Creamer or soy milk

1 whole cage-free egg or 2 egg whites

Pinch of salt

$\frac{1}{4}$ teaspoon pure vanilla extract

$1\frac{1}{2}$ ounces brandy or rum (optional)

Blend all the ingredients except the brandy or rum in the blender. Slowly add the brandy, if using. Pour into highball or collins glass and garnish with a mint leaf.

For grown-up tastes, with or without the alcohol:

## Bellini

2 ounces peach juice or nectar
   (I recommend Ceres brand)

4 ounces champagne

In a wine or champagne glass, pour in the peach juice and slowly add the champagne.

## Nonalcoholic Bellini

2 ounces sparkling mineral water, such as
   Pellegrino or Perrier

2 ounces peach juice or nectar (I recommend
   Ceres brand)

2 ounces Martinelli's Sparkling Cider

In a wine or champagne glass, combine the mineral water and peach juice. Slowly pour in the cider.

## TANGERINE MIMOSA

3 ounces tangerine juice

4 ounces champagne

In a wine or champagne glass, pour in the tangerine juice, then slowly pour in the champagne.

## STRAWBERRY DAIQUIRI

4 ounces natural unsweetened lemonade

1 banana or 4 ounces natural strawberry
purée

Over ice in a blender, combine the lemonade and strawberry purée. Blend and serve in a collins or rocks glass. The drink can also be shaken if you have a muddler. Garnish with a fresh cherry (not maraschino).

## CREAMSICLE

3 ounces orange juice (no pulp)

1½ ounces vanilla soy milk

1½ ounces vodka (optional)

Combine the orange juice, Vanilla soy milk, and vodka, if using, over ice. Shake and pour into a high-ball glass.

## PARTY IDEAS

- Hold an egg-coloring party the day before Easter. Have the gang over and get out the vinegar! Buy equal amounts of brown and white eggs for various Easter shades.
- After church services, invite your friends and their families for an Easter brunch and egg hunt.

## DECORATIONS

## NONNI'S EGG TREE

6 eggs

Egg dye

Ribbon

2 or 3 bare tree branches

Crack the eggs into 2 equal halves and carefully set aside the shells. Reserve the yolks and whites to make whatever dish you like. Wash the eggshells and remove the membrane. They should be completely clean.

Dye the eggshells in any fashion you like and let them dry. When dry, use a skewer to poke a hole at the top of each shell so you can pull the ribbon through.

Arrange the branches in a vase to look like a small tree. Tie the ribbons to the branches of the tree to make hanging egg ornaments.

## SCENTS

Spring scents—light, refreshing, and seasonal:

Tulip

Daffodil

Hyacinth

Lilac

Lily of the valley

Peony

Apple blossom

Rain

Chocolate

## ACTIVITIES AND GAMES

- Color eggs the day before, using both brown and white eggs for variety.
- Hunt for eggs. Use the colored eggs and hollow plastic eggs on the egg hunt. Do not fill the plastic eggs with the usual candy (unless it's healthy, of course) but with coins and/or coupons. (See For the Kids for suggestions.)
- Make permanently colored Easter eggs like the ones in Eastern Europe. First poke a hole at each end of an egg, then carefully blow out the contents of the egg. After it's empty, clean it off with a wet towel and let it dry. Now it's ready to be colored.

- Organize a field trip and make little baskets to bring to children and seniors in hospitals.
- Organize your own spring cleanup. Have everyone help with specific chores, then gather old toys and clothes to donate to the poor and homeless.
- The season of Lent is a time for reconciliation and forgiveness. Be the one to make the first gesture.

## PRIZES, GIFTS, AND PARTY FAVORS

Easter baskets with healthy candy and treats; books, games, puzzles, and stuffed animals for kids; recipe cards; certificates for field trips like Museum Day, Aquarium Day, and so on.

## MUSIC

| "White Rabbit" | Jefferson Airplane | Song |
| *Jesus Christ Superstar* | Various | Soundtrack |
| *Easter Parade* | Various | Soundtrack |
| *Godspell* | Various | Soundtrack |
| *Who Framed Roger Rabbit* | Various | Soundtrack |

## MOVIES

| *Easter Parade* | (1948–NR) |
| *Jesus Christ Superstar* | (1973–G) |
| *Godspell* | (1973–G) |
| *The Greatest Story Ever Told* | (1965–NR) |
| *Ten Commandments* | (1956–NR) |
| *The Last Temptation of Christ* | (1988–R) |
| *The Robe* | (1953–NR) |
| *Sign of the Cross* | (1932–NR) |
| *Life of Brian* | (1979–R) |

# Exercise and Calorie Chartz

| Activity | Calories Burned/Hour |
|---|---|
| Skipping | 326 |
| Hopping | 442 |
| Bunny hop | 342 |

## Ethnic Traditions

- Greece and Italy—Colorful eggs are baked into special breads.
- Norway—Easter eggs are rolled down slopes until all are cracked but one, which is declared the winner. The person who rolled the winning egg gets a prize.
- Germany, Switzerland, and Belgium—Children place nests in the grass so that the Easter bunny will fill them with eggs.
- Ireland—A meal of eggs at dawn on Easter breaks the fast of Lent.

Egg-rolling parties and egg hunts have been popular all over the world and have for many years been an annual event on the lawn of the White House.

## For the Kids

I love coloring eggs with my kids. I've carried on the Henner tradition, but without the artistic perfection that my uncle tried to inspire in all of us. We focus on quantity over quality, coloring about twelve dozen eggs: six dozen brown and six dozen white. Brown eggs provide a nice base for bringing out rich vivid colors, and white eggs are great for pastels.

On Easter Sunday, I always have a big brunch with lots of friends and a huge Easter egg hunt throughout the house and yard for the kids. The eggs we hide are a mixture of the hardboiled eggs we colored and hollow plastic eggs with money, little dime-store toys, healthy candies, or (my favorite) the coupons described on page 159–160, under "Activities and Games."

## For Couples

Hide plastic eggs all over the house, especially in creative, interesting places. In each egg write a note telling your partner what you will do for him/her. Let your imagination run wild! You can even dress like a bunny!

# Earth Day

I can't think of a better day to celebrate real food and good health than Earth Day! It's the perfect opportunity to go vegan for a day. If you don't want to go completely vegan, at least try some of the recipes in this chapter.

Spend the day eating only food that comes directly from the earth. Notice how much lighter you feel when you eat only real, rich, whole foods: salads, vegetables, and grains. And even if you overdo this kind of food, it is digested quickly and goes right through you. If eating like this is completely new to you, you may want to introduce these foods slowly. Your body may have to adjust to the process of cleaning out the junk, and these new foods may taste strange at first. But please give them more than just one try. The road to health is really about changing your palate and getting away from the extreme foods that so many people are addicted to, like salt, sugar, and chemicals. The trick with vegan food is to learn to taste the real flavors of the earth—not the lab! It's a shame we've gotten so far away from what is real that we have to relearn what we started with in the first place. But Earth Day is the perfect day to begin this journey.

## HISTORY, FACTS, AND FOLKLORE

Unless you're an extraterrestrial, Earth Day is everyone's celebration. Senator Gaylord Nelson came up with the idea in 1969, and it has gained momentum over the last three decades as the environment has been wasted by chemicals, overpopulation, and general disregard. Shut down your car, mind your spills and overflows, don't smoke in the woods, don't litter, protect the ozone, and love your Mother Earth. Unless you find access and accommodations on another planet, this is your home—and this is your holiday.

## RECIPES

# Henri's Best Vegetable Soup

Serves 6 (purple)

3 teaspoons soy margarine

1 large onion, chopped

6 organic celery stalks, chopped

1 cup organic carrots, peeled and chopped

1 32-ounce can diced tomatoes, drained

½ cup uncooked barley

3 teaspoons salt

1 tablespoon coarsely ground black pepper

2 bay leaves

2 quarts vegetable broth

1 cup chopped organic cabbage

1 cup organic fresh or frozen peas

2 cups or 1 15-ounce can tomato purée

1 teaspoon Tabasco sauce (optional)

In a large heavy soup pot over medium-high heat, sauté the margarine and the onion. Add the celery, carrots, tomatoes, barley, salt, pepper, and bay leaves and sauté about 10 minutes, or until the onion is translucent. Pour in the vegetable broth and cook until the barley is tender, about 30 to 40 minutes. Add the cabbage and peas and simmer 5 to 7 minutes, until the peas are cooked. Add the tomato purée and Tabasco, if using, bring to a boil, and serve.

# Moroccan Chickpea Soup Serves 6 (blue/green)

1½ cups dried chickpeas

1 35-ounce can organic whole tomatoes

1 large organic Spanish onion, finely chopped

2 small organic celery stalks, including leaves, finely chopped

3 tablespoons olive oil

1 teaspoon turmeric

1 teaspoon black pepper

½ teaspoon ground cinnamon

⅔ cup chopped fresh organic cilantro

2 tablespoons Bragg's Liquid Aminos

4 cups organic vegetable broth

1 cup dried lentils

2 ounces dried capellini (angel hair pasta), broken into 1-inch pieces

½ cup chopped fresh organic parsley

Salt

Place the chickpeas in a medium bowl and pour in water to cover by 2 inches. Soak the chickpeas 8 to 10 hours. Drain and rinse well. Transfer the chickpeas to a large saucepan and add 8 cups water. Bring to a boil over medium-high heat, then lower the heat and simmer, uncovered, until tender 1¼ to 1½ hours. Cool the chickpeas and drain, reserving 2½ cups of the cooking liquid. If you don't have enough liquid, add water to make up the difference. Coarsely purée the tomatoes in a food processor. In a 4-quart heavy pot over medium-low heat, cook the onion and celery in the oil, stirring occasionally, until softened, about 5 minutes. Add the turmeric, pepper, and cinnamon and cook, stirring, for 3 minutes. Stir in the tomato purée, ⅓ cup of the cilantro, the chickpeas, reserved chickpea cooking liquid, Bragg's, vegetable broth, and lentils. Bring to a boil, then reduce the heat and simmer, uncovered, until the lentils are tender, about 35 minutes. Stir in the pasta and cook, stirring, until tender, about 3 minutes more. Stir in the parsley, remaining ⅓ cup cilantro, and salt to taste.

# Mixed Green Salad with Arugula

Serves 4 (purple)

1 bunch organic butter lettuce, torn

1 bunch organic arugula, torn

1 head organic romaine lettuce, torn into bite-sized pieces

½ bunch fresh basil, cut into chiffonade

4 tablespoons olive oil

4 tablespoons red wine vinegar

Salt and pepper

In a large bowl, combine the butter lettuce, arugula, romaine, and basil. Whisk together the olive oil and vinegar in a small bowl. Add salt and pepper to taste. Toss the salad with the dressing and serve.

## Spicy Black Bean Salad

Serves 4    (blue/green)

1 15-ounce can black beans, rinsed and drained

3 tablespoons freshly squeezed organic lime juice (from about 1 fresh lime)

2 tablespoons olive oil

1 tablespoon red wine vinegar

1 teaspoon salt

$\frac{1}{2}$ teaspoon cayenne

2 scallions, chopped

$\frac{1}{4}$ cup chopped fresh organic cilantro

2 organic tomatoes, chopped

Place the beans in a medium ceramic or glass bowl. Mix in the lime juice, olive oil, vinegar, salt, and cayenne. Top with the scallions, cilantro, and tomatoes, but do not combine. Cover and refrigerate for at least 2 hours to let the flavors meld. Toss just before serving.

## Kasha with Cremini Mushrooms

Serves 6    (blue)

$1\frac{1}{2}$ cups uncooked kasha, medium granulation

3 teaspoons olive oil

9 ounces organic cremini mushrooms, sliced

1 onion, chopped

1 cup canned organic vegetable broth

1 tablespoon chopped fresh organic thyme, or 1 teaspoon dried thyme

$\frac{1}{4}$ teaspoon ground pepper

1 tablespoon chopped fresh organic flat-leaf parsley

In a heavy frying pan over medium-high heat, add the kasha, stirring for 2 to 4 minutes, or until slightly darkened. Remove from heat. In a large, nonstick frying pan over medium heat, add the olive oil, mushrooms, and onion and sauté until softened, about 3 to 5 minutes. In a small saucepan over medium heat, bring the broth and 2 cups water to a boil. Add the broth mixture to the mushroom mixture and stir in the kasha, thyme, and pepper. Reduce the heat to low, cover, and simmer for 8 to 10 minutes, or until the kasha is just tender and all the liquid is absorbed. Transfer to a serving platter and garnish with parsley.

# Sesame Quinoa with Tofu Serves 4 (blue)

2 8-ounce packages extra-firm tofu, drained

2 1/4 teaspoons olive oil

2 tablespoons sesame seeds

2 cups uncooked quinoa

3 cups vegetable stock

1/4 teaspoon salt

3/4 cup chopped organic green onions

2 tablespoons low-sodium tamari sauce

1/2 teaspoon black pepper

Place the tofu on several layers of heavy-duty paper towels; let stand 20 minutes to absorb as much liquid as possible. Cut into 1/2-inch cubes.

In a medium saucepan over medium heat, heat the oil. Add the tofu and sesame seeds and sauté 3 minutes, or until the tofu is golden. Remove the tofu mixture from the pan. Add the quinoa to the pan and cook 3 minutes, stirring frequently. Add the vegetable stock and salt; bring to a boil. Cover, reduce the heat, and simmer 20 minutes. Place the quinoa mixture in a large bowl. Add the tofu, green onions, tamari, and pepper; toss and serve.

# Couscous with Green and White Asparagus Serves 4 (purple)

1 1/2 cups vegetable stock

1 cup dried couscous

3/4 pound organic green and white asparagus
   spears, ends trimmed, cut in half
   (about 2 cups)

Kosher salt

Freshly ground black pepper

1/4 cup chopped organic arugula

2 teaspoons extra-virgin olive oil

In a medium saucepan over medium heat, bring the stock to a boil. Add the couscous, stir, and bring to a boil again. Remove from the heat immediately. Blanch the asparagus in a large pot of boiling water, then drain and transfer to a bowl filled with ice water. Season the couscous with salt and pepper to taste. Stir in the asparagus, cover, and let stand 5 minutes. Fluff the couscous with a fork and transfer to a bowl. Stir in the arugula and olive oil, season to taste with salt and pepper, and serve.

# Tofu Olive Wraps  serves 4  (green)

½ cup pitted kalamata olives

¼ cup pitted oil-cured black olives

½ teaspoon olive oil

2 cups boiling water

1 cup sun-dried tomatoes, packed without oil

1 pound organic extra-firm tofu, drained

1 cup ¼-inch-thick red onion slices,
    separated into rings

3 tablespoons balsamic vinegar

1 tablespoon white wine vinegar

2 tablespoons red wine vinegar

1 tablespoon honey

1 teaspoon chopped fresh organic rosemary

2 teaspoons Dijon-style mustard

¼ teaspoon sea salt

4 10-inch whole wheat flour tortillas

4 cups fresh organic watercress, trimmed
    (about 1 bunch)

Place the olives and oil in a food processor and pulse 2 or 3 times, or until minced. Set aside. To prepare the wraps, combine the water and sun-dried tomatoes in a bowl and let stand 30 minutes, or until soft. Drain, chop, and set aside. Cut the tofu lengthwise into quarters. Place the tofu slices on several layers of paper towels and cover with additional paper towels. Let stand about 20 minutes, or until barely moist.

Heat a large nonstick skillet coated with cooking spray over medium-high heat. Add the onion and sauté 5 minutes, or until lightly browned. Place in a bowl and stir in the balsamic vinegar. In a small bowl, combine the white wine vinegar, red wine vinegar, honey, rosemary, mustard, and salt.

Heat a large nonstick skillet coated with cooking spray over medium-high heat. Add the tofu and cook 6 minutes, browning on all sides. Stir in the vinegar mixture and cook 1 minute, or until the sauce thickens.

Warm the tortillas according to package directions. Spread 2 tablespoons of the olive paste evenly over each tortilla. Top each tortilla with 1 tofu piece, about ¼ cup sun-dried tomatoes, ¼ cup onion, and 1 cup watercress. Roll up and serve.

Five percent of summer air pollution in the United States comes from gas-powered lawn mowers.

Five percent of household water is used on the lawn.

It takes 27,000 gallons of water each week to maintain one acre of lawn.

Thirty-two million pounds of pesticides were used on U.S. lawns in 1994.
—Gristmagazine.com

# Orzo with Roasted Vegetables

Serves 6    (blue/green)

- 8 asparagus spears, ends discarded, cut into 1-inch pieces
- 1 organic zucchini, peeled and cut into 1-inch dice
- 1 organic squash, peeled and cut into 1-inch dice
- 1 organic red onion, peeled and cut into 1-inch dice
- 2 garlic cloves, minced
- ¼ cup plus ⅓ cup olive oil
- ½ pound orzo pasta
- ⅓ cup rice vinegar
- 2 teaspoons kosher salt
- 1 teaspoon freshly ground black pepper
- 4 scallions, minced (both white and green parts)
- ¼ cup toasted pine nuts
- 12 ounces firm tofu, cut into 1-inch cubes
- 10 fresh organic basil leaves, cut into chiffonade

Preheat the oven to 425°F.

On a large baking sheet, toss the asparagus, zucchini, squash, onion, and garlic with ¼ cup olive oil. Roast for 40 minutes, or until browned, turning once with a spatula. Meanwhile, in a large pot of boiling salted water, cook the orzo for 7 to 9 minutes, or until tender. Drain and transfer to a large serving bowl. Add the roasted vegetables to the pasta, scraping all the liquid and seasonings from the roasting pan into the pasta bowl.

For the dressing, in a small bowl, whisk together the rice vinegar, the remaining ⅓ cup olive oil, salt, and pepper and pour on the pasta and vegetable mixture. Let cool to room temperature, then add the scallions, pine nuts, tofu, and basil. Check the seasoning and serve at room temperature.

## Spinach with Garlic and Pine Nuts

Serves 4    (blue/green)

2 pounds fresh organic spinach, ends
    trimmed and discarded

1 1/2 teaspoons olive oil

2 teaspoons pine nuts

2 garlic cloves, chopped

Salt and pepper

Wash the spinach well and shake out the water. Heat a large saucepan over high heat and add the spinach. Cook for 2 to 3 minutes, or until tender, tossing frequently. Transfer the spinach to a colander and set aside.

Heat the saucepan over medium heat and add the olive oil. When the oil is hot, add the pine nuts and chopped garlic and cook until both are golden, about 2 minutes. Return the spinach to the saucepan, toss to combine, and cook until heated through, about 2 minutes. Add salt and pepper to taste.

## Sassy Rice Serves 2    (purple)

1 cup uncooked rice

1 medium Bermuda onion, chopped

3/4 teaspoon curry powder

1 small jalapeño pepper, finely chopped

2 medium tomatoes, chopped

1/2 cup diced bok choy

1 tablespoon chopped flat-leaf parsley

3 tablespoons chopped cilantro

Salt and pepper

In a medium saucepan over medium heat, add the rice, 2 cups water, onion, curry powder, jalapeño, tomatoes, and bok choy and simmer for about 20 minutes. When the rice starts to dry, add the parsley and cilantro. Add salt and pepper to taste, stir, and serve.

# Fruit Crisp  S e r v e s  4  ( y e l l o w )

3 organic peaches, peeled, quartered, and
   thinly sliced

1 organic mango, peeled, quartered, and
   thinly sliced

1 cup organic blueberries

$2/3$ cup whole wheat flour

$2/3$ cup rolled oats

3 tablespoons maple sugar

3 tablespoons milled sugar cane

$3/4$ teaspoon ground cinnamon

1 to $1\frac{1}{4}$ teaspoons grated nutmeg

$1/4$ teaspoon salt

5 tablespoons soy margarine, softened

Preheat the oven to 350°F.

Place the fruit in an ungreased 8 × 8-inch baking pan. In a medium mixing bowl, mix the remaining ingredients by hand or with two forks until the mixture is crumbly. Place the mixture on the top of the fruit and bake for 35 minutes, or until the top is golden brown.

# Apple-Oatmeal Crisp  S e r v e s  6  ( y e l l o w )

$2\frac{3}{4}$ pounds organic Granny Smith apples
   (7 medium), peeled, cored, and cut into
   $1/4$-inch slices

2 tablespoons fresh organic lemon juice

$3/4$ cup date sugar

2 tablespoons plus $1/3$ cup unbleached flour

$1/2$ cup old-fashioned oats

$1/2$ teaspoon ground cinnamon

6 tablespoons soy margarine, cut up

Preheat the oven to 425°F. In a large glass or ceramic baking dish, combine the apples, lemon juice, $1/2$ cup of the date sugar, and 2 tablespoons of the flour, tossing to coat. In a small bowl, stir together the oats, cinnamon, remaining $1/3$ cup flour, and remaining $1/4$ cup date sugar. With pastry blender or 2 knives used scissor-fashion, cut in the butter until the mixture resembles coarse crumbs. Sprinkle evenly over the apple mixture. Bake 30 to 35 minutes, or until the apples are tender and the topping is lightly browned. Place the dish on a wire rack and cool for 5 minutes before serving.

## BEVERAGES

- Wheat grass shots
- Vruit fruit and vegetable blend
- Fruit smoothies—try any combination of strawberry, mango, apple, banana, peach, grape, etc.
- Vegetable juices, either served in their purest form or mixed together: carrot, celery, spinach, beet, parsley, and so on. Add ginger for an extra kick.

## PARTY IDEAS

- A recycling party—Everyone brings a used item to be exchanged.
- Garden planting party—Each person brings herbs, flowers, or other plants, and together you take on the challenge of creating and planting a garden.
- Neighborhood beautification party—Organize a group to clean up your neighborhood or a neighborhood in need.
- Healthy food awareness potluck party—Ask your guests to bring a healthy vegan dish (and the recipe) to be sampled and exchanged.

## INVITATIONS

- Cards bearing the image of (or in the shape of) leaves, trees, or globes
- Seed packets with the party information written on the back label

## DECORATIONS

- Anything natural or recycled. Place leaves and branches or little green bonsai trees on the tables as centerpieces.

## SCENTS

Evergreen

Grass

Earth

Rain

Musk

## ACTIVITIES AND GAMES

- Have a contest and give an award to whoever makes the cleverest use of a recycled item.
- Create sculptures made out of old egg cartons, cans, paper rolls, string, corks, and so on. Throw an art show using recycled material.
- Play Jeopardy for a worthy cause—have each person contribute five or ten dollars and play for his or her favorite environmental charity.
- For the neighborhood beautification party, make cleaning teams with both children and grown-ups. The first group to fill up their bags with garbage and recyclables in the alloted time wins.

# Toasts

The subtlety of nature is greater many times over than the subtlety of the senses and understanding.
—SIR FRANCIS BACON

Keep your love of nature, for that is the true way to understand art more and more.
—VINCENT VAN GOGH

Here's to your health!

## PRIZES, GIFTS, AND PARTY FAVORS

- Recycled gifts—have each person bring something they like but no longer use—books, CDs, videocassettes, or clothes; subscriptions to magazines like *Vegetarian Times, Green,* or the *Utne Reader;* seeds and plants, vegan cookbooks, recipe cards, dried flower arrangements, globes, Resist-A-Balls, mud pack facials, natural oils.

## MUSIC

In addition to anything by Kenny Loggins (an environmentalist and a good friend of mine):

| | | |
|---|---|---|
| *Organic* | Joe Cocker | Album |
| *I Am* | Earth Wind & Fire | Album |
| *Down to Earth* | Ozzy Osbourne | Album |
| *Blue Earth* | Jayhawks | Album |
| *Earth, Sun, & Moon* | Love and Rockets | Album |
| *Back to Earth* | Cat Stevens | Album |
| *Live on Planet Earth* | The Neville Brothers | Album |
| *Somewhere Over the Rainbow* | Judy Garland | Album |
| *The Rainbow Children* | Prince | Album |
| *Earth* | Jefferson Starship | Album |
| *Heaven on Earth* | Belinda Carlisle | Album |
| *Earth Pressed Flat* | 10,000 Maniacs | Album |
| *Emergency on Planet Earth* | Jamiriquai | Album |
| *Earth & Sun & Moon* | Midnight Oil | Album |
| *Exit Planet Dust* | The Dust Brothers | Album |
| *What a Wonderful World* | Louis Armstrong | Album |

| | | |
|---|---|---|
| *Crystal Planet* | Joe Satriani | Album |
| *Planet Waves* | Bob Dylan | Album |
| *Songs for a Dying Planet* | Bob Dylan | Album |
| *Wild Planet* | B 52's | Album |
| *Eat a Peach* | Allman Brothers | Album |
| "Mercy Mercy Me" | Marvin Gaye | Song |

## MOVIES

| | |
|---|---|
| *Baraka* | (1992–NR) |
| *Koyaanisqatsi* | (1983–NR) |
| *The China Syndrome* | (1979–PG) |
| *The Day the Earth Stood Still* | (1951–NR) |
| *Soylant Green* | (1973–PG) |

## EXERCISE AND CALORIE CHART

| Activity | Calories Burned/Hour |
|---|---|
| Meditating | 170 |
| Cleaning up trash | 288 |
| Mud wrestling | 388 |
| Hiking | 422 |
| Gardening | 288 |

## FOR THE KIDS

- Plant a garden with your children. One of the best experiences I had was planting a vegetable garden with my kids. I'll never forget their expressions as they saw the plants grow from first sprout to vegetables that we could eat. There's no better way to teach your children about nature than to have them experience it firsthand through their own efforts.

## FOR COUPLES

Give each other a mud face and body massage. Buy mineral mud and clay at your local health store and play Tarzan and Jane's Beauty Spa for Lovers with an earthy treatment that will be as much fun to put on as it will to take off.

# Valentine's Day

*Chocolate Lovers' Hazelnut Macaroons,*
*Cupid's Chocolate Cake, and Chocolate Mousse*

# Chinese New Year

*Seared Tuna on a Bed of Asian Noodles, Honey-Glazed Mahimahi
with Gingered Snow Pea Stir-Fry, and Almond Cookies*

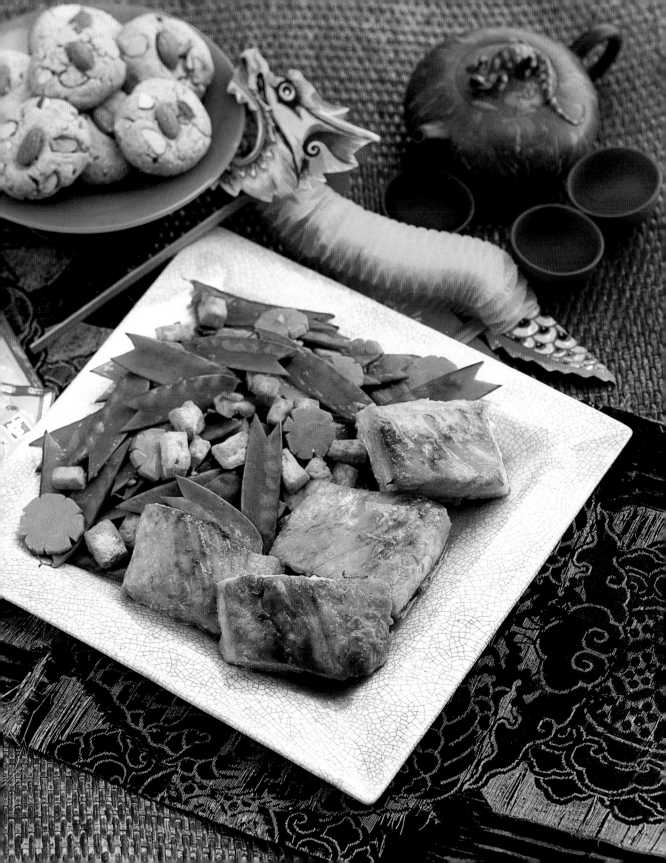

# Earth Day

*Couscous with Green and White Asparagus, Orzo
with Roasted Vegetables, and Fruit Crisp*

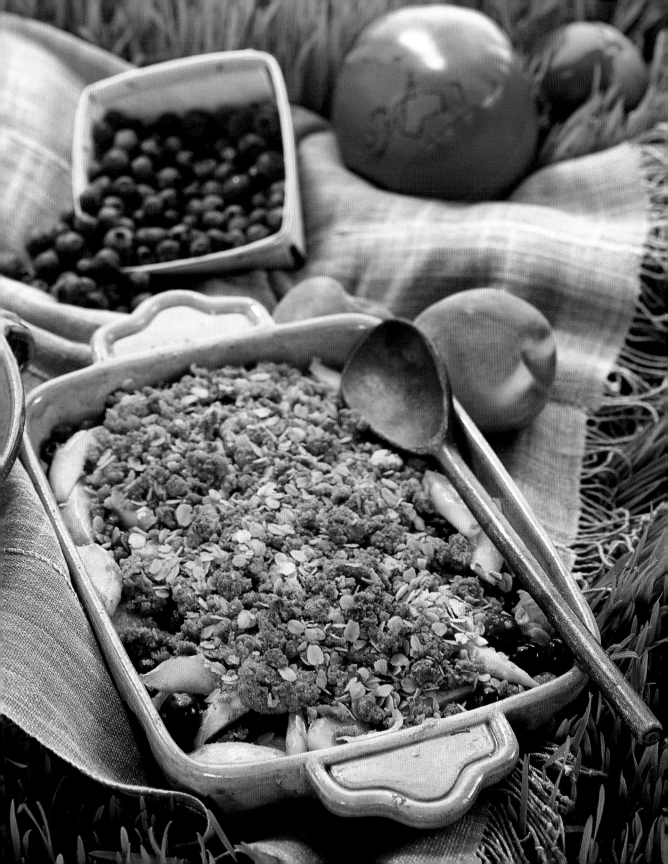

# Cinco de Mayo

*Guacamole and Chips, THM Margarita,*
*Mexican Gazpacho, and Hot Chili Salmon*

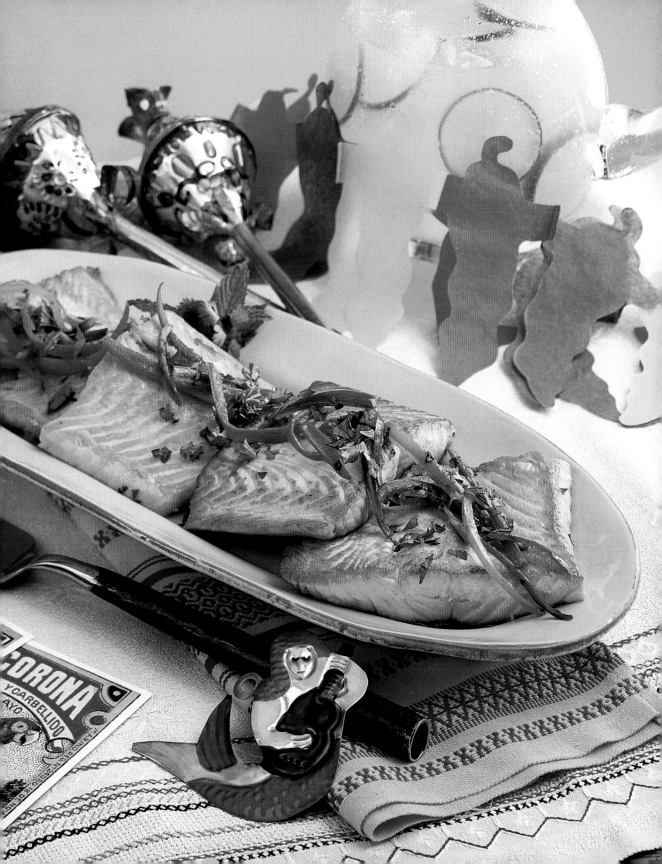

# Summer Picnic

*Barbecue Chicken with Homemade Sauce,
Blueberry Cobbler, Tuna Burgers,
and Southwest Corn Salad*

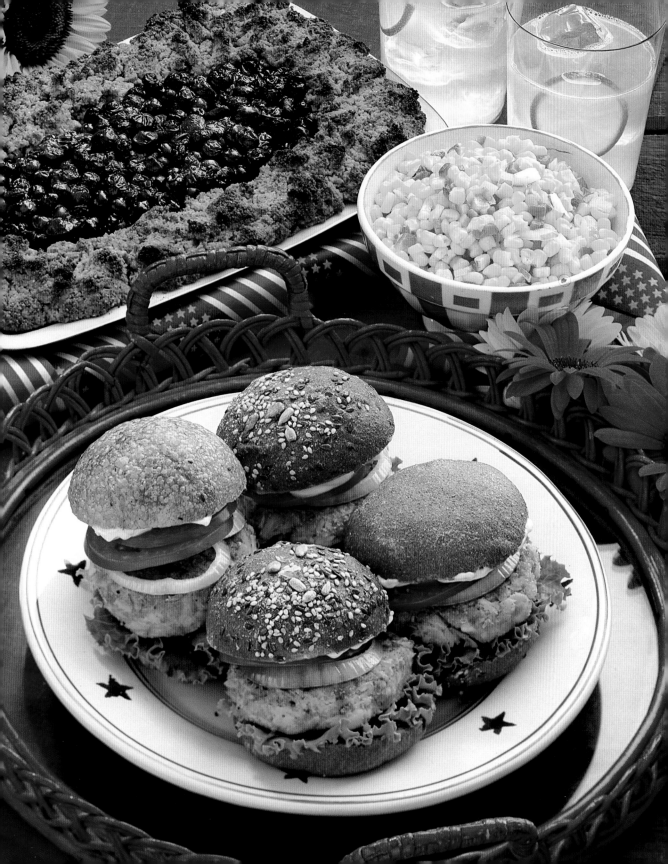

# Bastille Day

*Seared Halibut with Mushroom Vinaigrette,
Raspberry Jam Tart, and Salade Niçoise*

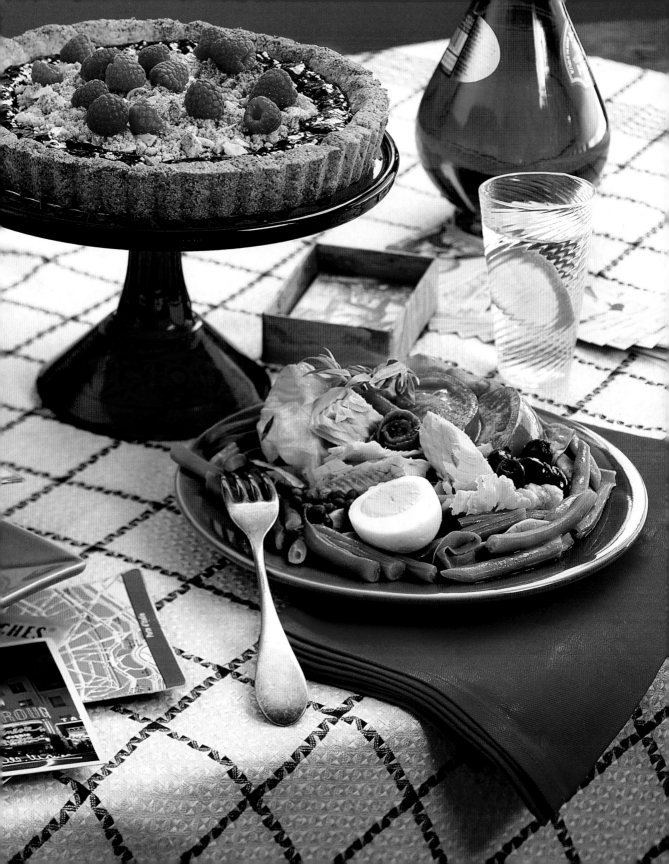

# Halloween

*Vegetable Bones with Brains, Witches' Hands,
Skeleton Fingers Dipped in Blood, and Creepy Spiders*

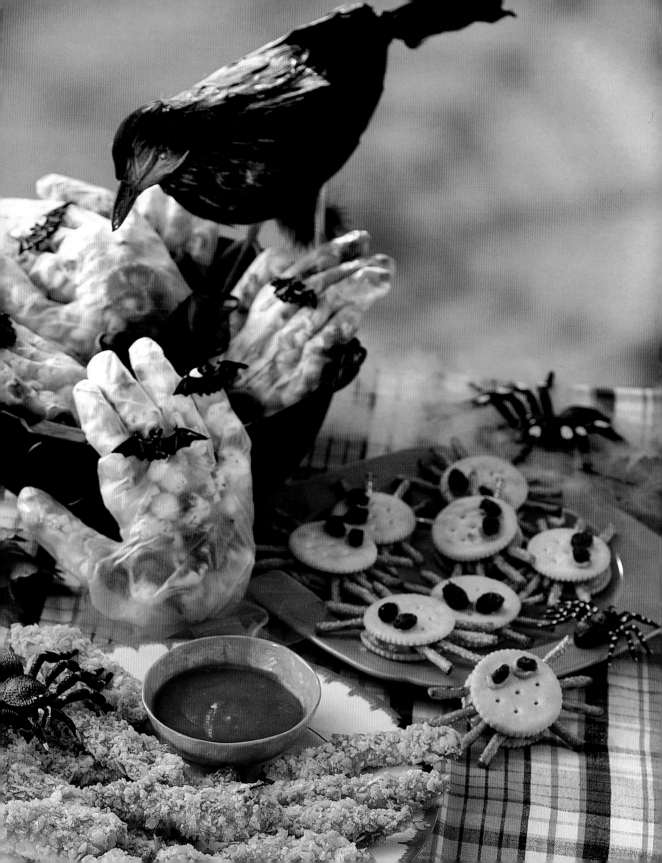

# Christmas

*Honey-Baked Winter Vegetables, Sweet Potato Biscuits,*
*Chocolate Almond Toffee Crunch, and Cornish Game Hens*

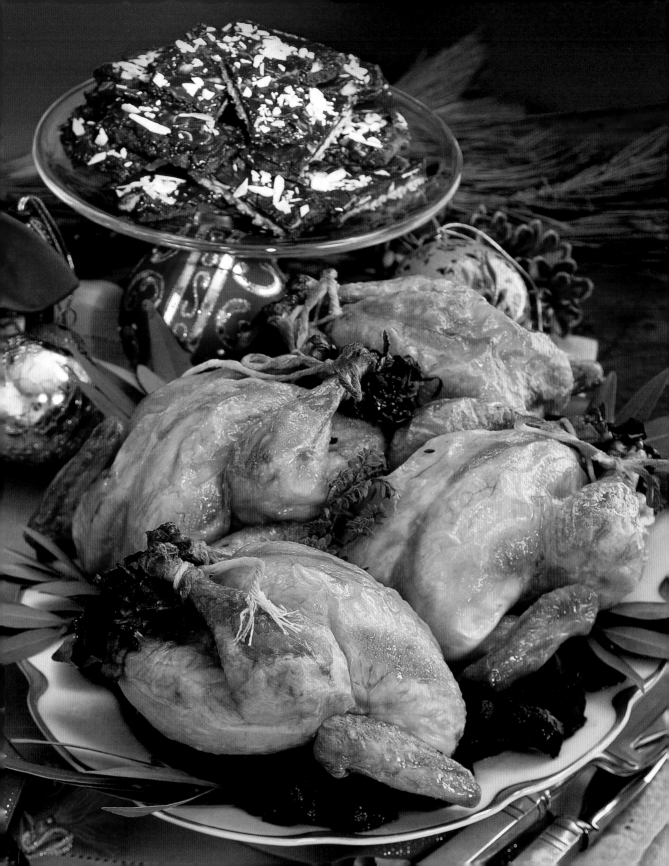

# Mardi Gras

*Seafood Gumbo, Crabmeat Salad*

# Cinco de Mayo

I wanted to include Cinco de Mayo in this book because I *love* Mexican food and culture. Even though the food can be heavy on dairy, meat, and lard, it bursts with so much flavor that it is worth the necessary substitutions to make the dishes THM-safe. Typical ingredients can include wonderfully nutrient-dense wet foods like jicama, tomatoes, tomatillos, and cilantro. By substituting for the less healthy stuff—replacing dairy with soy, cooking in nonhydrogenated vegetable oil, and substituting fish or chicken for beef—you'll have exciting, fun party food that is healthy, vibrant, and packed with nutrition. I eat Mexican food often, and I never gain weight or feel sick from it. Just make sure your ingredients are fresh and organic whenever possible, and most important—*no lard!*

## HISTORY, FACTS, AND FOLKLORE

Cinco de Mayo means May 5. It is not Mexican Independence Day, and it is not officially an American holiday either, but in my opinion it really should be. It commemorates the brave and impressive Mexican victory at the battle of Puebla, in which an army of 4,000 Mexican soldiers defeated 8,000 soldiers from the French Napoleonic army and their allies. This victory was significant in helping to fortify and preserve the countries of both Mexico *and* the United States. I had no idea!

At the time, the powerful French army, under Emperor Napoleon III, was trying to take advantage of two situations: Mexico's debt to France, and the preoccupation of the United States with its Civil War. The French moved in to collect Mexico's debt by force, which was really an excuse to overthrow the Mexican government and gain political advantage in the region. The French had been supplying the rebels of the Confederate Army against the Union, and the victory on May 5, 1862, prevented the French from continuing that support. This strengthened the Union Army and helped lead to the defeat of the Confederates and the end of the Civil War. After this victory, the United States was able to move to the Texas/Mexican border and support the Mexicans with weapons, ammunitions, and even some American soldiers to fight and eventually drive out the French. The American Legion of Honor marched in the victory parade in Mexico City.

It might be a historical stretch to credit the survival of the United States to the brave 4,000 Mexicans who faced an army twice as large in 1862. But who knows?

Mexicans never forget who their friends are, and neither do Americans. Cinco de Mayo is a great party day that celebrates freedom and liberty, two ideals that Mexicans and Americans have fought together to protect ever since. *Viva el Cinco de Mayo!*

## RECIPES
# Guacamole   Serves  8   (blue/green)

2 large ripe organic avocados

1 tablespoon minced organic red onion

1 teaspoon fresh organic chili, stemmed, seeded, and minced

1 tablespoon organic lime juice

1 tablespoon minced organic cilantro

Salt and pepper

Cut the avocados in half, saving one pit. Scoop out the avocado and mash it in a medium bowl. Add the onion, chili, lime juice, cilantro, and salt and pepper to taste. Tuck one pit inside the bowl of guacamole to keep the avocados from browning. Chill and serve with baked tortilla chips.

# Black Bean Dip Serves 10 (blue)

2½ 15-ounce cans organic black beans, drained

2 to 4 tablespoons vegetable stock

1 small white onion, minced

1 small organic tomato, seeded and chopped

1 teaspoon red wine vinegar

Chili powder

1 to 2 tablespoons soy sour cream

Place 2 cups of the black beans in a food processor or blender. Add enough vegetable stock so you are able to purée them into a smooth, slightly chunky texture. Lightly mash the remaining beans with a fork. Combine with the puréed beans and the onion, tomato, vinegar, and chili powder to taste. If the dip is too thick, stir in some soy sour cream to achieve the right texture. Serve with baked tortilla chips.

# Avocado and Tomatoes Serves 4 (blue)

2 large ripe Hass avocados, peeled and pitted

3 large organic tomatoes

1 teaspoon olive oil

2 teaspoons red wine vinegar

1 tablespoon soy Parmesan cheese

Salt and coarsely ground pepper

Cut the avocados and tomatoes into similar bite-sized pieces. In a small bowl, mix them together gently. Whisk together the olive oil and vinegar. Pour the dressing over the avocados and tomatoes. Sprinkle the soy Parmesan over the salad. Add salt and pepper to taste.

# Roasted Corn Salsa Serves 6 (blue)

6 cups organic corn kernels

3 tablespoons plus 1 teaspoon olive oil

1 small organic red onion, diced

¼ cup finely chopped organic cilantro

3 tablespoons balsamic vinegar

2 teaspoons salt

Preheat the oven to 450°F.

In a medium bowl, toss the corn in 1 teaspoon of the olive oil. Spread the corn on a foil-lined baking sheet and roast until the kernels begin to brown slightly, about 15 minutes. Remove from the oven and cool. Place the remaining ingredients in a bowl, add the corn, and mix.

## Halibut and Coconut Ceviche

Serves 6 to 8     (blue/green)

1 pound halibut fillets, skin removed

¾ cup fresh lime juice

½ cup cream of coconut

2 mild red chili peppers, seeded
    and chopped

¼ cup organic cilantro leaves

Sea salt

Cracked black pepper

Organic lettuce leaves for garnish

Cut the fish into thin sashimi-style slices. Place the fish in a glass or ceramic bowl with ½ cup of the lime juice and refrigerate for 2 hours. Combine the fish with the cream of coconut, peppers, the remaining ¼ cup of lime juice, cilantro, and salt and pepper to taste. Chill for up to 4 hours before serving. Place a lettuce leaf on each plate, top with the ceviche, and serve.

## Nachos   Serves 8     (green/yellow)

1 8-ounce bag baked corn tortillas chips

2 cups grated soy Cheddar cheese

1 cup canned organic pinto beans, heated
    and drained

½ cup chopped green chili peppers

½ cup Mexican Sauce (see recipe page 184)

8 fresh organic tomato slices

8 fresh organic avocado slices

2 tablespoons soy sour cream

Preheat the oven to 350°F.
    Spread the chips on a platter. Sprinkle 1 cup of the soy cheese over them. With a large spoon, drop dollops of cooked beans randomly over the chips. Sprinkle on the chopped green chilies. Spoon on Mexican sauce to taste. Add the remaining 1 cup soy cheese and top with sliced tomatoes. Place in the oven until the soy cheese melts, about 5 minutes. Garnish with the sliced avocados and soy sour cream.

# Corn Soup with Cilantro <small>Serves 10 (blue)</small>

2 teaspoons olive oil

1 Spanish onion, coarsely chopped

2 to 3 garlic cloves, finely chopped
  or pressed

½ teaspoon cayenne (optional)

6 large ears of corn (approximately 4 cups
  of kernels)

1 tablespoon Bragg's Liquid Aminos

7 or 8 cups vegetable stock

¼ cup chopped fresh cilantro for garnish

Heat a large stockpot over medium-low heat and add the oil. When the oil is hot, add the onion, garlic, and the cayenne, if desired. Cook for 15 minutes, or until the onion and garlic are softened. Raise the heat to high, add the corn kernels, Bragg's, and stock, and bring to a boil. Reduce the heat to low and cook, partially covered, for 25 minutes. Transfer half of the solids to a blender or food processor fitted with a steel blade and purée. Return the purée to the soup and stir. Garnish each serving with fresh cilantro.

# Mexican Gazpacho <small>Serves 6 (blue)</small>

6 large organic ripe tomatoes, peeled,
  seeded, puréed, and strained

2 cups vegetable stock

½ cup fresh lime juice

1 medium organic cucumber, peeled, seeded,
  and finely chopped

2 Anaheim chili peppers, stemmed, seeded,
  and finely chopped

4 organic scallions, trimmed and minced

1 large garlic clove, minced or pressed

2 tablespoons chopped fresh organic cilantro

2 tablespoons olive oil

Salt

1 medium organic avocado, peeled, pitted,
  and coarsely chopped

In a large bowl, stir together the tomatoes, vegetable stock, lime juice, cucumber, chilies, scallions, garlic, and cilantro. Cover and refrigerate for several hours or overnight, until very cold. Just before serving, stir in the olive oil and add salt to taste. Ladle the soup into individual bowls and garnish each bowl with the chopped avocado.

## Tostados Serves 4 (green)

4 whole wheat or corn tortillas

2 cups Refried Pinto Beans, warmed (see recipe page 184)

1½ cups Mexican Brown Rice, warmed (see recipe page 183)

2 cups Mexican Sauce (see recipe page 184)

8 organic lettuce leaves, shredded

1 organic avocado, peeled, seeded, and diced

1 cup salsa

Soy cheese (optional)

Preheat the oven to 350°F.

Lay the tortillas on the oven rack and bake until crispy, about 3 to 5 minutes for whole wheat and 10 to 12 minutes for corn. Spread a thin layer of beans, rice, and Mexican sauce on each tortilla. Top with lettuce, avocado, salsa, and soy cheese, if using.

## Hot Chili Salmon Serves 4 (blue)

2 to 3 tablespoons peanut oil

4 large organic green chili peppers, seeded and shredded

4 large organic red chili peppers, seeded and shredded

3 tablespoons shredded organic ginger

4 8-ounce salmon fillets

¼ cup chopped fresh organic parsley

½ cup chopped fresh organic mint leaves

⅔ cup chopped fresh organic cilantro leaves

2 tablespoons organic lime juice

In a large frying pan over high heat, heat the oil. Add the green and red chilies and the ginger and sauté for 5 to 7 minutes, or until the ingredients are crisp. Remove from the pan with a slotted spoon and drain on absorbent paper. Set aside. Using the same frying pan and oil, over medium heat, cook the salmon for 2 minutes on each side, or until cooked to your liking. In a large bowl, toss the chilies and ginger with the parsley, mint, and cilantro. Place the salmon on serving plates, top with the chili mixture, and drizzle the lime juice over all.

# Chopped Salad Serves 4 (blue)

2 medium organic carrots, chopped

½ pound organic white mushrooms,
trimmed and chopped

1 medium organic zucchini, trimmed and
chopped

1 organic yellow squash, trimmed and
chopped

1 small organic jicama, peeled and chopped

15 organic radishes, trimmed and chopped

4 organic roma tomatoes, chopped

¼ cup white wine vinegar

Salt and pepper

½ teaspoon Dijon-style mustard

1 teaspoon coriander seeds

1½ teaspoons crushed cilantro

¾ cup extra-virgin olive oil

8 large organic lettuce leaves, torn

1 large organic avocado, pitted, peeled, and
chopped

In a large bowl, combine the carrots, mushrooms, zucchini, yellow squash, jicama, radishes, and tomatoes, set aside. In a food processor, combine the vinegar, ¾ teaspoon salt, mustard, coriander, and cilantro and mix, slowly drizzling in the oil until a smooth texture forms. Toss a small amount on the vegetable mixture, enough to coat. Toss the vegetables with the lettuce and avocado and add more dressing to taste. Season to taste with salt and pepper and serve.

## Portobello Quesadillas with Salsa

Serves 12 (green)

1½ cups chopped organic Italian plum
   tomatoes

⅓ cup chopped organic Spanish onion

1 jalapeño pepper, seeded (optional)

1 tablespoon fresh organic lime juice

¼ teaspoon kosher salt

¼ teaspoon freshly ground black pepper

2 cups ¼-inch-thick sliced portobello
   mushrooms (about 1 pound)

1 to 2 tablespoons olive oil

1 cup shredded soy Cheddar cheese (4 ounces)

8 8-inch whole wheat tortillas

¾ cup soy sour cream

To prepare the salsa, combine the tomatoes, onion, jalapeño (if using), lime juice, salt, and pepper in a medium bowl. Refrigerate until ready to use. To prepare the quesadillas, in a large sauté pan over medium heat, sauté the mushrooms in the olive oil for 6 minutes, or until tender. Sprinkle 2 tablespoons of the soy Cheddar cheese over each of 4 tortillas; top each with ½ cup mushrooms, 2 tablespoons soy cheese, and another tortilla. Lightly coat the top of the tortillas with cooking spray. Heat a sauté pan coated with cooking spray over medium-high heat. Place 1 quesadilla in the pan and cook 2 minutes on each side, or until the tortillas are lightly browned. Set aside and keep warm. Repeat with the remaining quesadillas. Cut each quesadilla into 6 wedges. Serve with the salsa and soy sour cream.

## Burritos Serves 4 (green)

4 whole wheat flour tortillas

1 cup warm refried beans (from a 15-ounce
   can)

2 cups sliced and cooked organic chicken
   breast or 2 cups firm tofu slices

2 cups Mexican Sauce (see page 184)

½ organic avocado, peeled and sliced

1 organic tomato, diced

4 organic red-leaf lettuce leaves

½ teaspoon salt

½ teaspoon freshly ground black pepper

Warm the tortillas, beans, chicken, and sauce. Spread out the tortillas on a work surface. Place a strip of refried beans down the center of each. Add the chicken or tofu, avocado, tomato, and lettuce. Season with the salt and pepper. Drizzle some Mexican sauce over each burrito. Fold the bottom quarter of each tortilla up and then roll the tortilla into a cylinder.

# Arroz con Pollo Serves 6 (blue)

1 3-pound organic free-range chicken, cut up

½ cup olive oil

1 large white onion, chopped

1 garlic clove, crushed

½ teaspoon crushed red pepper

2½ teaspoons salt

½ teaspoon pepper

2 cups uncooked basmati rice

2 to 3 teaspoons saffron threads

1 15-ounce can Italian plum tomatoes, undrained

1 15-ounce can organic chicken broth

1 15-ounce can organic petit peas

1 4-ounce bottle pimientos

Preheat the oven to 350°F.

In a Dutch oven, brown the chicken in the oil about 7 minutes on each side. Remove and place on a plate. Add the onion, garlic, and red pepper and cook until golden brown, about 3 minutes. Add the salt, pepper, rice, and saffron and cook until the rice is lightly browned, about another 3 minutes. Add the tomatoes, chicken broth, and the browned chicken and cook over medium heat until the liquid comes to a boil. Cover and put in the oven for 1 hour. After 1 hour, add ½ cup water and sprinkle the top with the peas and pimientos. Bake, uncovered, for 20 minutes more. Fluff the rice with a fork and serve.

# Mexican Brown Rice Serves 8 (purple/blue)

2 cups uncooked organic long-grain brown rice

2 medium organic hothouse tomatoes

1 small Spanish onion

1 garlic clove, minced

1 jalapeño pepper (optional)

3 tablespoons olive oil

4 cups vegetable stock

¼ teaspoon salt

½ cup fresh organic cilantro leaves, chopped

Put the rice in a large bowl of water and soak about 20 minutes. Drain and rinse. Using a food processor, purée the tomatoes, onion, garlic, and pepper, if using. In a medium pot, heat the oil over medium heat. Add the rice and cook until the grains become translucent, about 5 minutes. Add the puréed mixture and cook about 5 minutes, until no longer wet. Add the stock and salt and bring to a boil. Reduce the heat to low. Cover and cook without disturbing until the liquid is absorbed and the rice is tender, about 17 to 20 minutes. Fluff the rice with a fork. Cover the pot and set aside for 15 minutes. Garnish with the cilantro and serve immediately.

## Refried Pinto Beans  Serves 8  (blue)

2 cups organic pinto beans

1/3 cup olive oil

1 large Spanish onion, chopped

1 1/2 teaspoons salt

1/2 teaspoon freshly ground black pepper

1/3 cup vegetable broth

1/4 cup chopped cilantro

In a medium saucepan, bring 2 quarts of water to a boil. Add the beans and reduce to a simmer. Cover and cook for about 1 1/2 hours. Test a couple of beans; they should be creamy inside. With a potato masher, mash the beans with the cooking liquid until creamy.

In a medium saucepan over medium-high heat, add the olive oil. Sauté the onion, salt, and pepper until the onion is golden brown, about 10 minutes. Add the mashed beans and vegetable broth. Cook until most of the liquid has evaporated, about 10 minutes. Garnish with the cilantro and serve immediately.

## Mexican Sauce  Makes 5 cups  (blue)

1 cup chopped onions

1/4 cup tamari sauce

8 teaspoons Bragg's Liquid Aminos

1/4 cup chili powder

1 teaspoon cumin

4 1/2 cups vegetable broth

1/4 cup arrowroot

8 teaspoons whole wheat flour

Cook the onions in 2/3 cup of water until they are tender. Add the tamari, Bragg's, chili powder, cumin, and broth and bring to a boil. In a measuring cup or small bowl, mix the arrowroot and flour in 1/3 cup of water. Slowly add this mixture to the simmering sauce, stirring until the sauce begins to thicken. Cook over low heat, stirring occasionally, about 25 to 30 minutes.

## BEVERAGES
## THM MARGARITA

4 ounces organic fruit juice–sweetened
  lemonade (I recommend R.W. Knudsen's or
  Santa Cruz lemonade)

1½ ounces tequila (optional)

1 tablespoon fresh, natural, unsweetened
  lime juice

¼ orange or 1 tablespoon orange juice

Lime wedge for garnish

Combine the lemonade, tequila, if using, lime juice, and orange juice over ice. Shake, blend, or stir, then pour into a rocks glass (salted rim optional). Garnish with the lime wedge.

## THM TEQUILA SUNRISE

6 ounces orange juice

1½ ounces tequila (optional)

1 tablespoon organic unsweetened cranberry
  juice

Orange slice and fresh cherry for garnish

Over ice in a highball glass, pour the orange juice, tequila, if using, and cranberry juice. Don't stir, just serve with the orange slice and fresh cherry (not maraschino).

## SOMBRERO
*Warning: not lo-cal!*

2 ounces Silk Coffee Soylatte

2 ounces Silk Vanilla Creamer or soy milk

1½ ounces vodka (optional)

Grated nutmeg or ground cinnamon
  (optional)

Combine the soylatte, soy milk, and vodka, if using, over ice. Shake or stir, then pour into a rocks glass. Sprinkle with the nutmeg or cinnamon, if using.

## SANGRIA

1 bottle Cabernet Sauvignon or
   nonalcoholic red wine

8 ounces orange juice

3 ounces organic fruit juice–sweetened
   lemonade (I recommend R.W. Knudsen's
   or Santa Cruz lemonade)

1 orange, sliced

8 ounces sparkling mineral water
   (such as Pellegrino or Perrier)

Lemon twists and fresh cherries for
   garnish

In a large pitcher or punch bowl, combine the wine, orange juice, lemonade, and orange over ice. Stir in the mineral water just before serving. Garnish with the lemon twists and fresh cherries (not maraschino).

## PARTY IDEAS

- Celebrate Mexican culture with history, music, art, dancing, food, piñatas, paper flowers, limbo, chips and salsa, and healthy margaritas.
- Have an adult or one of the kids dress up as a Mexican border guard to greet guests as they arrive to make them feel as if they are entering a new country.

## INVITATIONS

Postcards of Mexican art or tourist spots with a quirky rhyme about Cinco de Mayo:
Frida Kahlo skipped her tweezers
Margaritas in the freezer
Chips and salsa ain't enough
Come on by and show your stuff
We're celebrating Cinco de Mayo!

## DECORATIONS

- Lace paper flags, sombreros, and maracas
- Red, white, and green streamers and balloons
- Mexican flags and travel posters
- Inexpensive Mexican marionettes—kids can put on a puppet show with them later.
- Make paper flowers. You'll need an assortment of red, white, and green tissue paper and a bunch of pipe cleaners. Cut the tissue paper into 10- to 15-inch squares. For each flower,

stack six sheets, alternating the colors. Fold back and forth from end to end like you would for a fan. Twist one end of a pipe cleaner around the center of the folds. Then spread the folds out back and forth, pulling up toward the center in the shape of a flower. The remaining pipe cleaner is the stem. This activity is a lot of fun for kids.

## SCENTS

Coconut
Pineapple
Banana
Ocean
Avocado

# Toasts

To freedom, and the borders we cross to get here.

To freedom, Frida, and Fritos.

To Mexico.

To pesos and possibilities.

Salud (Cheers).
—SUZANNE CARNEY

## ACTIVITIES AND GAMES

- *Do the limbo!* It's important to play fun, lively Mexican music during this game to add to the excitement and atmosphere. You need two people to hold a long stick or broom at each end and one person to act as judge and master of ceremonies. Players line up to take turns trying to maneuver their bodies under the stick, arching their backs, bending backward, and making sure they don't fall or touch the bar. If they do either, they're out of the game. After everyone in the line has gone through, the bar is lowered a few inches and the process starts again. The winner is the person who has cleared the bar at the lowest point without touching or falling. This is one game in which children and very limber adults have the advantage.
- *Break a piñata.* Get them at a party store, or make your own. Blindfold each child one at a time and place him or her right in front of the piñata. Turn them three times, then let 'em swing. Make sure the other children are well out of swinging range. Instead of using candy, fill the piñatas with little toys or healthy treats made without sugar or dairy.

   Years ago I was on *The Donny and Marie Show* with my boys. One of the other guests made a piñata. When it burst open, Donny handed my son Nicky, who was four at the time, a package of M&Ms. Nicky responded, "No thank you, I don't eat sugar." Kids will eat healthy food if you are consistent in giving it to them. As I am always saying, "If you build it, they will come."
- *Plan a field trip to a museum that features Mexican art.* Learn the styles of Jose Clemente Orozco, Diego Rivera, David Alfaro Siqueiros, and Frida Kahlo.

· If you live near Mexico, go south of the border for the day. Tijuana, Juarez, and even Olvera Street in downtown Los Angeles are always a blast. Or spend the day celebrating in the nearest Mexican community.

## PRIZES, GIFTS, AND PARTY FAVORS

Sombreros, marionettes, castanets, mini bongo drums, little trumpets, maracas, colorful scarves, silver jewelry, little rings, bracelets, necklaces, beaded craft kits, gift certificates to a Mexican restaurant; Mexican food baskets filled with chips, salsas, bean dips, rice, taco shells, guacamole, tortillas, Mexican corn bread, piñatas of different shapes, Mexican sun replicas, Mexican folk music tapes and CDs, Spanish language tapes, Mexican blankets, leather wallets and change purses, tambourines.

## MUSIC

In addition to anything by the Gypsy Kings, Jesse Cook, or Menudo:

| | | |
|---|---|---|
| *A Mexico* | Julio Iglesias | Album |
| *Seashores of Old Mexico* | Merle Haggard and Willie Nelson | Album |
| *Viva* | Percy Faith | Album |
| *The Mexican* | Various | Soundtrack |
| *My Spanish Heart* | Chick Corea | Album |
| *Buena Vista Social Club* | Buena Vista Social Club | Soundtrack |
| *Kiko* | Los Lobos | Album |
| *Canciones de Mi Padre* | Linda Ronstadt | Album |
| *Mexican American Border Music, Vol. 1, 1928–1958* | Various Artists | Album |
| *Mexican Love Songs, Vol. 2* | Various Artists | Album |

## MOVIES

| | |
|---|---|
| *Like Water for Chocolate* | (1992–R) |
| *The Milagro Bean Field War* | (1988–R) |

## EXERCISE AND CALORIE CHART

Rent a video that teaches Mexican folk dances. Learning them will be great exercise.

| Activity | Calories Burned/Hour |
| --- | --- |
| Flamenco dancing | 370 |
| Tango | 320 |
| Mexican hat dance | 353 |
| Hitting a piñata (papier mâché) | 246 |
| Hitting a piñata (clay) | 376 |

## FOR THE KIDS

· Paint like the masters. Set up a table with everything kids need to paint using watercolors: paints, water, paper, aprons, newspaper, masking tape, and a place for them to hang their masterpieces. For inspiration, set out a book of the masters of Mexican art.

· Teach your kids the Mexican hat dance. But first, have them make their own Mexican hats. Set up an arts and crafts table and give each child a plain straw hat to decorate. Each child can create his or her own colorful hat for the festival. Have them do a traditional hat dance with their new creations.

· Have the kids make their own Mexican smiling sun out of colored clay. Set up a table with a variety of colored clays so they'll have a lot to play with. It's best to use the kind of clay that hardens by air or baking so that they can keep them for souvenirs.

## FOR COUPLES

Play Viva Zapata Meets the Seductive Peasant Girl. All you need is a sexy, lacy peasant skirt and an off-the-shoulder peasant blouse for her and a really big sombrero for him. Light some candles. Put on some soft Mexican guitar music, and start your own revolution. If you two are the intellectual, socialist, bohemian type, try Diego Rivera and Frida Kahlo instead. Same outfits, smaller sombrero.

# Mother's Day/
# Father's Day

**W**hat better way to honor your mother and father than by devoting the entire day to improving their health? Start the day by sharing a fun, healthy activity, like going for a walk, swim, or bike ride or playing tennis or golf. After that, prepare a healthy, great-tasting meal for them. Here's your chance to try something new. If they don't usually eat like this, be patient. Remember that old habits die hard, so it might take them a little while to adjust to this style of eating. Trust me—if you can get them started (especially while showing great interest yourself), they'll be on their way to a healthier lifestyle. If they're always been resistant to health food, don't even tell them what it is. Parents hate to admit they've been eating the wrong foods, or even worse, feeding you the wrong foods. Parents and health food can be just like Mikey's brothers and Life cereal. They don't want to try anything that's supposed to be good for them. So don't tell your parents until they've eaten and enjoyed the meal. Tell them it's a recipe from Europe or something. It's trick your parents day!

It's great to spend this day really listening to your parents. You may want to set up a tape player or video recorder and tape them talking about their lives and family history. Write down a list of questions beforehand, and make sure one of the topics you cover is family *health* history. Ask about aunts, uncles, grandparents, and great-grandparents. This can be useful for uncovering problem family health areas that may need to be addressed. And one last thing—if they haven't done so recently, encourage them to make an appointment with a physician for a complete physical. Perhaps you should make an appointment for yourself on the same day and make it a family field trip! Take responsibility for your health, too. After all, you may be someone's mother or father yourself.

## HISTORY, FACTS, AND FOLKLORE
### Mother's Day

Every spring in ancient Rome, a festival was held to honor Rhea, the great mother of the gods. The Christians honored the Virgin Mary, the mother of Jesus. And during the Civil War, Americans unofficially set aside a day for mothers. In 1914 President Woodrow Wilson officially proclaimed the second Sunday in May to be Mother's Day. (Such a good boy, that Woodrow!)

### Father's Day

The first Father's Day was observed on June 19, 1910, in Spokane, Washington. The idea started with Sonora Smart Dodd, who wanted to honor her father, a man who raised six children by himself after his wife died in childbirth. Eventually President Lyndon Johnson proclaimed the third Sunday of June to be Father's Day. (And the price of neckties soared!)

It took the all-male U.S. Congress longer to acknowledge Father's Day than it took them to recognize Mother's Day. The reason: they feared voters would think it was too self-serving.
—BRIAN L. FOUST

## HENNER FAMILY TRADITIONS AND STORIES
One of my favorite childhood memories was our ritual every Sunday morning, when all six kids would pile onto my parents' bed. We'd wake them up and jump on their bed like a trampoline. After that we'd all go to mass and come home to a big Sunday breakfast. But on Mother's and Father's Day, we would bring our parents breakfast in bed and give them a day off from the trampoline.

I'll never forget my two favorite Mother's and Father's Day gifts, which I gave when I was eight. Both gifts tell you what my parents were like. I gave a pair of kelly green satin opera gloves to my glamorous Lana Turner look-a-like mom and a book of jokes and toasts to my charming Clark Gable–lookin', James Cagney–talkin' dad.

# Light and Hearty Chicken Soup

Serves 4    (blue)

- 8 cups organic chicken broth
- 2 tablespoons Bragg's Liquid Aminos
- 2 8-ounce skinless, boneless chicken breast halves, trimmed of fat
- 2 large organic carrots, peeled and sliced into 1/4-inch rounds (about 2 1/2 cups)
- 2 organic celery stalks, chopped
- 1 small organic fennel bulb, peeled and very thinly sliced
- 1/2 cup chopped organic escarole
- 1 cup cooked organic Great Northern beans
- Kosher salt and freshly ground black pepper

In a 3-quart soup pot over medium heat, bring the broth to a simmer. Add the Bragg's and chicken, and poach until opaque and firm, about 10 minutes. Transfer to a plate. Add the carrots and celery to the broth and cook until fork-tender, about 10 minutes. Add the fennel, escarole, and beans and simmer for another 10 minutes. Shred the chicken into 1-inch strips with your hands. Add to the pot and simmer until the chicken is heated through, about 2 minutes. Season to taste with the salt and pepper.

# White Bean Salad with Basil

Serves 4    (blue)

- 2 16-ounce cans small white cannellini beans, drained and rinsed
- 1/2 small red onion or 1/4 Vidalia onion, coarsely chopped
- 2 teaspoons olive oil
- 1 tablespoon balsamic vinegar
- 1 teaspoon chopped fresh organic basil
- 5 organic cherry tomatoes, halved
- Kosher salt and freshly ground black pepper

In a medium serving bowl, combine all the ingredients except the salt and pepper. Let sit at room temperature for 1 hour while the flavors blend. Add the salt and pepper to taste. Serve at room temperature.

Mother's Day/Father's Day

## Seared Ahi Tuna with Arugula Salad

Serves 4    (purple)

- 4 6-ounces Ahi tuna steaks about ¾ inch thick)
- 1½ teaspoons freshly ground black pepper
- ¾ teaspoon kosher salt
- 2 tablespoons olive oil
- 2 tablespoons red wine vinegar
- 8 cups fresh organic arugula leaves, washed and dried
- 2 cups fresh organic endive, sliced thinly

Sprinkle the tuna with 1 teaspoon of the pepper and ¼ teaspoon of the salt and set aside. In a large nonstick skillet over medium-high heat, heat 1 tablespoon of the oil and add the tuna steaks. Cook 2 minutes on each side, or until desired degree of doneness.

In a large bowl, whisk together the remaining ½ teaspoon pepper, remaining ½ teaspoon salt, remaining 1 tablespoon oil, and the vinegar. Add the arugula and endive and toss well. Place about 2 cups salad on each of 4 plates. Top each serving with 1 tuna steak and serve immediately.

# Wild Mushroom Stew Serves 4 (blue)

4½ cups quartered shiitake mushrooms
(about 8 ounces)

4½ cups quartered cremini mushrooms
(about 8 ounces)

1 8-ounce package button mushrooms,
quartered

1 tablespoon plus 1½ teaspoons olive oil

2 cups thinly sliced organic leeks (about 2
medium)

1 cup chopped fennel (about 1 small bulb)

1 cup 1-inch-thick sliced carrots

¾ teaspoon salt

2 cups vegetable stock

2 tablespoons low-sodium tamari sauce

½ teaspoon minced fresh organic tarragon

½ teaspoon chopped fresh organic thyme

1 teaspoon agave sweetener

1 14½-ounce can chopped organic tomatoes,
drained

1 tablespoon arrowroot

Preheat the oven to 450°F.

To prepare the stew, combine all the mushrooms and 1 tablespoon of the oil in a single layer on a jelly roll pan. Bake the mushrooms for 30 minutes, stirring once, until tender and browned.

In a Dutch oven over medium heat, heat 1½ teaspoons of the oil. Add the leeks, fennel, and carrots and cook 5 minutes, or until the carrots are softened. Sprinkle the leek mixture with ¼ teaspoon salt. Cover, reduce the heat, and cook 10 minutes. Uncover and add the mushroom mixture, stock, tamari, tarragon, thyme, agave, and tomatoes. Bring to a boil. Reduce the heat and simmer 5 minutes, or until all the vegetables are tender. Stir in the remaining ½ teaspoon salt.

In a small bowl, combine the arrowroot and 1 tablespoon water. Stir the arrowroot mixture into the mushroom mixture and cook 1 minute more, to a nice thick stew texture. Serve hot.

## Chicken with Olives and Capers

Serves 10    (green)

*BETH EVIN HEFFNER*

4 2½-pound chickens, quartered

1 head of garlic, cloves peeled and finely
   puréed

¼ cup dried oregano

Coarse salt and freshly ground black pepper

½ cup red wine vinegar

½ cup olive oil

1 cup pitted prunes

½ cup pitted Spanish green olives

½ cup capers, with a bit of juice

6 bay leaves

1 cup packed maple sugar

1 cup white wine

½ cup finely chopped Italian parsley

In a large bowl, combine the chicken quarters, garlic, oregano, salt and pepper to taste, vinegar, olive oil, prunes, olives, capers with juice, and bay leaves. Cover and let marinate in the refrigerator overnight.

Preheat the oven to 350°F.

Arrange the chicken in a single layer in one or two large, shallow baking pans and spoon the marinade evenly over it. Sprinkle the chicken pieces with the sugar and pour the white wine around them.

Roast the chicken for 50 minutes to 1 hour, basting frequently with the pan juices. The chicken is done when the thigh pieces yield clear liquid when pricked with a fork at their thickest. With a slotted spoon, transfer the chicken, prunes, olives, and capers to a serving platter.

Moisten with a few spoonfuls of pan juices and sprinkle generously with the parsley. Pass the remaining pan juices in a gravy boat.

# Snapper in Parchment Serves 4 (blue)

1 leek, julienned, green leaves reserved

2½ pounds snapper, filleted, skinned, and
    cut into 2 pieces

2 teaspoons olive oil

Salt and pepper

6 thin organic lemons slices

2 tablespoons capers

6 fresh organic thyme sprigs

Paprika

2 tablespoons white wine

2 tablespoons chopped fresh organic parsley

4 fresh organic rosemary sprigs

Preheat the oven to 400°F.

Have ready a sheet of parchment paper, approximately 16 × 24 inches, depending on the size of the fillets. Place 2 leek leaves next to each other in the center of the parchment paper, making a bed for the snapper. Brush each fillet with 1 teaspoon of olive oil and season to taste on both sides with salt and pepper. Lay the fish on top of the leek greens. Top the fish with the julienned leeks, lemon slices, capers, and thyme. Sprinkle a little paprika and salt and pepper on top. Pour the white wine and add parsley and rosemary over the fish. To wrap the fish, fold the two long ends together and roll the top closed like a burrito. Place the wrapped fish on a baking sheet and bake for 20 to 25 minutes, until the fish flakes.

# Caramelized Corn with Shallots

Serves 4 (blue)

1 tablespoon soy margarine

4 ears of fresh organic corn, kernels shaved
    from the cob (about 3 cups)

4 large organic shallots, cut into ¼-inch
    slices

Pinch of Sucanat

Kosher salt and freshly ground black pepper

2 tablespoons minced fresh organic thyme
    leaves

In a large sauté pan over medium heat, melt the margarine. Add the corn, shallots, Sucanat, and salt and pepper to taste. Cook, stirring occasionally, until the corn is caramelized, about 5 minutes. Stir in the thyme and cook 5 minutes more, or until all the flavors are combined. Season to taste with salt and pepper.

## Pasta with Fresh Vegetable Tomato Sauce

Serves 6 (purple)

*SUSAN ROMITO*

- 1 tablespoon olive oil
- 2 small onions, diced
- 2 carrots, diced
- 1 small eggplant, diced
- Salt and freshly ground black pepper
- ¼ cup minced parsley
- 2 28-ounce cans peeled or crushed tomatoes, undrained
- 1¼ cups vegetable broth
- 2 small zucchini, cut in half lengthwise, sliced into ½-inch circles
- ¼ cup basil, cut into chiffonade
- 1 pound dried pasta

In a large saucepan over medium-high heat, add the oil, onions, carrots, and eggplant and sauté until lightly browned, about 5 to 7 minutes. Add salt and pepper to taste and the parsley. Stir in the tomatoes in their juice and the broth and simmer 10 minutes over low heat, breaking up the tomatoes with the back of a spoon. Add the zucchini and basil and cook another 5 minutes, or until the zucchini is tender.

Fill a large stockpot over high heat with water and add 1 teaspoon salt. When it comes to a boil, drop in the pasta and cook according to package directions. Top the pasta with the sauce and serve.

## Apple Crisp with Macadamia Nuts

Serves 6 (yellow)

- ¼ cup unbleached white flour
- ½ cup Sucanat
- 2 tablespoons maple sugar
- 2 tablespoons chopped macadamia nuts
- ⅛ teaspoon ground cinnamon
- 2½ teaspoons chilled soy margarine
- 5 cups peeled thinly sliced organic Rome apples
- 2 tablespoons all-natural, no-sugar-added apricot preserves

Preheat the oven to 375°F.

Combine the flour, Sucanat, maple sugar, chopped nuts, and cinnamon in a medium bowl. Cut in the soy margarine with a pastry blender until the mixture resembles coarse meal. Set aside. In an 8-inch square baking dish coated with cooking spray, place the apple slices. Drop the preserves by teaspoonfuls on top and sprinkle evenly with the flour mixture. Bake for 35 minutes, or until bubbly and golden.

# Perfect Pudding Cake · Serves 9 · (yellow)

1 cup flour

2 teaspoons baking powder

¼ teaspoon salt

1 cup Sucanat

¼ cup plus 2 tablespoons unsweetened
  cocoa powder

1½ tablespoons instant coffee substitute
  (such as Roma)

1 cup boiling water

½ cup rice milk or soy milk

3 tablespoons canola oil

1 teaspoon vanilla extract

2¼ cups vanilla soy ice cream

Preheat the oven to 350°F.

Spay an 8-inch square pan with cooking spray.

In a large bowl, combine the flour, baking powder, salt, ⅔ cup of the Sucanat, ¼ cup of the cocoa, and the coffee substitute. In a small bowl, combine the soy milk, oil, and vanilla. Add the soy milk mixture to the flour mixture, stirring well until a smooth batter forms, about 2 minutes. Spoon the batter into the prepared pan.

In a small bowl, combine the remaining ⅓ cup Sucanat and 2 tablespoons cocoa. Sprinkle the Sucanat/cocoa mixture over the batter. Pour the boiling water over the batter. Do not stir. Bake for 30 minutes, or until the cake springs back when touched lightly in center. Serve warm, topped with the soy ice cream.

## Mother's Day

$212 million—value of shipments of Mother's Day cards in 1997, up from $148 million in 1992. For the sake of comparison, shipments of Mother's Day cards exceeded those of Easter cards ($116 million) but lagged somewhat behind Valentine's Day cards ($277 million) and considerably behind Christmas cards ($571 million).—U.S. Census Bureau

## Father's Day

There are more collect calls on Father's Day than any other day of the year.

## Toasted-Hazelnut Cake with Chocolate Glaze Serves 8 (yellow)

*MARYANN HENNINGS*

### CAKE:

1²/₃ cups hazelnuts

¼ cup matzo cake meal

1 cup Sucanat

4 large organic eggs, separated, at room temperature

¼ teaspoon salt

### GLAZE:

1 cup grain-sweetened chocolate chips

3 tablespoons soy margarine

3 tablespoons Sucanat

Preheat the oven to 350°F, and grease a 9-inch springform pan.

Lay the hazelnuts on a baking sheet and toast them until golden brown, about 5 minutes. Rub the hot toasted nuts in a kitchen towel to remove some of the skins, then cool them completely.

Pulse the nuts, cake meal, and ¼ cup of the Sucanat in a food processor until the nuts are very finely chopped; be careful not to process into a paste. In a large bowl with an electric mixer on high speed, beat the egg yolks and ½ cup of Sucanat until pale and very thick, about 3 to 5 minutes. In another bowl with cleaned beaters on high speed, beat the egg whites with the salt until soft peaks form. Gradually beat in the remaining ¼ cup of Sucanat until the whites just hold stiff, glossy peaks. In three batches, alternately fold the nut mixture and the whites into the yolk mixture.

Spoon the batter into the prepared springform pan and smooth the top. Bake in the middle of the oven until golden and a tester comes out clean, about 35 minutes. Cool in the pan on a rack 3 minutes, then loosen the edge with a knife and remove the side of the pan. Cooled completely, the cake will sink slightly in center. Invert the cake onto a rack set over a shallow baking pan. Carefully loosen the bottom of the pan and remove.

To make the glaze, in a small, heavy saucepan over low heat, combine the chocolate chips, 3 tablespoons water, the margarine, and Sucanat, whisking until smooth, about 5 minutes. Pour the warm glaze over the cake, allowing it to coat evenly and drip down the sides. Chill until the glaze is set, about 5 minutes.

### PARTY IDEAS

- Serve breakfast in bed.
- Have the kids cook dinner for Mom or Dad.
- Throw a work party—Mom or Dad decide what jobs need to be done around the house, and the kids do the jobs without complaining.

### INVITATIONS

- Send special invitations made from your children's craft projects. Include a memory written by each family member.
- Have your children (their grandchildren) write up a menu of what will be served at the dinner or brunch.

# Toasts

Mothers hold their children's hands for just a little while . . . and their hearts forever.

We have toasted our sweethearts,
Our friends and our wives,
We have toasted each other
Wishing all merry lives.
Don't frown when I tell you
This toast beats all others,
But drink one more toast, boys—

A toast to—*our mothers*.

To our fathers' sweethearts—our mothers.

Here's to mothers: the guideposts to heaven.

There are two lasting bequests we can give our children: One is roots. The other is wings.
— HODDING CARTER, JR.

Here's to every man here, may he be what he thinks himself to be.

## DECORATIONS

Decorate the house with some of your mother's or father's favorite things. Include their favorite flowers, balloons and candles in their favorite colors, and any memorabilia that would really appeal to them. If you can't decorate the whole house, decorate a special area that is theirs, such as their office or workspace.

## SCENTS

Any scent that reminds you of your mother or father. For me it will always be the smell of Oil of Olay for my mom and the smell of Vitalis for my dad.

Rose
Other floral
Homemade bread
Cookies

## ACTIVITIES AND GAMES

- Have everyone in the family write something about their mother or father. Edit the material into an essay and read it at dinner.
- Tape the members of your family and create a videotaped tribute to your parents. This is especially wonderful to do if you can't be with them on that day. These tapes usually become valuable items for the family archives.
- Organize your parents' photos or tapes. Categorize and label them, and if you're really clever, take them to an editing house and have them transferred onto video or CD and scored with your parents' favorite music from the era of your tape.
- Clean or paint the house, or take their car in for a wash.
- Rent or buy your mother's or father's favorite classic movie.
- Create a trivia game about famous moms or dads, or even better, make up a Jeopardy board based on what you know about your mom or dad and play with the rest of the family.

Mother's Day/Father's Day

- Tape-record your parents' stories so you will be able to hear them in their words for years to come. Interview them and ask them what life was like when they were little, or what it was like when they became parents.
- Enjoy a fun sport or physical activity together, even if it's just a walk around the block.

## PRIZES, GIFTS, AND PARTY FAVORS

- Homemade presents: handprints, picture frames with current photos
- Treat your mom or dad to a luxury spa day. Make them feel special by giving them a gift certificate for a massage, facial, Reflexology, herbal wrap, or all the above. Keep them company and get a treatment for yourself, too.
- For daughters, get mother-daughter makeovers together. Make dual appointments for a haircut/style and manicure, and celebrate together the joy of looking your best. On the way home you'll probably be asked to be in a Pond's commercial. You know—the kind in which you can't tell who is the mother and who is the daughter.
- Put together a health basket. Turn your mom and dad on to the latest in alternative healing, organic fruits and vegetables, herbs, and recipes. Give them the wealth of health.
- Give your parents a health club membership. These can be pricey, so pitch in with siblings if you have to. If they use it, this can be one of the greatest gifts for improving their health. Also consider getting them a treadmill if a health club is not their style.
- Buy ballroom dance lessons for Mom and/or Dad. Even if they are divorced or widowed, this is a great chance for them to brush up, go steppin' out, get exercise, make new friends, or spark a new romance.

## MUSIC

Music inspires some very powerful memories, and for Mother's Day or Father's Day the musical possibilities are endless. You can find your parents' favorite music or music from the day they became parents or even the most popular love songs nine months before they became parents. My parents have been gone for many years now, but their favorite songs, "And I Love Her" and "Fly Me to the Moon," take me right back.

## For Mom

| | | |
|---|---|---|
| "And I Love Her" | Beatles | Song |
| Atom Heart Mother | Pink Floyd | Album |
| Mother Lode | Loggins & Messina | Album |
| Wildwood Pickin' | Mother Maybelle Carter | Album |
| Mother's Milk | Red Hot Chili Peppers | Album |
| Mama's Big Ones | Mama Cass | Album |
| I Got Those Ol' Kosmic Blues Again, Mama | Janis Joplin | Album |

| | | |
|---|---|---|
| *Throw Mama from the Train* | Various | Soundtrack |
| *Tell Mama* | Etta James | Album |
| *Mama Tried* | Merle Haggard and The Strangers | Album |

## For Dad

| | | |
|---|---|---|
| "Fly Me to the Moon" | Frank Sinatra | Song |
| *Dad Loves His Work* | James Taylor | Album |
| *Father of the Bride* | Various | Soundtrack |
| *Child Is Father to the Man* | Blood, Sweat & Tears | Album |
| *My Father's Eyes* | Amy Grant | Album |
| *Tribute to My Father* | Hank Williams, Jr. | Album |
| *Big Bad Voodoo Daddy* | Big Bad Voodoo Daddy | Album |
| *Daddy-O! Daddy* | Woody Guthrie | Album |
| *Songs Our Daddy Taught Us* | Everly Brothers | Album |
| *Big Daddy* | John Cougar-Mellencamp | Album |

# MOVIES

## Mother's Day

| | |
|---|---|
| *I Remember Mama* | (1948—NR) |
| *The Stepmother* | (1971—R) |
| *Mother* | (1996—PG-13) |
| *Bye Bye Birdie* | (1963—NR) |
| *Two Women* | (1960—R) |
| *'Night Mother* | (1986—PG-13) |
| *Psycho* | (1960—NR) |
| *Terms of Endearment* | (1983—PG) |
| *The Joy Luck Club* | (1993—R) |
| *Mother Wore Tights* | (1947—NR) |
| *Big Mama* | (2001—PG-13) |

# Mother's Day/Father's Day

| | |
|---|---|
| *Throw Mama from the Train* | (1987–PG-13) |
| *Gypsy* | (1962–NR) |
| *Stella Dallas* | (1937–NR) |
| *Imitation of Life* | (1934–NR; 1959–NR) |
| *Mommy Dearest* | (1981–PG) |
| *Mildred Pierce* | (1945–NR) |
| *Now Voyager* | (1942–NR) |
| *I Could Go On Singing* | (1963–NR) |
| *Lolita* | (1962–NR; 1997–R) |
| *Tugboat Annie* | (1933–NR) |
| *Stepmom* | (1998–PG-13) |

## Father's Day

| | |
|---|---|
| *I Never Sang for My Father* | (1970–PG) |
| *Lies My Father Told Me* | (1975–PG) |
| *On Golden Pond* | (1981–PG) |
| *Father of the Bride* | (1950–NR; 1991–PG) |
| *The Champ* | (1931–NR; 1979–PG) |
| *Godfather I and II* | (1973, 1974–R) |
| *Kramer vs. Kramer* | (1979–PG) |
| *Papa's Delicate Condition* | (1963–NR) |
| *Life with Father* | (1947–NR) |
| *The Easy Way* | (1952–R) |
| *Father Goose* | (1964–R) |
| *Mrs. Doubtfire* | (1993–PG-13) |
| *Mr. Mom* | (1983–PG) |
| *Hole in the Head* | (1959–NR) |
| *Big Daddy* | (2000–PG-13) |
| *Cheaper by the Dozen* | (1950–NR) |

| | |
|---|---|
| *Indiana Jones and the Last Crusade* (with Sean Connery) | (1989—PG-13) |
| *Bachelor Father* | (1931—NR) |
| *Father's Day* | (1997—PG-13) |
| *Father's Little Dividend* | (1951—NR) |
| *Houseboat* | (1958—NR) |
| *Jazz Singer* | (1927—NR, 1953—NR, 1980—PG) |
| *Father Was a Fullback* | (1949—NR) |
| *Remarkable Mr. Pennypacker* | (1959—NR) |
| *Courtship of Eddie's Father* | (1963—NR) |
| *Oh Dad, Poor Dad, Mama's Hung You in the Closet and I'm Feeling So Sad* | (1967—NR) |
| *Field of Dreams* | (1989—PG) |
| *3 Men and a Baby* | (1987—PG) |
| *Nothing in Common* | (1986—PG) |
| *I Am Sam* | (2001—PG13) |
| *Table for Five* | (1983—PG) |
| *John Q* | (2002—PG-13) |

## EXERCISE AND CALORIE CHART

Do an activity with Mom or Dad—take a walk, play tag, dance around the house to Mom's favorite music, from Mozart to Madonna, from Mantovani to Metallica.

| Activity | Calories Burned/Hour |
|---|---|
| Walking | 176 |
| Playing tag | 363 |
| Dancing around the house | 320 |
| Bowling | 186 |
| Running bases | 289 |

# Mother's Day/Father's Day

## CELEBRITY HOLIDAY STORIES

It was Father's Day 1963, and I had to break the news to my dad. He had encouraged me all my growing up to get an education, go to college, and make something of myself. Accordingly, I managed through three schools to get a degree in history and psychology, took the law boards, picked a law school, and was now about to break my father's heart.

"Dad," I said, "I don't want to be a lawyer anymore. I think I want to be an actor. . . . He, who had been an elephant trainer on the Ringling Circus in the years before World War II and who was proud to have worked the Center Ring with his 'Bulls,' didn't miss a beat. . . . "I think you can do that, Bob," he said.

He pulled for me for the next thirty-four years in the certainty that I would make it. Some Father's Days are better than others.

**ROBERT FORSTER**

## FOR THE KIDS

My favorite gifts from *my* children over the years have been:

- Handprints and foot outlines: from ages zero to five, I have traced my boys' hands and feet on their Mother's Day cards and saved every card. It's amazing to watch their little hands and feet grow over the years.
- Plaster of Paris hands and feet. You can buy a kit that takes a mold of your child's fist or foot and makes a plaster replica.
- A planter made out of one of their shoes.
- Various crafts painted and glazed at a pottery-making store.
- Frames with pictures or poems

And recently, they took a camera and snapped pictures throughout the day in order to document our day together.

## FOR COUPLES

Buy a romantic weekend getaway for your parents. Pick a place where they can exercise, eat well, and enjoy being together.

# Summer Holidays

I decided to combine the three big summer holidays—Memorial Day, Fourth of July, and Labor Day—because they are similar and connected in so many ways. Together they unofficially mark the beginning, middle, and end of summer. The food, activities, and weather are pretty similar, and they all have a patriotic American theme that tells us it's time to honor our heritage, gather the kids, family, and friends together, toss around a Frisbee, stay cool, and enjoy a great picnic and barbecue. Like most holidays, these three usually lead to too much eating and beer drinking. This is really unfortunate, because these are the easiest holidays to make healthy. The weather is ideal for lots of fun, fat-burning activities and exercise. And produce is at its freshest. Ripe, whole fruits and vegetables are bursting with flavor and nutrients. What could be better than a piece of ripe, juicy watermelon on a hot summer day?

You've got all the ingredients you need to plan a healthy holiday strategy. To start, try limiting your consumption of heavy barbecued meats, and skip the red meat steaks completely. Consider barbecued salmon or halibut, and if you're having chicken, make that your one and only concentrated food.

And most important, enjoy lots of fun games and exercise. Just remember to drink plenty of fresh water and pace yourself. This is one day when you have no excuse not to exercise. You'll be surrounded by friends and family and kids who can't sit still, and you probably won't want to drink much alcohol or eat too much because the sports and games will be too much fun to interrupt. Pretend you're planning the Olympics, and make a big deal about the competition by awarding cute prizes, but make sure you always keep it friendly. If you're not the competitive type, you can always ride bikes, fly a kite, take a walk in the park, or do swing or square dancing.

So pump up the volleyball, fill the water cooler, and peel the papaya. You're going to have the coolest, healthiest summer holidays ever!

## HISTORY, FACTS, AND FOLKLORE
### Memorial Day

While almost all other holidays were started by an event or a single person's need to commemorate some specific figure, the need for survivors and descendants to honor veterans has been almost too prevalent to pinpoint in terms of who started it or how it began. Memorial Day is the call of many to honor the vast numbers of people who died; a collective effort for an endless event, the loss of men and women in service.

Memorial Day was officially proclaimed on May 5, 1868, and observed on May 30, 1868, when Arlington National Cemetery decorated the graves of both Union and Confederate soldiers. The symbolism of wearing a red poppy on this day comes from the poem "In Flanders Field," which likens the splash of red color to the blood shed by soldiers on so many fields.

### Fourth of July

This is the day our nation was born in 1776. "Happy birthday, United States of America! You look marvelous, considering you're more than two hundred and twenty-seven years old."

July 4, 1776, marks the signing of the Declaration of Independence by the Continental Congress in Philadelphia, Pennsylvania. The first signature was by the Congress president, John Hancock, who declared, "I wrote it large enough for King George to read it without his spectacles!"

At the time, the Revolutionary War was in full swing, and the members of the Continental Congress representing the thirteen colonies decided it was time to break the ties with England. They had many grievances, but the main one was "taxation without representation." By June 1776, efforts to end the conflict were hopeless, and the Congress decided to draft an official Declaration of Independence. A committee was formed that included John Adams, Benjamin Franklin, and Thomas Jefferson. John Adams was most passionate about the cause but took a back seat due to his unpopularity in Congress. Thomas Jefferson was chosen to write the first draft. Even John Adams considered him to be the best man for the job. Adams once said, "Jefferson writes ten times better than anyone in Congress." By coincidence, both Jefferson and Adams died exactly fifty years after the signing, on July 4, 1826.

## Labor Day

Labor Day began as a pro-worker parade in New York in 1882 and quickly became a very popular event. By 1884, it had become a state holiday in Colorado, New York, New Jersey, and Massachusetts. In 1886 the U.S. Congress declared the first Monday of each September a national holiday in honor of the working class. Canada celebrates Labor Day on the same day.

## HENNER HOLIDAY TRADITIONS AND STORIES

When I was a kid, summer holidays meant one thing: the potluck-barbecue-luau-and-treasure-hunt at the Howard Johnson's Motor Lodge swim club. Back then, my family would often take impromptu twenty-four-hour summer vacations. Our parents would pile the eight of us into our 1961 pea-green Chevy station wagon with wood-look side paneling and check us into a fun motel somewhere in Chicago for the night. One day we stumbled onto the Howard Johnson's Motor Lodge near O'Hare, and it was love at first sight! By morning, we were annual members of the swim club and remained members for the following ten years. During that decade, we spent nearly every rainless summer day swimming, making friends, and sampling the twenty-eight flavors of Howard Johnson's ice cream. The best three days of the year were the blowout potluck picnics every Memorial Day, Fourth of July, and Labor Day. Every guest would contribute at least one dish. My mother's dishes were German potato salad and Greek pilaf made with Mrs. Grass's Noodle Soup. I always thought it looked like rice and rubber bands. One woman always brought a gigantic hollowed-out watermelon filled with melon balls and lime sherbet. That was always the centerpiece of the buffet table. For all three holidays, the theme was usually a luau. Anything Hawaiian was popular then, especially in Chicago. There were always a swim meet and treasure hunt for the kids. The lifeguards would scatter coins throughout the pool, and we would fight it out for the quarters and silver dollars. My brother Tommy always cleaned up, because he was the only kid who could reach the bottom of the deep end—twelve feet—and it really went to his head. He thought he was Lloyd Bridges.

Those Howard Johnson's pool party picnics defined the summer holidays of my childhood. The potluck theme is great for diffusing responsibility for an overwhelmed host. Consider doing that at your next summer holiday party. Request that everyone prepare a holiday dish that's THM safe. Your holiday will be healthier and more balanced, and you'll be doing your part to spread the wealth of health to your family and friends.

For a patriotic bonus, you can always get one of your kids to sing my specialty number from the picnic talent show—the Betsy Ross song my uncle Dan wrote to the tune of "Ballin' the Jack":

First you take some stripes and you sew 'em up tight,
Seven of 'em red and the other six white,
Then take thirteen stars and here's what you do,
Sew 'em in a circle on a background of blue.

The stripes will remind us of the colonies
Every time we see Old Glory wavin' in the breeze.
The stars will represent the thirteen Union States
When it comes to makin' flags, I'm one of the greats.

While talkin' on the hotline, here's what Washington said,
"For tolerance and valor, we will use the red,
For innocence and purity, we'll use the white,
For vigilance and justice, the blue seems right."

Now sewin' Stars and Stripes may not be your bag,
But like Georgie said to me, and I don't brag,
"I tell ya, Betsy baby, it ain't no drag,
That's sure what I call designin' a flag!"

## RECIPES
# Avocado Dressing Serves 4 to 6 (blue)

1 ripe avocado, peeled, pitted, and mashed

1 teaspoon honey

½ teaspoon Bragg's Liquid Aminos

1 tablespoon Nayonnaise

¼ cucumber, seeded and finely diced

1 tomato, finely diced

2½ tablespoons finely chopped
   yellow onion

¼ teaspoon onion powder

8 cups mixed greens, washed and dried

In a medium bowl, mash the avocado with the honey, Bragg's, and Nayonnaise. If needed, add a little water to thin the avocado mixture. Stir in the diced cucumber, tomato, onion, and onion powder. Serve over the mixed greens.

# Sugar Snap Pea and Cucumber Salad

Serves 8    (blue)

1 pound organic sugar snap peas, trimmed

2 tablespoons chopped toasted walnuts

1 tablespoon vegetable broth

1 tablespoon walnut oil

1½ teaspoons white wine vinegar

1 tablespoon chopped fresh organic
    dill weed

Salt and pepper

1 English cucumber, halved lengthwise and
    cut crosswise into ¼-inch-thick slices

In a large saucepan over medium-high heat, cook the peas in salted water until tender and bright green, about 2 to 3 minutes. Drain and transfer to a bowl of ice water. When cold, drain well and pat dry. Mash the walnuts to a paste with a mortar and pestle. In a small bowl, whisk together the walnut paste, broth, oil, vinegar, and dill until blended. Season to taste with salt and pepper. In a large bowl, toss the walnut mixture with the peas and cucumber until the vegetables are coated and serve.

# Southwest Corn Salad Serves 8    (blue)

*JO TAYLOR*

2 1-pound bags super sweet frozen cut corn
    (no sugar added)

1 small red onion, finely diced

1 roasted red pepper, finely diced

¼ cup chopped cilantro

¼ cup apple cider vinegar

¼ cup extra-virgin olive oil

Salt and freshly ground black pepper

Blanch the corn for 1 minute in a large pot of boiling water. Place in a bowl of ice water for another minute to cool. Drain and set aside. In a large bowl, mix the corn, onion, pepper, and cilantro. In a small jar with a lid, put the vinegar and oil and shake until well combined. Pour the dressing into the corn mixture and toss. Season to taste with salt and pepper.

## Fresh Corn Salad Serves 10 (blue)

5 tablespoons extra-virgin olive oil

8 cups fresh organic corn kernels
   (10 to 12 ears)

1½ teaspoons salt

½ teaspoon freshly ground black pepper

1 small red onion, thinly sliced

3 organic scallions, white and green parts,
   thinly sliced

2 tablespoons cider vinegar

1 teaspoon balsamic vinegar

1 cup julienned organic sweet basil

Heat 3 tablespoons of the oil in a large skillet over medium heat. Add the corn, salt, and pepper, and cook for 5 minutes, or until just cooked and no longer starchy. Remove from the heat. Stir in the red onion, scallions, cider and balsamic vinegars, and the remaining olive oil. Allow the salad to cool; stir in the basil before serving. Serve cold or at room temperature.

## Ginger-Jalapeño Slaw Serves 6 (purple)

*SUZANNE PALUMBO*

¼ cup seasoned rice vinegar

2 tablespoons extra-virgin olive oil

2 teaspoons peeled grated fresh ginger

½ teaspoon sea salt

2 jalapeño peppers, seeded and minced

1 pound cabbage, thinly sliced (about 6 cups)

½ pound red cabbage, thinly sliced
   (about 3 cups)

3 medium carrots, finely shredded (about
   1½ cups)

2 green onions, thinly sliced

1 cup thinly sliced kale

In a large bowl, mix the vinegar, oil, ginger, salt, and jalapeño peppers until well blended. Add the remaining ingredients and toss well. Refrigerate, covered, for 1 hour before serving.

# Four-Bean Salad   S e r v e s   6   t o   8     ( b l u e / g r e e n )

*S U Z A N N E   P A L U M B O*

1 pound green beans, trimmed and cut into
  1½-inch lengths

½ 16-ounce box or bag frozen shelled
  soybeans (known as edamame or sold as
  sweet beans by Sno Pack)

3 tablespoons extra-virgin olive oil

¼ cup balsamic vinegar

¼ cup red wine vinegar

1 tablespoon Sucanat

1½ teaspoons sea salt

¼ teaspoon black pepper

1 15-ounce can black soybeans, rinsed and
  drained

1 15-ounce can kidney beans, rinsed and
  drained

1 small red onion, finely diced

In a 12-inch skillet, heat ½ inch of water to boiling over high heat. Add the green beans and cook 5 minutes, or until crisp-tender. Place the frozen soybeans in a colander and drain the green beans over the soybeans. Rinse with cold water until cool; drain well.

In a large bowl, whisk together the oil, vinegars, Sucanat, sea salt, and pepper. Add the green beans, both soybeans, kidney beans, and onion and toss to combine. Let stand 1 hour to allow the flavors to blend or refrigerate until ready to use.

## Uncle Charlie's Bean Salad

Makes 2 quarts    (green)

*SUSAN ROMITO*

2 15-ounce cans cut string beans, drained

2 15-ounce cans cut wax beans, drained

1 15-ounce can red kidney beans, drained
   and rinsed

1 onion, finely chopped

1 green pepper, finely chopped

3 celery stalks, finely chopped

1 teaspoon sea salt

$\frac{1}{2}$ cup Sucanat, or to taste

$\frac{1}{3}$ to $\frac{2}{3}$ cup vegetable oil

$1\frac{1}{2}$ cups apple cider vinegar

In a large bowl, combine all the beans, the onion, green pepper, and celery. In a small bowl, mix together the salt, Sucanat, oil, and vinegar. Toss the dressing with the salad and serve.

## Uncle Charlie's Potato Salad

Makes 5 pounds    (blue/green)

*SUSAN ROMITO*

5 pounds small potatoes

$\frac{1}{2}$ cup cider vinegar

1 tablespoon salt

3 tablespoons Sucanat

2 tablespoons oil

1 medium onion, grated

Dash of white pepper

Nayonnaise or Vegenaise (optional)

In a medium saucepan over medium heat, boil the potatoes until done, about 40 minutes. To test for doneness, pierce a potato with a matchstick. If the potato falls off when the matchstick is lifted, it is done. Drain.

In a small saucepan, bring $\frac{1}{2}$ cup water and the vinegar to a boil. In a large bowl, combine all the other ingredients except the Nayonnaise. Add the water and vinegar mixture and mix well. Cool. Add the Nayonnaise, if using, to taste before serving.

# Marinated Potato Salad  Serves 4  (green)

*SUZANNE PALUMBO*

¾ pound tiny whole new potatoes

¾ cup vinaigrette or oil and vinegar
   dressing (I like Annie's Tuscany)

1 13-ounce can artichoke hearts, drained
   and halved

1 small red or yellow pepper, cut into strips

6 cherry tomatoes, halved

½ small red onion, thinly sliced

¼ cup halved pitted ripe or kalamata olives

¼ cup chopped fresh Italian parsley

Cook the potatoes in boiling water for 15 to 20 minutes, or until tender. Drain well; cut into quarters. Add the remaining ingredients and toss gently to mix. Cover and chill for 4 to 24 hours, stirring occasionally.

# Curried Tuna Salad  Serves 4  (blue w/o raisins/green with raisins)

½ cup plain soy yogurt

½ cup Vegenaise or Nayonnaise

1 tablespoon freshly squeezed organic
   lemon juice

1 to 2 tablespoons mild curry powder

2 7-ounce cans tuna packed in water,
   drained and flaked

¼ cup pickle relish

½ cup raisins (optional)

2 tablespoons minced green onion,
   including some green tops

¼ cup oven-toasted or raw cashew nuts

Minced fresh organic Italian parsley

In a small bowl, combine the soy yogurt, Vegenaise, lemon juice, and curry powder. Blend well and set aside.

In a larger bowl, combine the tuna, pickle relish, raisins (if using), onions, and toasted nuts. Stir in the soy yogurt dressing to taste. Transfer to a serving bowl or mound on a platter or individual plates and sprinkle with the parsley.

# Grilled Vegetable Sandwich

Serves 8     (green)

**SANDWICH:**

- 4 organic zucchini, sliced into ¼-inch-thick strips
- 4 organic yellow squash, sliced into rounds
- 4 red onions, sliced into ½-inch strips
- 1 or 2 small portobello mushrooms, sliced into ½-inch strips
- 6 tablespoons olive oil
- Salt and pepper
- 16 slices Italian or thick whole-grain bread

**PESTO MAYO:**

- ¾ cup Vegenaise or Nayonnaise
- 1 8-ounce package prepared dairy-free pesto
- 16 thin slices soy mozzarella cheese (optional)

Heat the grill. Brush the vegetables with the olive oil and season to taste with salt and pepper. Grill the vegetables until they are soft and have grill marks. Generously spray the bread slices with olive oil spray and grill until toasted. Combine the Vegenaise or Nayonnaise and pesto to create a pesto mayo. Assemble the sandwiches with the soy mozzarella (if using), vegetables, and pesto mayo.

# Grilled Polenta with Vegetables

Serves 6     (purple/blue)

*SUSAN ROMITO*

- 1 organic polenta roll, plain or with basil or garlic
- 2 teaspoons olive oil
- 1 yellow pepper, sliced
- 1 red pepper, sliced
- 1 orange pepper, sliced
- 1 large red onion, sliced
- 1 sweet potato, sliced
- 2 large zucchini, sliced

Heat the grill. Slice the polenta, brush with the olive oil, and grill 3 to 5 minutes on each side. Set aside and keep warm. Toss the vegetables lightly with olive oil in a large bowl. Grill 5 to 7 minutes, or until the desired crispness is achieved. Chop the vegetables and serve over the polenta.

# Barbecue Chicken with Homemade Sauce

Serves 4    (blue/green)

*BEV POWELL*

1 onion, minced

2 garlic cloves, minced

2 tablespoons olive oil or
   Earth Balance margarine

¼ teaspoon salt (optional)

1 tablespoon chili powder

2 tablespoons molasses

2 tablespoons Sucanat

2 to 4 tablespoons maple syrup (optional,
   if you want more sweetness)

4 tablespoons balsamic or other vinegar

4 tablespoons vegetarian Worcestershire
   sauce

1 cup fruit juice–sweetened catsup

1 teaspoon Tabasco or your favorite
   hot sauce

1 pound organic free-range chicken legs
   and breasts, washed and dried

In a medium saucepan over high heat, sauté the onion and garlic with the olive oil or margarine until soft. Add the remaining ingredients (except for the chicken) and 2 cups water. Mix well (or blend in a blender for a few seconds). Simmer the sauce over medium-low heat for 30 to 60 minutes, or until it reaches the desired thickness. Cool. In a large bowl, cover the chicken with the sauce on all sides and marinate for 1 hour, refrigerated and covered. Grill on medium-high heat, turning for 15 to 20 minutes on each side, until the chicken is cooked.

## Tuna Burgers  serves 4  (green)

MARYANN HENNINGS

3 tablespoons plus ¼ cup Vegenaise

1 tablespoon Dijon-style mustard

1 egg white

2 6-ounce cans albacore tuna packed
  in water, drained and flaked

½ cup bread crumbs

¼ cup finely chopped organic
  Spanish onion

4 whole grain hamburger buns,
  split

4 organic lettuce leaves

4 slices organic tomato

4 thin slices organic red onion

In a medium bowl, combine 3 tablespoons Vegenaise, mustard, and egg white and stir well. Add the tuna, ¼ cup of the bread crumbs, and the Spanish onion and stir well. Divide the mixture into 4 equal portions, shaping each into a 4-inch patty. Press the remaining ¼ cup bread crumbs evenly onto both sides of the patties. Coat a large nonstick skillet with cooking spray and place over medium-high heat until hot. Add the patties, cover, and cook 3 minutes. Carefully flip the patties and cook 3 or 4 minutes more, or until golden brown. Spread the remaining ¼ cup Vegenaise on the buns, add lettuce, tomato, and onion, and serve.

If you wish to grill, do not press the bread crumbs into the patties. Instead, brush with olive oil and grill on high heat 5 to 7 minutes on each side, or until the desired doneness is attained.

## Maple Corn Bread  serves 10  (yellow)

2⅓ cups yellow cornmeal

1 cup unbleached flour

4 teaspoons baking powder

1¼ teaspoons salt

½ cup (1 stick) chilled soy margarine, cut
  into ½-inch pieces

1⅓ cups soy cream or soy milk

4 large cage-free eggs

¾ cup pure maple syrup

Preheat the oven to 375°F. Butter a 9-inch square metal baking pan.

Combine the cornmeal, flour, baking powder, and salt in a food processor; blend 5 seconds, or until combined. Add the margarine and process until the mixture resembles coarse meal. In a large bowl, whisk together the soy cream or soy milk, eggs, and maple syrup. Add the cornmeal mixture and stir just until evenly moistened (do not overblend). Transfer to the prepared pan. Bake until the corn bread is golden and cracked on top and a tester inserted into the center comes out clean, about 45 minutes. Cool the bread in the pan on a rack.

# Balsamic Mixed Vegetable Roast

Serves 12 (blue)

2 medium organic eggplants, unpeeled, cut crosswise into ¼-inch-thick rounds

2 teaspoons salt

1 cup extra-virgin olive oil

⅓ cup balsamic vinegar

½ teaspoon freshly ground black pepper

1½ pounds zucchini, washed, dried, and cut on the bias into ¼-inch rounds

3 large red onions, sliced into ¼-inch rounds

2 medium red bell peppers, cored, seeded, and cut into ¾-inch squares

2 medium yellow bell peppers, cored, seeded, and cut into ¾-inch squares

6 large heads of endive, cored, halved, and quartered lengthwise

Place a layer of paper towels over a baking sheet. Arrange the eggplant on top in a single layer. Sprinkle with 1 teaspoon of the salt and let stand for 30 minutes. Pat dry.

Preheat the oven to 450°F.

In a small bowl, whisk together the olive oil, vinegar, remaining salt, and pepper. Set aside.

Divide the eggplant, zucchini, red onions, peppers, and endive between two large baking sheets with sides. Gently mix the vegetables with three quarters of the blended oil and vinegar. Place one baking sheet on the bottom oven rack and the second on the middle rack. Roast the vegetables 20 minutes, turning them once and rotating the pans between the shelves after 10 minutes. The vegetables should be crisp when they are done.

Arrange the vegetables in colorful bunches on a round or oval platter. Sprinkle the vegetables with salt and pepper and drizzle with the remaining dressing. Serve at room temperature.

# Fourth of July Smoothie Cake

Serves 10 to 12    (yellow)

*SUSAN ROMITO*

**FIRST LAYER:**

- 1 15-ounce can lite coconut milk
- 2 bananas
- 2 apples, peeled and cored
- 2 cups frozen or fresh pitted dark cherries

**SECOND LAYER:**

- 2 bananas
- 2 peaches
- 2 cups apple cider
- 2 cups frozen or fresh blueberries

Line a Bundt pan with plastic wrap. Blend the coconut milk, bananas, and apples together in a blender or food processor. If you have an ice cream maker and a lot of time, you can start to freeze the blended mixture in the ice cream maker to make it a little creamier. If not, it can be used as is; it will just be a little more icy when done. Pour the mixture into the pan, then sink the frozen dark cherries evenly around the pan into the "batter." Place it in the freezer for 2 to 3 hours, or until firm.

Blend the bananas, peaches, and cider, again using an ice cream maker if desired, and pour on top of the first layer. Sink the blueberries into this layer and freeze for 4 hours, or until frozen through.

To unmold, invert the pan on a serving plate, remove the pan, and peel off the plastic wrap.

For a fancier cake, you can place sliced fruit and/or slivered almonds or other nuts in a pattern in the pan before pouring the first layer.

# Blueberry Cobbler with a Cornmeal Crust

Serves 8 (yellow)

*MARYANN HENNINGS*

## CRUST:

1 cup unbleached flour

2½ cups cornmeal

¾ cup date sugar

½ cup maple sugar

6 teaspoons baking powder

½ teaspoon salt

1¼ cups soy cream

12 tablespoons (1½ sticks) soy margarine, melted and cooled

2 cage-free eggs, lightly beaten

## FILLING:

10 cups organic blueberries, washed and picked over

¾ cup Sucanat

Juice from ½ organic lemon

½ teaspoon grated nutmeg

½ teaspoon ground cinnamon

Preheat the oven to 425°F.

Place the flour, cornmeal, sugars, baking powder, and salt in a large bowl and whisk together. Make a well in the center of the mixture. In another bowl, mix together the soy cream, melted margarine, and beaten eggs. Pour the liquid mixture into the dry mixture and combine until the batter comes together.

To make the filling, in a bowl, toss the blueberries with the Sucanat, lemon juice, nutmeg, and cinnamon. Put the mixture into an 9 × 13-inch square baking dish. Dollop the crust batter by spoonfuls around the edges of the dish. Bake for 35 minutes, or until the dough is golden brown and the berries are bubbling. Serve warm with soy ice cream.

## Oatmeal Coconut Squares with Chocolate Chips
Makes 16 squares (yellow)

5 tablespoons soy margarine, melted and cooled, plus more for the pan

1 cup old-fashioned rolled oats

½ cup whole wheat flour

½ cup maple sugar

½ cup Sunspire grain-sweetened chocolate chips

½ cup sweetened flaked coconut

¼ teaspoon baking powder

¼ teaspoon salt

1 large organic egg

½ teaspoon vanilla extract

Preheat the oven to 350°F. Line a 9-inch square metal baking pan with a 12- to 14-inch-long sheet of foil, letting the excess hang over the sides, and margarine the foil inside the pan.

In a large bowl, toss together the oats, flour, maple sugar, chips, coconut, baking powder, and salt. In another bowl, beat the melted margarine, egg, and vanilla with a fork. Stir into the oat mixture until combined. Spoon the batter into the baking pan, patting evenly. Bake in the middle of the oven until set, about 25 minutes. Remove from the pan by lifting the ends of the foil. Cool on a rack, then cut into 16 squares.

## Watermelon Roll
Serves 8 to 10 (yellow)

MARY BETH BORKOWSKI

*I have had neighborhood kids knock on my door in the summer to see if I have any of this in the freezer.*

1 quart plus 1 pint vanilla flavor Soy Delicious or Soy Dream, softened

Green food coloring

½ cup Tropical Source dairy-free grain-sweetened chocolate chips

3 pints raspberry Soy Dream frozen dessert, softened

In a large mixing bowl, blend 1 quart of vanilla frozen dessert with several drops of green food coloring. Using a spatula or large spoon, spread the "ice cream" up the sides of a rounded 3-quart bowl. Freeze approximately 1 hour, or until firm.

With a clean spoon, spread the softened pint of vanilla Soy Delicious over the top of the green layer. Freeze another hour.

Mix the chocolate chips into the softened raspberry "ice cream." Fill the center of the bowl with the raspberry mixture and freeze until just ready to serve. Before serving, turn over onto a large round serving plate. A towel moistened with warm water can be rubbed on the outside of the bowl to loosen the dessert, if necessary.

Dip a pastry brush into a small bowl of food coloring mixed with water and "paint" the watermelon stripes on the outside of the dessert. Cut into slices and serve.

# Apple Pie  Serves 10    (yellow)

Pastry Crust (recipe follows)

²⁄₃ cup Sucanat

2 tablespoons unbleached flour

½ teaspoon ground cinnamon

⅛ teaspoon salt

3 pounds cooking apples (9 medium),
    peeled, cored, and thinly sliced

1 tablespoon fresh lemon juice

1 tablespoon soy margarine, cut up

Prepare the dough as directed through chilling. Preheat the oven to 425°F.

In a large bowl, combine the Sucanat, flour, cinnamon, and salt. Add the apples and lemon juice; toss to combine.

Roll out the bottom crust as directed and place it in the pie plate. Spoon the filling into the piecrust plate and dot with the soy margarine. Roll out the top crust as directed, place it on top of the filling, and make a decorative edge.

Bake 20 minutes, then turn the oven down to 375°F. Bake 1 hour more, or until the filling is bubbly in the center. If necessary, cover the pie loosely with foil during the last 20 minutes of baking to prevent overbrowning. Cool the pie on a wire rack 1 hour to serve warm or cool completely to serve later.

## PASTRY CRUST FOR APPLE PIE
Makes crust for 1 pie

2¼ cups unbleached flour

½ teaspoon salt

¾ cup (1½ sticks) cold soy margarine,
    cut up

4 to 6 tablespoons ice water

In large bowl, mix together the flour and salt. With a pastry blender or two knives used scissor fashion, cut in the margarine until the mixture resembles coarse crumbs. Sprinkle in the ice water, 1 tablespoon at a time, mixing lightly with a fork after each addition, until the dough is just moist enough to hold together.

Shape the dough into 2 disks, one slightly larger than the other. Wrap each in plastic wrap and refrigerate 30 minutes or overnight. If chilled overnight, let stand at room temperature 30 minutes before rolling.

On a lightly floured surface, with a floured rolling pin, roll the larger disk into a 12-inch round. Roll the dough round gently onto a rolling pin and ease into the pie plate. Trim the edge, leaving a 1-inch overhang. Reserve the trimming for decorating the pie, if you like. Fill the piecrust.

Roll the remaining disk into a 12-inch round. Cut a ¾-inch circle out of the center and cut 1-inch slits to allow the steam to escape during baking; center over the filling or make a desired pie top. Fold the overhang under and make the desired decorative edge.

Bake the pie as directed in the recipe.

# Quick and Easy Ice Cream Sandwiches

Serves 6     (yellow)

12 large sugar- and dairy-free soft oatmeal
   cookies

1 pint whole soy vanilla ice cream

1 cup grain-sweetened semisweet chocolate
   chips

Place the oatmeal cookies upside down on a parchment-lined cookie sheet. Place the soy ice cream in the bowl of a stand mixer and, using the paddle attachment, gently stir until the ice cream is spreadable. Using an offset spatula, cover the bottom of 6 of the oatmeal cookies with ¼ cup each of the ice cream. Place an oatmeal cookie on top and gently press down. Place the ice cream sandwiches in the freezer for 30 minutes, or until the ice cream is firm. Gently roll the outside edge of each sandwich in the chocolate chips. Return the sandwiches to the freezer to harden for 30 minutes, or until ready to serve. Before serving, let the sandwiches stand at room temperature for no more than 5 minutes to soften.

## BEVERAGES

- Summer smoothies—Blend your favorite fruit with Soy Delicious ice cream or Rice Dream ice cream. Add a fresh fruit garnish and little parasols to make it summery and fun.
- Fresh-squeezed orange juice and grapefruit juice—or make fresh-squeezed lemonade with stevia or agave nectar instead of sugar.
- Sizzle buster spritzers—Mix freshly squeezed juices with sparkling mineral water for natural spritzers bursting with flavor. Crush ice and add fresh fruit for a slushy thirst-quenching summer taste.
- Floating dreams—Make your own natural floats using sarsaparilla or fruit juice–sweetened root beer with Soy Delicious or Rice Dream vanilla ice cream
- Apple cider crush—Mix apple juice, apple cider, and crushed ice to make a mock spicy non-alcoholic rum-free beverage of colonial days. Add some grated nutmeg and a fresh cinnamon stick for flavor.
- Knudsen natural sodas—Garnish with real fruit.
- Spring water, natural or carbonated—Garnish with fresh fruits, especially raspberries, strawberries, or blueberries, for a patriotic flair.
- Patriotic soy shake—Mix raspberries, blueberries, and soy ice cream in a blender with crushed ice and whip it up. Add a small flag and real fruit garnish for a yummy American treat!

For grown-up tastes, here are THM versions (no sugar, no chemicals) of famous cocktails. The alcohol, of course, is optional.

## THM STRAWBERRY MARGARITA

4 ounces organic fruit juice–sweetened
  lemonade (I recommend R.W. Knudsen's or
  Santa Cruz lemonade)
1½ ounces tequila (optional)
1 tablespoon fresh, natural, unsweetened
  lime juice
2 tablespoons fresh strawberry purée
Lime wedge for garnish

Over ice, combine the lemonade, tequila (if using), lime juice, and strawberry purée. Shake, blend, or stir, then pour into a rocks glass (salted rim optional). Garnish with a wedge of lime and serve.

## MOONLIGHT SONATA

2½ ounces organic fruit juice–sweetened
  lemonade (I recommend R.W. Knudsen's
  or Santa Cruz lemonade)
1½ ounces vodka (optional)
1 tablespoon unsweetened natural
  cranberry juice
1 tablespoon grape juice

Combine the lemonade, vodka (if using), and cranberry and grape juice. Shake with ice, then strain into a martini glass and serve.

## SUMMER SANGRIA

1 bottle Pino Grigio or
  nonalcoholic white wine
8 ounces orange juice
3 ounces organic fruit juice–sweetened
  lemonade (I recommend R. W. Knudsen's
  or Santa Cruz lemonade)
1 orange, sliced
8 ounces sparkling mineral water, such as
  Pellegrino or Perrier
Lemon twists and fresh cherries

In a large pitcher or punch bowl, combine the wine, orange juice, lemonade, and orange over ice. Just before serving, stir in the mineral water. Garnish with the lemon twists and fresh cherries (not maraschino).

## Piña Colada

6 ounces all-natural Lakewood piña colada juice (could also use 3 ounces natural pineapple juice and 3 ounces coconut juice instead of piña colada juice—I recommend R. W. Knudsen's)

2 ounces White Wave Silk Soymilk Creamer

2 ounces rum (optional)

Over ice, combine the piña colada juice, soy milk creamer, and rum, if using. Shake or blend, then pour into a tall Collins or pint-size glass and serve.

## Banana Daiquiri

4 ounces natural unsweetened lemonade

1 banana or 4 ounces natural banana nectar

Fresh cherry for garnish

2 ounces rum (optional)

In a blender, combine the lemonade and banana over ice. Blend and serve in a Collins or rocks glass (it can also be shaken if you have a muddler). Garnish with the cherry (not maraschino).

## Sex on the Beach

4 ounces orange juice

4 ounces natural peach juice or 2 ounces natural peach nectar (I recommend Ceres brand)

1½ ounces vodka (optional)

1 tablespoon natural unsweetened cranberry juice

Over ice, combine the orange and peach juices, vodka (if using), and cranberry juice. Shake or blend and serve in a Collins or highball glass.

## THM Tequila Sunset

6 ounces grapefruit juice

1½ ounces tequila (optional)

1 tablespoon natural grape juice

Orange slice and fresh cherry for garnish

Over ice in a highball glass, pour the grapefruit juice, tequila (if using), and grape juice. Don't stir, just serve with the orange slice and fresh cherry (not maraschino).

## THM Kamikaze

3 ounces organic fruit juice–sweetened lemonade (I recommend R. W. Knudsen's or Santa Cruz lemonade)

1½ ounces vodka (optional)

1 tablespoon fresh, natural, unsweetened lime juice

¼ orange or 1 ounce orange juice

Over ice, combine the lemonade, vodka (if using), and lime juice. Squeeze in the orange juice. Shake or stir, then pour into a rocks glass and serve.

Interestingly enough, the most common drinks from 1776 were beer, wine, and cocktails made with dark and light rums mixed with fruit juice. Our forefathers probably drank more than we do. Washington, Franklin, and Jefferson were supposedly all boozers, but Adams was not. Please don't follow their example. They really had no choice. Beer was considered a healthy substitute for water because of the poor sanitary standards of the time. Only the most destitute drank water. We, however, have the luxury of clean water, decaffeinated iced teas, and fresh juices. There is no excuse for drinking sugary soft drinks and diet sodas full of chemicals when we have such an assortment of healthy beverages available.

## INVITATIONS

### General

- Small flag-shaped cards with party information written on the white stripes
- Beach party invitation with information written on the bottom of a kid-size flip-flop
- Red, white, and blue Frisbee with party information written on it

### Memorial Day

- Mini wreath card
- Heart-shaped flags with details

### Fourth of July

- Glittery fireworks card made on black construction paper with glitter and glue
- Get a calligraphy pen and a copy of the Declaration of Independence off the Internet or

from a history book and write out the invitations so they look similar to the original document. Make as many photocopies as you need. This requires some artistic skill, but it doesn't have to be perfect. If you can't do it, just use a John Hancock–like font on the computer. It's available in Microsoft Word and most other word processing programs. You can start the invitation by saying something like, "When in the course of human events it becomes necessary for friends and family to put their work aside . . . and party—"

## Labor Day

- "Eatin' and Neatin' Up Day" invitations with a barbecue and broom on the front of the card. BYO broom or rake or dust cloth.

## DECORATIONS

### General

Anything that symbolizes the United States: flags, Uncle Sam, bald eagle, Statue of Liberty, White House, and so on. Go to a party supply store and buy an assortment of red, white, and blue balloons, crepe paper, ribbon, construction paper, and anything else that will work. You can't go wrong here. Tie the ribbon or balloons on chairs or table centerpieces. Drape the crepe paper from tree to tree or even around the basketball hoop. It doesn't matter. Use your own artistic eye here and have a blast doing it.

### Memorial Day

Red poppies, fatigue wear, and camouflage patterns on the walls or on the tables.

### Fourth of July

Parchment paper and feather pens on each table, assorted colored strings hanging from the ceiling, or beach umbrellas, to resemble fireworks.

### Labor Day

Dust cloth napkins, union signs.

## SCENTS

The following scents are inspirational for all three summer holidays:

Fresh-cut grass
Thunderstorm
Rain
Summer flowers
Any floral fragrance:
    Hydrangea
    Rose
    Freesia
    Honeysuckle

# Toasts

## Memorial Day

To those gone but not forgotten. And to those forgotten but not gone.
—SHOE COMIC

A man's feet should be planted in his country, but his eyes should survey the world.
—GEORGE SANTAYANA

## Fourth of July

Here's to the health of Columbia, the pride of the earth,
The Stars and Stripes—drink the land of our birth!
Toast the army and navy, who fought for our cause,
Who conquered and won us our freedom and laws.

## Labor Day

Well done is better than well said.
—BENJAMIN FRANKLIN

Plumeria
Lavender
Sweet pea
Magnolia
Wisteria
Cucumber
Peach
Citrus—tangerine, grapefruit, orange, lemon, lime
Berries—raspberry, strawberry, blueberry
Honeydew melon
Watermelon

## ACTIVITIES AND GAMES

### Memorial Day

- Talk to a veteran for a real war story. Find out what it was like to be involved in the armed forces, what their job entailed, and what they did to help protect our nation.
- With your kids, create a miniature memorial to a soldier who served in battle, a friend, relative, ancestor, or even an Unknown Soldier representing all soldiers. Use little flags, construction paper, beads, Styrofoam, glue, pipe cleaners, and garbage bag ties to make little floral arrangements.
- Go to the bookstore or library and find a book containing the diary of a soldier who fought in combat for our country. You'll find these in the young readers' section, and they are usually fascinating. Read passages aloud with your family.

# Summer Holidays

## Fourth of July

- Make your own child-safe fireworks "show" using glitter, glue, and a sketchbook. Flip the pages to make them "explode."
- Hold a decathlon or pentathlon with events like lawn darts, water balloon toss, Frisbee toss, golf chipping, bocce ball, dodgeball, handball, croquet, soccer, badminton, table tennis, running bases, beanbag toss, horseshoes, shuffleboard, relay races, swimming races, treasure hunt, and tether ball. It doesn't matter which events you choose. Kids especially love to participate in competitive events that have an Olympic-like feel to them, and adults with a youthful spirit do too. The key is to keep score and award prizes so it feels like an important event. Be careful, though, not to hurt feelings here. You always have to be aware of how competitions like this are affecting the kids who are not winning.

## Labor Day

- Write down all the chores to be done for the day, red cards for more grown-up chores, blue cards for kids, and white cards for either kids or adults. Everyone takes turns picking a card for a specific chore to be performed. The one who completes his tasks first wins a prize. After all the labors are finished, playtime can begin. But don't forget the after-playtime cleanup chores!
- Labor for the people who can't labor. Do a chore for an elderly person or someone else who needs help in your neighborhood. Volunteer to clean his or her house, cut the grass, grocery shop, and so on. Do this with your children, and help them discover what is important in life.

## PRIZES, GIFTS, AND PARTY FAVORS

### Memorial Day

Dog tags, a donation to a veterans' group, poppy plants.

### Fourth of July

Red, white, and blue anything: bead making, bracelets, pencils, stickers; U.S. map puzzle, fireworks stickers, historical cutout books, American flags, history books, biographies of Adams, Jefferson, or Franklin.

### Labor Day

Cleaning supplies—brooms, mops, dust rags, garden gloves; organizational supplies—boxes, hangers, mini tool kits.

## MUSIC

There is so much patriotic music, from John Philip Sousa to Aaron Copland to the Andrews Sisters, that the only problem is choosing what to listen to. The following selections are for the specific holidays.

## Memorial Day

| | | |
|---|---|---|
| *Remembrance;*<br> *A Memorial Benefit* | George Winston | Album |
| *Memorial* | Glenn Miller | Album |
| *Memorial* | Ledbelly | Album |
| *War* | U2 | Album |

## Fourth of July

| | | |
|---|---|---|
| *Songs of Freedom* | Bob Marley | Album |
| *Chimes of Freedom* | Bruce Springsteen | Album |
| *Freedom* | Neil Young | Album |
| "Fourth of July" | Jackson Browne | Song |
| *Made in America* | Blues Brothers | Album |
| *America* | Johnny Cash | Album |
| *America Rocks: Kids* | Schoolhouse Rock | Album |
| *Breakfast in America* | Supertramp | Album |
| *America* | Boys Choir of Harlem | Album |
| *Greatest Hits* | America | Album |
| *Captain America* | Jimmy Buffett | Album |
| *Freedom of Choice* | Devo | Album |
| *Freedom Highway* | Staple Singers | Album |
| *The Freedom Sessions* | Sara McLaughlan | Album |
| *At Liberty* | Elaine Stritch | Album |

## Labor Day

| | | |
|---|---|---|
| "She Works Hard for the Money" | Donna Summer | Song |
| "Take This Job and Shove It" | Waylon Jennings | Song |
| "Nine to Five" | Dolly Parton | Song |
| "Covergirl" | Ru Paul | Song |
| "We Can Work It Out" | The Beatles | Song |

## MOVIES

### Memorial Day

| | |
|---|---|
| *Best Years of Our Lives* | (1946–NR) |
| *Coming Home* | (1978–R) |
| *Hollywood Canteen* | (1944–NR) |
| *The Deer Hunter* | (1978–R) |
| *From Here to Eternity* | (1953–NR) |
| *Hope and Glory* | (1987–PG-13) |
| *Three Came Home* | (1950–NR) |
| *Pearl Harbor* | (2001–PG-13) |
| *Patton* | (1970–PG) |

### Fourth of July

| | |
|---|---|
| *Yankee Doodle Dandy* | (1952–NR) |
| *Born on the Fourth of July* | (1989–R) |
| *1776* | (1972–G) |
| *Independence Day* | (1996–PG-13) |
| *Miss Firecracker* | (1989–PG) |
| *Picnic* | (1955–NR) |
| *Cat on a Hot Tin Roof* | (1958–NR) |
| *Hope Floats* | (1998–PG-13) |

### Labor Day

| | |
|---|---|
| *Norma Rae* | (1979–PG) |
| *Pajama Game* | (1964–NR) |
| *Hoffa* | (1992–R) |
| *Tucker: A Man and His Dream* | (1988–PG) |
| *How to Succeed in Business Without Really Trying* | (1967–NR) |
| *On the Waterfront* | (1954–NR) |

| | |
|---|---|
| *Silkwood* | (1983–R) |
| *Nine to Five* | (1980–PG) |
| *Working Girl* | (1988–R) |
| *Secret of My Success* | (1965–NR; 1987–PG-13) |
| *Career Opportunities* | (1991–PG-13) |
| *Modern Times* | (1936–NR) |
| *Swing Shift* | (1984–PG) |
| *Desk Set* | (1957–NR) |

## EXERCISE AND CALORIE CHART

| Activity | Calories Burned/Hour |
|---|---|
| Marching | 246 |
| Playing tag | 363 |
| Swimming | 394 |
| Running bases | 289 |
| Throwing Frisbee | 211 |
| Skipping | 326 |
| Three-legged race | 354 |
| Water balloon fight | 261 |

## FOR THE KIDS

- Organize your own parade. Construct costumes of the colonial days and use your bikes, wagons, and scooters as floats. Make homemade drum sets with coffee cans and spoons, and use paper towel rolls as horns. Learn different songs to sing and play.
- Explain to the kids what the stars and stripes represent on the American flag, and tell them they are each the ruler of a new country. Have them design their own flags using crayons and construction paper.
- Pull the kids aside and tell them the story of how the Declaration of Independence was drafted and signed. Then let them go off on their own to construct a play to perform for the adults. This works really well if they watch a movie like *1776* first.
- Consider dressing up your youngest child as Uncle Sam, and have him or her greet your guests when they arrive.

## FOR COUPLES

### Memorial Day

Memorial Day lends itself to several scenarios. You can play:
- The Night Before Going Off to War
- The Soldier and the Nurse
- Coming Home
- Burt Lancaster and Deborah Kerr, Ben Affleck and Kate Beckinsale, or even Alan Alda and Jamie Farr

### Fourth of July

- Bring a sleeping bag instead of a blanket. Lie under the sky and watch the fireworks above as you have your own fireworks below.
- Dress up as Betsy Ross and George (the original Dubya). Imagine what she had to do to get that flag gig! And remember to tidy up before Martha gets home.

### Labor Day

- Modify the house cleanup listed in "Activities and Games." On a series of red, white, and blue cards, write "lovers' chores." White cards are for poetry and sweet talk, and as the color of the card gets hotter, the activity on the card is more passionate. See how long you can linger in the blue section or, if you're feeling particularly frisky, go straight to red! If you play your cards right, you'll be satisfied. (And if you don't, love's labors may be lost!)

# Bastille Day

French cuisine goes way beyond the heavy meats, butter, cream, and sugar we often associate with it. None of those health robbers are necessary to have an exciting French cultural experience. Every time I've visited France I've actually lost weight because of the fabulous fruits, vegetables, grains, legumes, and tasty fish dishes that are so plentiful. And there's so much to look at in France that you can spend your whole day walking in an attempt to see it all.

I once spent two *fantastique* months in the south of France shooting the film *Grand Larceny* for Showtime. It was one of the healthiest, most productive times of my life because of the incredible food I enjoyed every day—and I never once had sugar or butter or cream. You can totally re-create the French experience without the heavy stuff, and you'll love it! The French are known for their sense of style and appreciation of beauty. It's easy for them; after all, they're living in France! But even though you're not in France, focus on the beauty around you as you celebrate Bastille Day. Take a walk in the park, downtown, or even around the mall and view life as a *individus Français.* That's not Wal-Mart ahead. It's Galéries Lafayette!

## HISTORY, FACTS, AND FOLKLORE

First things first: Marie Antoinette did not say, "Let them eat cake." She was beheaded for political reasons, but that statement is hearsay.

Le Bastille was a prison in Paris where political prisoners were kept. Anyone who unsurped the absolute power of the king of France was thrown in. The king's dictum was up there with God's own. A hard pill to swallow today, but back then a very common one.

It was those enlightened eighteenth-century philosophers who helped give birth to a new regime. Remember René Descartes—"I think, therefore I am"? You may say the French became enlightened to the fact that the king of France was not God, nor can he parlay his will. So . . . good-bye king!

However, the king and his courtiers did not leave amicably, so the people stormed the Bastille to release anyone being punished within his jurisdiction. Bastille Day is named for a prison, an ideal, a movement—and a good reason to have a healthy, enlightened party approach today.

# French Onion Soup Gratinée

Serves 8 (green)

- 8 cups onions (½ red onion, ½ Maui onion), cut into thin half circles
- 2 tablespoons olive oil
- 1 tablespoon flour
- 1 cup red wine
- 3 to 5 vegetable bouillon cubes
- 1 baguette, sliced 1 inch thick and toasted until golden
- 16 slices Soyco rice milk Swiss cheese
- ¼ cup Soyco rice milk Parmesan cheese

Preheat the oven to 425°F.

In a large pot, slowly sauté the onions in the oil over very low heat until they are translucent, about 20 minutes. Sprinkle on the flour and blend completely. Add 6 cups water and the wine and simmer over medium-low heat for 10 minutes. Add the bouillon cubes one at a time, tasting the broth after each one has dissolved. Pour the soup into individual oven-safe bowls. Lay the slices of bread on top of the soup, using as many slices as needed to cover the tops. Lay 2 slices of rice milk Swiss cheese on top of the bread and sprinkle with rice milk Parmesan cheese. Put the bowls into skillet pans that have handles to make them easier to retrieve from the oven. Cook for 10 minutes, or until the cheese has melted. Serve immediately. Be careful; the bowls will be very hot.

# Three-Bean Salad with Mustard-Tarragon Dressing Serves 8 (blue)

**SALAD:**

> 2 teaspoons salt
>
> 8 ounces organic green beans, ends removed, cut into 1½-inch pieces
>
> 1 15-ounce can cannellini beans, drained
>
> 1 15-ounce can kidney beans, drained
>
> 1 small red onion, diced

**DRESSING:**

> ⅓ cup red wine vinegar
>
> 1½ tablespoons Dijon-style mustard
>
> 1½ teaspoons honey
>
> 2 tablespoons chopped fresh organic tarragon
>
> ¼ teaspoon salt
>
> ¼ teaspoon pepper
>
> ¼ cup canola oil

For the salad, in a medium saucepan, add the salt and 2 cups water and bring to a boil. Add the green beans and simmer for 5 minutes, or until the beans are tender but still slightly crunchy. Drain the water from the pan and immediately fill the saucepan with ice water. This will stop the beans from cooking and also give them a bright color. Drain the beans from the ice water and in a large bowl, mix them with the cannellini beans, kidney beans, and red onion.

In a small bowl, combine the ingredients for the dressing. Toss with the beans and serve.

# Chopped Salad with Tarragon

Serves 8    (purple/blue)

2 organic red onions, diced

4 medium organic tomatoes, diced

1 organic hothouse cucumber, halved
  lengthwise and diced

1/2 cup quartered pitted kalamata olives

1 small head of organic red-leaf lettuce
  leaves, stacked and sliced into 1/4-inch
  strips, then halved crosswise

1 garlic clove, minced

2 tablespoons tarragon vinegar

3 teaspoons Dijon-style mustard

1 tablespoon organic lemon juice

1/3 cup olive oil

Freshly ground black pepper

1 teaspoon chopped fresh organic tarragon

In a large bowl, combine the onions, tomatoes, cucumber, olives, and lettuce and toss with your hands until evenly distributed. In a small bowl, combine the garlic, vinegar, mustard, and lemon juice. Whisk in the oil in a stream until well blended. Season to taste with pepper.

To serve, gather a handful of salad and gently drop it onto a salad plate, forming a pyramid. Sprinkle with the dressing and top with the fresh tarragon.

## Salade Niçoise Serves 12 (green)

¾ cup olive oil

¼ cup tarragon vinegar

3 tablespoons Dijon-style mustard

1 organic garlic clove, finely minced

Salt and pepper

2 tablespoons chopped organic tarragon

¼ pound organic green beans

2 large heads of organic Boston or Bibb
   lettuce, washed, leaves left whole

3 hard-boiled organic eggs, peeled and
   halved

2 7-ounce cans Italian tuna, drained and
   flaked

3 tablespoons tiny capers

½ cup Niçoise olives

1 2-ounce tin rolled anchovy fillets

4 ripe organic tomatoes, quartered,
   tossed with 2 tablespoons vinaigrette

In a small bowl, whisk together the olive oil, vinegar, mustard, garlic, salt and pepper to taste, and tarragon. Blanch the green beans in boiling salted water for 3 to 5 minutes. Refresh in ice water and drain. Toss with 2 tablespoons of the vinaigrette.

In a large bowl, toss the lettuce leaves with 2 tablespoons of the dressing. Arrange the leaves on a deep round platter. Make a concentric circle of the green beans. Put the flaked tuna in a mound in the center. Sprinkle the capers and olives around it. Put the rolled anchovy fillets on top. Garnish with egg and tomatoes. Spoon the remaining dressing over the whole salad and serve at once.

# Seared Halibut with Portobello Mushroom Vinaigrette Serves 4 (blue)

*MaryAnn Hennings*

1 pound organic portobello mushrooms, stems discarded, caps sliced ½ inch thick

6 tablespoons extra-virgin olive oil

1 cup vegetable broth

1 tablespoon rice vinegar

1 tablespoon balsamic vinegar

1 tablespoon organic minced shallots

¾ teaspoon kosher salt

Pepper

1½ pounds baby spinach

2 tablespoons (¼ stick) soy margarine

4 1¼-inch-thick pieces halibut fillet (1½ pounds total), skinned

To prepare the mushroom vinaigrette, in a 12-inch heavy skillet over medium-high heat, cook the mushrooms in 1 tablespoon of the oil, stirring occasionally, until softened, about 5 minutes. Add the broth and simmer until the mushrooms are tender, about 5 minutes. With a slotted spoon, transfer the mushrooms to a plate, cover, and keep warm. Boil the liquid in the skillet until reduced to about ⅓ cup. Transfer to a bowl and cool. Whisk in 3 tablespoons oil, the vinegars, shallots, salt, and pepper to taste.

In a large saucepan over medium-high heat, bring 2 cups water to a boil. Add half the spinach and cook, covered, until the leaves are wilted, 1 to 2 minutes more. Drain well in a colander, pressing on the spinach with a large spoon. Return the spinach to the pan and stir in the margarine and salt and pepper to taste. Cover and keep warm. Pat the fish dry and season to taste with salt and pepper. In a heavy 12-inch skillet over medium-high heat, heat the remaining 2 tablespoons oil until hot but not smoking. Cook the fish until golden, about 3 to 4 minutes on each side. Arrange the fish, spinach, and mushrooms on four large plates or bowls. Spoon the mushroom vinaigrette over each serving.

## Chicken Paillards with Balsamic Vinaigrette and Wilted Greens

Serves 8 (purple)

4 skinless, boneless chicken breasts, halved, trimmed of fat and membranes

2 to 3 garlic cloves

1 teaspoon Dijon-style mustard

4 tablespoons balsamic vinegar

6 tablespoons olive oil

Salt and pepper

8 cups assorted organic salad greens

Flatten each breast into paillards by pounding them between two pieces of wax paper with a mallet or rolling pin. You can make them paper-thin or as thick as ¼ inch.

Place the garlic, mustard, balsamic vinegar, and olive oil in a blender or a food processor fitted with a steel blade. Blend until the mixture starts to thicken. Add salt and pepper to taste.

Place the paillards in a large shallow ceramic or glass container and pour about ¼ cup of the marinade over them. Cover and let them sit at room temperature no longer than 1 hour, or refrigerate for 4 hours or overnight. Refrigerate the remaining vinaigrette.

Heat a large nonstick or cast-iron skillet over high heat. Remove as much of the marinade as possible from the paillards and discard. When the skillet is hot, add the 2 paillards, reduce the heat to medium, and cook for about 1 to 2 minutes per side, depending on the thickness of the chicken. Repeat with the remaining paillards.

Serve the hot paillards, whole or shredded, over the greens, which will wilt. Drizzle the remaining vinaigrette over the paillards. Add salt and pepper to taste.

## French Mustard Mixed Vegetables

Serves 4 (purple)

½ cup carrots, cut into 1½-inch slices

1½ cups cauliflower florets

1½ cups broccoli florets

2¼ tablespoons Dijon- mustard

2¼ tablespoons honey

½ teaspoon dried dill weed

In a steamer over simmering water, steam the carrots for 10 minutes, or until tender. Add the cauliflower and broccoli and steam until barely tender, about 10 minutes. In a small bowl, combine the mustard, honey, and dill weed to make a smooth sauce. Mix the sauce with the cooked vegetables and stir. Serve hot.

# Beets with Raspberry Vinegar

Serves 6    (blue)

12 medium organic beets, trimmed, washed, and peeled

3 tablespoons soy margarine

2 tablespoons raspberry vinegar

Salt and freshly ground black pepper

Place the beets in a large saucepan and cover with water. Bring to a boil over medium-high heat, then lower the heat and simmer, uncovered, until the beets are just tender. Drain and return the beets to the saucepan. Add the soy margarine and raspberry vinegar. Cook over low heat until the soy margarine is melted and the beets are lightly glazed, about 5 minutes. Season to taste with salt and pepper and serve at once.

# Chocolate Soufflé    Serves 8    (yellow)

*MaryAnn Hennings*

1¼ cups plus 2 tablespoons Florida evaporated cane sugar

¼ cup flour

1 teaspoon Roma instant grain drink powder (coffee alternative)

1 cup soy milk

2 tablespoons (¼ stick) soy margarine, softened

5 1-ounce squares unsweetened baking chocolate, coarsely chopped

4 large organic cage-free egg yolks

2 teaspoons vanilla extract

6 large organic cage-free egg whites

¼ teaspoon salt

Preheat the oven to 350°F. Grease eight 6-ounce ramekins or custard cups, or one 2-quart soufflé dish; sprinkle with 2 tablespoons of the sugar.

In a 3-quart saucepan, combine the remaining 1¼ cups sugar, the flour, and the Roma powder. Gradually stir in the soy milk until blended. Cook over medium heat, stirring constantly, until the mixture thickens and boils. Boil, stirring, for 1 minute. Remove the saucepan from the heat. Stir in the margarine and chocolate until smooth. With a wire whisk, beat in the egg yolks until well blended. Stir in the vanilla. Cool to lukewarm, stirring the mixture occasionally.

In a large bowl, with the mixer at high speed, beat the egg whites and salt until stiff peaks form. With the rubber spatula, gently fold one third of the beaten whites into the chocolate mixture. Fold the chocolate mixture gently back into the remaining whites. Pour into the prepared ramekins or soufflé dish. (If using individual ramekins, place in a jelly roll pan for easier handling.)

Bake the ramekins or the soufflé dish 20 to 25 minutes. The centers of the soufflés will still be glossy. Serve immediately.

Bastille Day

# Raspberry Jam Tart with Almond Crumble

Serves  8    ( y e l l o w )

2 cups sliced natural almonds

²/₃ cup date sugar

½ cup plus 2 tablespoons (1¼ sticks) cold
   soy margarine, cut into pieces

1¼ cups flour

¼ teaspoon salt

2 tablespoons cage-free egg, beaten

1 cup organic fruit-sweetened raspberry jam

Preheat the oven to 400°F.
   Reserve ¼ cup almonds in a bowl to use as a topping. Finely grind the remaining almonds with the date sugar in a food processor. Add the margarine, flour, and salt and process until the mixture resembles sand. In a small bowl, mix 1 cup of the flour mixture with the reserved almonds. Add the egg to the remaining flour mixture and pulse until the mixture begins to clump together.

Transfer the mixture from the processor to a 9-inch round tart pan with a removable bottom. Press the mixture with floured fingers onto the bottom and up the sides of the pan and bake in the middle of the oven for 15 minutes, or until golden.

   Meanwhile, stir the raspberry jam to loosen. Rub the reserved almond mixture between your palms to form small clumps. Spread the jam over the baked crust. Sprinkle the almond mixture over the jam and bake for 15 minutes more. Cool the tart in the pan on a rack. Loosen the crust from the side of the pan with a knife before serving.

## BEVERAGES

- French lemonade with lavender
- Kir royale
- THM Orangina: mix freshly squeezed orange juice with sparkling mineral water
- French wine and champagne (the best in the world!)

## PARTY IDEAS

A French party celebrating Bastille Day and everything French—food, art, music, history, and so on.

## INVITATIONS

- Shape your invitations like a guillotine and write the details of the party within a cartoon bubble coming from the severed head of Marie Antoinette. "Off with your head if you don't come to my party!"
- Find blank greeting cards with famous French paintings on the front. Look for cards with works by Claude Monet, Paul Cézanne, Vincent van Gogh, Henri de Toulouse-Lautrec, and Edward Degas.

# Toasts

To Louis, Marie, and Versailles
The cake we never ate
The tears we'll have to cry
The love we'll never forget
And Jean-Paul Sartre
With his eternal Why?
—SUZANNE CARNEY

A votre sante (Cheers).

If the French were really smart, they'd speak English.
—WILFRED SHEED

## DECORATIONS

Eiffel Tower hats; berets; red, white, and blue French flags; French painter palettes, watercolors, and paints.

## SCENTS

French lavender
French lilac
French vanilla
French bakery
Seaside
Wine
French roast coffee
Chocolate mousse
Rosé

## ACTIVITIES AND GAMES

- Hold French waiter races. You'll need lots of plastic champagne glasses and a waiter or bartender's tray for each constestant. Set it up like a regular race, but the runners must carry glasses full of champagne on their trays. If a glass drops, they are out. Spilling a little is okay, though. Contestant must add a glass to their tray every time they return to the starting station. The winner is the first player to finish the course with the predetermined amount of glasses—usually around five to ten—without dropping or tipping any. I suggest buying cheap champagne for the race, since most of it will end up on the ground. You could use water, too, or Perrier, but Perrier costs more than some cheap champagnes!
- Learn French folk songs.
- Play French painter in the Montmartre district and paint each other's portraits. It'll be fun seeing how you portray your friends.
- Play French charades.

Bastille Day

# Bastille Day

- Play Beatles French. Write out Beatles tunes in French and see who can guess what they are in English.

## PRIZES, GIFTS, AND PARTY FAVORS

Trivia questions on Enlightenment quotes, ideas, philosophers, etc. The winner—the enlightened one—gets a candle and a book about Voltaire; French language tapes, berets, potpourri, French country fabrics, sachets, lingerie, eau de toilette.

## MUSIC

| | | |
|---|---|---|
| *Eternelle: The Best of Edith Piaf* | Edith Piaf | Album |
| *Chansons, Accordions, Croissants: 25 Original French Accordion Songs* | Various Artists | Album |
| *I Love Paris* | Various Artists | Album |
| *April in Paris* | Count Basie | Album |
| *Last Mango in Paris* | Jimmy Buffett | Album |
| *Hot Night in Paris* | Phil Collins | Album |
| *Les Misérables* | Various | Soundtrack |
| *The French Album* | Céline Dion | Album |
| *French Kiss* | Various | Soundtrack |

## MOVIES

| | |
|---|---|
| *A Man and a Woman* | (1986—PG) |
| *A Tale of Two Cities* | (1935—NR) |
| *Quills* | (2001—R) |
| *Les Misérables* | (1998—PG-13) |
| *Before Sunrise* | (1995—R) |
| *Dangerous Liaisons* | (1988—R) |
| *The Art of Love* | (1965—NR) |
| *Killing Zoe* | (1994—R) |
| *Marat Sade* | (1966—NR) |
| *Rendezvous in Paris* | (1996—NR) |

| | |
|---|---|
| *French Kiss* | (1995—PG-13) |
| *Funny Face* | (1957—NR) |
| *The Scarlet Pimpernel* | (1935—NR) |
| *French Postcards* | (1979—PG) |
| *Can Can* | (1960—NR) |
| *Frantic* | (1957—NR; 1988—R) |
| *The French Connection* | (1971—R) |
| *Moulin Rouge* | (2001—PG-13) |

## EXERCISE AND CALORIE CHART

Learn or teach the can-can, one of the most energetic aerobic dances ever. Dance like a Rockette, and you have a good start!

| Activity | Calories Burned/Hour |
|---|---|
| Can-can | 493 |
| Kissing | 125 |
| French kissing | 165 |

## FOR COUPLES

Get a short black slit skirt, a tight striped T-shirt, and a beret for her and a black jacket, top hat, and watercolor set for him and play Irma la Douce Meets Toulouse-Lautrec. If you really want this to be authentic, he should do everything on his knees. You know . . . because Lautrec was very short—not what *you're* thinking!

## Midsummer Night's Eve

Just what we all need—a sexy, romantic holiday to break up the long hot summer. Imagine eating under the stars with all your lovely, lusty friends looking for a summer romance, and well...you get the picture. But remember—nothing kills romance more than a bloated stomach. How many times have you gone out to eat a big meal with your honey, come home, and said, "Ohhh! It's too bad we didn't fool around *before* dinner. Let's just hang and watch cable."

# Midsummer Night's Eve

If romance is the theme of the evening, I suggest a proper food-combining strategy, because bloating, belching, and gurgling do *not* go with the dance of love. Tonight you've got to make sure your stomach is working efficiently. It's easy. Just follow the proper food-combining rules given in the first chapter. You can have savory, sexy food without being stuffed. And remember this, too: vegetarians taste better!

## HISTORY, FACTS, AND FOLKLORE

Shakespeare's play *A Midsummer Night's Dream* takes off on the practices of midsummer night, the night before June 24, which involve merrymaking, various superstitions and folk customs, dances, pageants, and revels.

More than any other night of summer, midsummer night suggests enchantment and witchcraft. To an Elizabethan audience, the word *midsummer* called to mind a kind of madness and hysteria, a belief in the delusions of the mind due to a bout of great heat.

## RECIPES
# Panzanella Salad Serves 8 (blue)

4 cups day-old Italian bread, cut into
  ½-inch cubes

⅓ cup pine nuts

½ cup plus 1 teaspoon olive oil

1 tablespoon capers, drained

2 teaspoons minced garlic

1 teaspoon diced anchovy fillets

¼ cup red wine vinegar

¼ cup chicken or vegetable broth

3 to 4 tomatoes, seeded and diced

1 to 2 cucumbers, peeled, seeded, and diced

1 to 2 red onions, thinly sliced

½ cup diced mixed red bell and yellow bell
  pepper

¼ cup pitted kalamata olives

¼ cup fresh basil, cut into chiffonade

Salt and pepper

Lay the bread cubes on a baking sheet and toast under the broiler about 5 to 7 minutes, until golden, turning often. Set aside.

In a sauté pan over medium-high heat, toast the pine nuts in 1 teaspoon of the olive oil, stirring often, about 5 minutes. Watch carefully or else they will burn. Mash the capers, garlic, and anchovies into a smooth paste with a mortar and pestle. Transfer the paste to a mixing bowl and whisk in the remaining ½ cup olive oil, the vinegar, and the broth. Add the toasted bread cubes and toss thoroughly. Add the tomatoes, cucumbers, onions, peppers, toasted pine nuts, olives, and basil. Season to taste with salt and pepper and toss all ingredients until blended. Let the salad sit for at least 5 minutes before serving. Serve at room temperature. (If not using immediately, refrigerate without the dressing.)

# Tomato, White Bean, and Basil Salad

Serves 4    (blue)

4 beefsteak tomatoes, sliced or diced

1 15-ounce can white beans, drained

1 small can anchovy fillets, drained (optional)

12 fresh organic basil leaves, cut into chiffonade

2 tablespoons red wine vinegar or balsamic vinegar

2 tablespoons olive oil

Salt and pepper

Place the tomatoes, beans, and anchovies, if using, in a large, shallow plate or bowl and sprinkle with the basil. Sprinkle with the vinegar and oil and add salt and pepper to taste.

# Saffron Pasta Serves 4    (green)

*MARY BETH BORKOWSKI*

1 teaspoon saffron strands

8 ounces organic fettuccine

12 tablespoons (1½ sticks) Earth Balance margarine

¾ cup Silk soy creamer

1 tablespoon arrowroot powder or cornstarch

1 cup cooked shelled edamame

Salt and pepper

Chopped fresh parsley

Soak the saffron strands in ¼ cup of water for 30 minutes. In a large pot of boiling salted water, cook the fettuccine until al dente, according to the package directions. In a large sauté pan over medium heat, melt the margarine. Stir in the soy creamer. Line a small strainer with cheesecloth or a paper towel and strain the saffron water into the cream mixture. In a small bowl, mix the arrowroot with ¼ cup water and whisk it into the cream mixture. Cook until thickened, about 2 to 3 minutes. Add the pasta to the pan. Toss to coat the pasta with the sauce and season to taste with salt and pepper. Add the edamame and toss again. Top with the chopped parsley.

## Cannellini Beans and Tuna Salad

Serves 6 (green)

1½ cups dried cannellini beans

1 teaspoon salt, or as needed

3 6-ounce cans tuna packed in olive oil, drained

1 small red onion, thinly sliced

¼ cup extra-virgin olive oil

2 tablespoons red wine vinegar

2 tablespoons chopped fresh Italian parsley

Salt

Freshly ground black pepper

6 thick slices country bread, toasted or lightly grilled (optional)

Place the beans in a small, deep bowl and pour in enough cold water to cover by at least 4 inches. Let the beans soak in a cool place or the refrigerator at least 12 hours or up to 1 day. Drain the beans and transfer them to a 3-quart saucepan. Pour in enough water to cover by three fingers. Bring to a boil over high heat. Lower the heat and simmer until the beans are tender, 1½ to 2 hours, adding a little water from time to time to keep the beans completely covered. Remove the beans from the heat, stir in the salt, and let stand until cool. Drain the beans and transfer them to a large serving bowl. Add the tuna, red onion, olive oil, vinegar, and parsley. Toss gently to keep the tuna in big pieces. Add salt if necessary and pepper to taste. Toss gently and serve with the bread if you like.

## Simple and Elegant Chicken

Serves 4 (blue)

*BETH EVIN HEFFNER*

¾ cup halved pitted green olives

½ cup chopped Italian parsley

2 tablespoons grated lemon zest

8 ounces cherry tomatoes

2 tablespoons extra-virgin olive oil

Sea salt and cracked black pepper

1 chicken, cut into 8 pieces

4 garlic cloves, peeled and halved

Preheat the oven to 400°F.

Soak the olives in cold water for 5 minutes and drain. In a medium bowl, combine the olives, parsley, lemon zest, tomatoes, olive oil, and salt and pepper to taste. Place the chicken in a 9×12-inch baking dish, skin side up, with half a garlic clove under each piece. Spoon the olive-tomato mixture over the chicken to cover evenly. Drizzle more olive oil over the chicken and bake until the chicken is golden, 45 to 55 minutes. Place on serving plates, drizzle with the pan juices, and serve.

# Grilled Scallops with Mixed Greens

Serves 4    (blue)

12 large sea scallops

Kosher salt

Freshly ground black pepper

1/2 teaspoon Dijon-style mustard

1 teaspoon mirin

1 teaspoon fresh organic lemon juice

1 tablespoon extra-virgin olive oil

1 teaspoon walnut oil

1 teaspoon boiling water

4 cups organic mixed greens (baby spinach,
  arugula, and mâche)

1/4 cup coarsely chopped fresh organic
  basil leaves

1 1/2 teaspoons chopped fresh organic
  tarragon

Soak four 6-inch bamboo skewers in water for at least 5 minutes. Spray a ridged cast-iron stove-top griddle or outdoor grill with nonstick cooking spray and preheat it on high. Season the scallops with salt and pepper and thread 3 onto each of the skewers. Cook the scallops until slightly firm and almost cooked through, about 1 or 2 minutes on each side. Remove and set aside.

In a small food processor or blender, combine the mustard, mirin, lemon juice, and a pinch of salt and pepper. With the machine running, add the oils in a stream, then add the boiling water and blend well, about 10 seconds more. In a large mixing bowl, toss the mixed greens and the dressing, reserving about 2 teaspoons of dressing. Divide the lettuces evenly among four plates. Arrange 3 scallops on each plate, drizzle with the reserved dressing, top with the basil and tarragon, and serve.

# Glazed Carrots   Serves 6   (blue)

1 1/2 pounds organic carrots, peeled and
  cut into 1/2-×2-inch strips

Salt

2 to 4 teaspoons maple sugar

2 tablespoons vegetable oil

Put the carrots in a large sauté pan and add enough water to cover them. Add salt to taste, the maple sugar, and the oil and bring to a boil over medium heat. Simmer, uncovered, about 25 minutes, or until the thickest carrot pieces are very tender. If too much liquid remains in the pan, continue cooking over medium-low heat, shaking the pan often, 2 or 3 more minutes, or until the sauce thickens to your taste.

## Green Beans with Shiitake Mushrooms

Serves 8    (blue)

6 tablespoons (³/₄ stick) soy margarine

8 ounces fresh shiitake mushrooms,
   stemmed, caps sliced

2 shallots, chopped

2 garlic cloves, minced

2 pounds slender green beans, trimmed

²/₃ cup vegetable broth

Salt and pepper

In a large nonstick skillet over medium-high heat, melt 3 tablespoons of the soy margarine. Add the mushrooms and sauté until tender, about 5 minutes. Transfer the mushrooms to a medium bowl. Melt the remaining 3 tablespoons margarine in the same skillet. Add the shallots and garlic and sauté until tender, about 2 minutes. Add the green beans and toss to coat with the margarine. Pour the broth over the green bean mixture. Cover, lower the heat, and simmer until the liquid evaporates and the green beans are crisp-tender, about 10 minutes. Stir in the mushrooms. Season to taste with salt and pepper, transfer to a platter, and serve.

## Oven-Roasted Potatoes Serves 8    (blue)

*Susan Romito*

5 pounds Yukon Gold potatoes, unpeeled,
   cut into 1-inch pieces

5 pounds waxy potatoes, unpeeled, cut
   into 1-inch pieces

3 onions, chopped

4 garlic cloves, minced

2¹/₂ teaspoons dried rosemary

2 teaspoons sea salt

Pepper

Spike seasoning

3 tablespoons olive oil

Preheat the oven to 400°F.
   In a large roasting pan (the size for a big turkey), place the potatoes, onions, and garlic. Crumble the rosemary on top and sprinkle on the salt and pepper and Spike seasoning to taste. Drizzle on the olive oil and toss to mix. Roast for about 1 hour, stirring every 15 minutes, until the potatoes are cooked through. Note: The potatoes will be cooked but not crispy.

# Lentils and Roasted Leeks

Serves 4      (blue / green)

- 4 organic leeks, washed and halved lengthwise
- 4 organic tomatoes, halved
- 4 tablespoons olive oil
- Sea salt
- Cracked black pepper
- 2 garlic cloves, sliced
- 2 15-ounce cans lentils
- ½ cup chopped organic flat-leaf parsley
- 3 tablespoons mirin

Preheat the oven to 350°F.

Place the leeks cut side up on a baking sheet and top with the tomatoes, also cut side up. Drizzle with 2 tablespoons of the olive oil and sprinkle with salt and pepper. Bake for 40 minutes, or until the leeks and tomatoes are soft. In a frying pan over medium heat, heat the remaining 2 tablespoons of olive oil and cook the garlic for 1 minute, or until soft. Add the lentils and simmer over low heat for 20 minutes to let the flavors come together. To serve, place the leeks and tomatoes on serving plates. Stir the parsley, mirin, and salt and pepper to taste into the lentils. Spoon the lentils over the leeks and tomatoes and serve.

The average American's vocabulary is around 10,000 words—15,000 if you are REALLY smart. Shakespeare had a vocabulary of more than 29,000 words.
— Bedford Companion to Shakespeare

## Double-Trouble Chocolate Bundt Cake

Serves 16    (yellow)

2¼ cups unbleached all-purpose flour

1½ teaspoons baking soda

½ teaspoon baking powder

¾ cup unsweetened cocoa

1 teaspoon espresso coffee powder or Roma
   grain drink

¾ cup hot water

2 cups Sucanat

⅓ cup vegetable oil

2 large organic egg whites

1 large organic egg

1 square (1 ounce) unsweetened chocolate,
   melted

2 teaspoons vanilla extract

½ cup soy cream

salt

Preheat the oven to 350°F. Grease a 12-cup Bundt pan. On sheet of wax paper, mix the flour, baking soda, baking powder, and salt. In a 2-cup measuring cup, mix the cocoa, espresso coffee powder, and hot water until thoroughly blended, then set aside. In a large bowl with the mixer at low speed, beat the Sucanat, oil, egg whites, and whole egg until blended. Increase the speed to high and beat for about 2 minutes, until creamy. Reduce the speed to low and beat in the cocoa mixture, chocolate, and vanilla. Add the flour mixture alternately with soy cream, beginning and ending with flour mixture. Beat just until combined, scraping bowl occasionally with rubber spatula.

Pour the batter into the prepared pan and bake 45 minutes, or until a toothpick inserted in the center of the cake comes out clean. Cool 10 minutes in the pan on a wire rack. With a small knife, loosen the cake from side of pan and invert it onto a wire rack. Cool completely.

Meanwhile, prepare the Mocha Glaze. Place the cake on a cake plate and pour the glaze on the cooled cake, letting it run down the sides. Allow the glaze to set before serving.

## MOCHA GLAZE

¼ teaspoon espresso coffee powder or
   Roma grain drink

2 tablespoons hot water

3 tablespoons unsweetened cocoa

1 cup grain-sweetened chocolate chips

¾ cup soy cream

In a medium bowl, combine the espresso coffee powder or Roma grain drink and the hot water and stir until dissolved. Stir in the unsweetened cocoa. Into the 1-cup measuring cup that holds the chocolate chips, pour the soy cream until it reaches just below the 1 cup mark. In a double boiler, stir together all the ingredients until melted. Cool completely.

Healthy Holidays

# Chocolate Icebox Cookies

Makes 2 dozen cookies (yellow)

⅔ cup unbleached flour

½ cup unsweetened cocoa

1 teaspoon baking powder

½ teaspoon salt

¾ cup soy margarine (1½ sticks), softened

¼ cup maple sugar

¾ cup Sucanat

4 ounces semisweet chocolate chips, melted
  and cooled

1 teaspoon vanilla extract

1 large organic egg

On a sheet of wax paper, stir together the flour, cocoa, baking powder, baking soda, and salt. In a large bowl, with the mixer at medium speed, beat the soy margarine, maple sugar, and Sucanat until light and fluffy. Beat in the chocolate and vanilla. Beat in the egg. Reduce the speed to low and beat in the flour mixture until well combined. Divide the dough in half. On separate sheets of wax paper, shape each piece of dough into a 12 × 1½-inch log. Wrap each log in the wax paper and freeze overnight.

Preheat the oven to 350°F. Keeping the second log in the freezer, cut 1 log into scant ¼ inch thick slices. Place the slices 1 inch apart on two large, ungreased cookie sheets. Bake 10 to 11 minutes, rotating sheets between upper and lower racks halfway through baking, until baked but soft in the center. Cool the cookies on the cookie sheets on wire racks for 1 or 2 minutes. Remove from the cookie sheets and cool completely. Repeat with the second log.

## BEVERAGES
- Spring water
- Lemonade (I recommend R. W. Knudsen's) with honey and raspberries
- Lavender tea
- Champagne

## PARTY IDEAS
A romantic picnic or al fresco dinner party.

## INVITATIONS
- Send each invitation as a scroll with the party information and a map showing people how to find the picnic spot.
- Write the information on hand-painted fans (signifying summer heat/madness) and include a passage from the play *A Midsummer Night's Dream*, such as "What masque? What music? How shall we beguile the lazy time, if not with some delight?"

# Midsummer Night's Eve

## DECORATIONS

Hang caged lovebirds and chandeliers from the trees. Arrange throw rugs and sofas in a wooded area. Buy an old-fashioned record player from Restoration Hardware and play old music. String up a hammock. Dress the children like fairies and sprites.

## SCENTS

Clover
Tangerine
Bergamot
Jasmine
Lilac
Sandalwood

## ACTIVITIES AND GAMES

- Hire a photographer to take portraits of your guests frolicking in the woods.
- Hire actors to do a scene from *A Midsummer Night's Dream.*
- Have children put on a play in their fairy costumes.
- Have a dancer come to teach Renaissance dance to the group, and hire musicians to accompany them.
- Give pony rides.
- Create your own version of the Memory game. Ask each guest to submit five photos per person. Make two cheap copies of each and laminate them. Place them facedown and have people take turns choosing the pairs.

## PRIZES, GIFTS, AND PARTY FAVORS

Because it is an evening marked by long light, merry chaos, no rules, and ethereal yet heightened pleasures:

- Send each guest a copy of his or her photographic portrait or candid party photo with a sprig of rosemary to remember the evening. If you framed the invitation, make sure the photo fits the frame.
- Make a tea of lavender and Saint-John's-wort in small sachets to brew and drink on the *last* day of summer. Any of the following herbs are a token of midsummer's festivities: mistletoe, vervain, heartsease, lavender, and Saint-John's-wort.

## MUSIC

- Elizabethan minstrel music
- New age music, such as Brian Eno, Enya, Kitaro, Indian ragas

# Toasts

Over hill, over dale,
Through bush, through brier,
Over park, over pale,
Through flood, through fire,
I do wander everywhere,
Swifter than the moon's sphere;
And I serve the Fairy Queen,
To dew her orbs upon the green.
—SHAKESPEARE

. . . Love is not love
Which alters when it alteration finds,
Or bends with the remover to remove.
O, no! It is an ever-fixed mark,
That looks on tempests and is never shaken.
It is the star to every wandering bark,
whose worth's unknown, although his height be
    taken.
—SHAKESPEARE

My bounty is as deep boundless as the sea. My
    love as deep;
The more I give to thee, the more I have, for both
    are infinite.
—SHAKESPEARE

Love comforteth like sunshine after rain.
—SHAKESPEARE

Love sought is good, but given unsought is
better.
—SHAKESPEARE

Hand in Hand with fairy grace,
We will sing and bless this place.
—SHAKESPEARE

Love is the answer, but while you're waiting for
the answer, sex raises some pretty good
questions.
—WOODY ALLEN

## MOVIES

| | |
|---|---|
| *A Midsummer Night's Sex Comedy* | (1982—PG) |
| *Much Ado about Nothing* | (1993—PG-13) |
| *Bob and Carol and Ted and Alice* | (1969—R) |
| *Picnic* | (1955—NR) |
| *Indian Summer* | (1993—PG-13) |
| *Miami Rhapsody* | (1995—PG-13) |
| *Beach Blanket Bingo* | (1965—NR) |
| *LA Story* | (1991—PG-13) |

Midsummer Night's Eve

# Midsummer Night's Eve

## EXERCISE AND CALORIE CHART

| Activity | Calories Burned/Hour |
|---|---|
| Dancing | 320 |
| Romping through the woods | 212 |
| Frolicking and/or gamboling | 258 |

## Elizabethan Insults

BY MATTHEW A. LECHER

Combine one word from each of the columns below, preface with "Thou," and thus shalt thou have the perfect insult. Let thyself go—mix and match to find a barb worthy of the Bard!

| Column 1 | Column 2 | Column 3 |
|---|---|---|
| artless | base-court | apple-john |
| bawdy | bat-fowling | baggage |
| beslubbering | beef-witted | barnacle |
| bootless | beetle-headed | bladder |
| churlish | boil-brained | boar-pig |
| cockered | clapper-clawed | bugbear |
| clouted | clay-brained | bum-bailey |
| craven | common-kissing | canker-blossom |
| currish | crook-pated | clack-dish |
| dankish | dismal-dreaming | clotpole |
| dissembling | dizzy-eyed | coxcomb |
| droning | doghearted | codpiece |
| errant | dread-bolted | death-token |
| fawning | earth-vexing | dewberry |
| fobbing | elf-skinned | flap-dragon |

| | | |
|---|---|---|
| froward | fat-kidneyed | flax-wench |
| frothy | fen-sucked | flirt gill |
| gleeking | flap-mouthed | foot-licker |
| goatish | fly-bitten | fustilarian |
| gorbellied | folly-fallen | giglet |
| impertinent | fool-born | gudgeon |
| infectious | full-gorged | haggard |
| jarring | guts-griping | harpy |
| loggerhead | half-faced | hedge-pig |
| lumpish | hasty-witted | horn-beast |
| mammering | hedge-born | hugger-mugger |
| mangled | idle-headed | jolthead |
| mewling | ill-breeding | lewdster |
| paunchy | ill-nurtured | lout |
| pribbling | knotty-pated | maggot-pie |
| puking | milk-livered | malt-worm |
| puny | motley-minded | mammet |
| quailing | onion-eyed | measle |
| rank | plume-plucked | minnow |
| reeky | pottle-deep | miscreant |
| rougish | pox-marked | moldwarp |
| saucy | reeling-ripe | mumble-news |
| spleeny | rough-hewn | nut-hook |
| spongy | rude-growing | pigeon-egg |
| surly | rump-fed | pignut |
| tottering | shard-borne | puttock |
| unmuzzled | sheep-biting | pumpion |
| vain | spur-galled | ratsbane |

## Elizabethan Insults (cont.)

| Column 1 | Column 2 | Column 3 |
|----------|----------|----------|
| venomed | swag-bellied | scut |
| villainous | tardy-gaited | slut |
| warped | tickle-brained | varlot |
| wayward | toad-spotted | wagtail |

# Columbus Day

I know Columbus was Italian, but he sailed for Spain, one of my favorite countries. And although it's not common to throw Columbus Day parties, after reading through this chapter, I'm sure you'll want to throw one of your own. I'll never forget the wonderful experience I had eating and celebrating with the Castilian people while I was filming *Rustler's Rhapsody* in Spain in 1984. Columbus Day offers a great opportunity to share that experience with you.

I got in the best shape of my life while in Spain. I not only walked everywhere every day I was there, but I also learned to appreciate eating smaller portions because of the Spanish tradition of serving tapas. Tapas are small amounts of food placed on dishes throughout your meal. Many people have heard of tapas, but not as many know their origin. The word *tapas* is actually the plural of *tapa,* which means "cover." Tapas were invented in the Andalusian wine-making region of southern Spain, where it is customary to place a saucer on top of a glass of wine in order to keep the little fruit flies out of the wine. Originally, a small amount of food was placed on the dish to help attract clients to the wine bar. Tapas are now found in the smallest of bars in the tiniest of villages. The dishes vary from simple to complex, hot to cold, and include fish, vegetable dishes, and desserts.

Eating this way is a great way to get healthy, because you are never stuffed after dining slowly on small amounts of food. I had tapas everywhere in Spain and had fun tasting a little bit of everything instead of a lot of something!

## HISTORY, FACTS, AND FOLKLORE

Although Columbus made four voyages to what would become North America and visited many islands, he never actually walked on soil that later became the United States, and he died in 1506 never knowing that he had found a new continent.

For decades, American history books and schoolteachers told us that Columbus discovered America. That must have been amusing to the Native Americans, whose ancestors were here long before Columbus. Also, very little was mentioned about the Nordic explorers who had traveled down the eastern coast of Canada thousands of years earlier.

Today Columbus Day is celebrated more appropriately. Columbus did discover the existence of a New World for Europeans and began an enormous change in globalization. And the focus on this holiday now is more about this change in globalization and less about Columbus himself.

Many Latin American countries celebrate this day as Día de la Raza (Day of the Race). This day celebrates the Spanish heritage of the Latin American peoples with brightly colorful fiestas.

# Gazpacho Serves 4 (purple)

- 2 cups vegetable broth
- ½ large red bell pepper, chopped
- 1 large cucumber, peeled, seeded, and chopped
- 3 cups lightly packed chopped romaine lettuce
- ⅓ cup chopped fresh cilantro
- 1 cup cooked corn kernels
- ½ large Bermuda onion, chopped
- 1 tablespoon olive oil
- 2 tablespoons red wine vinegar
- ½ teaspoon Bragg's Liquid Aminos

Place all the ingredients in a food processor and purée, working in batches, if necessary. Chill before serving.

# Garlicky Mushrooms Serves 6 to 8 (purple/blue)

- 3 garlic cloves, minced
- 2 tablespoons olive oil
- 1½ tablespoons flour
- 1 cup vegetable broth
- Dash of red pepper flakes
- 2 tablespoons minced parsley
- 2½ teaspoons fresh lemon juice
- ¾ pound white button mushrooms

In a medium sauté pan over medium heat, sauté the garlic in 1 tablespoon of the olive oil until almost browned, about 4 minutes. Remove from the heat and whisk in the flour. Return to the heat and cook over low heat for 2 minutes, or until a smooth paste forms. Slowly add the broth, red pepper flakes, parsley, and lemon juice.

In a separate sauté pan over medium heat, sauté the mushrooms in the remaining 1 tablespoon olive oil until browned. Add the mushrooms to the sauce and serve.

## White Beans with Vinaigrette Sauce

S e r v e s   4     ( b l u e )

1 cup dried white beans

1 red pepper, minced

½ medium onion, minced

5 small canned anchovies, minced (optional)

6 tablespoons red wine vinegar

Salt and pepper

2 teaspoons olive oil

Soak dried beans in a bowl of cold water overnight. Drain. In a medium saucepan over low heat, boil the beans in 7 cups of water until they are tender, about 1½ hours. Drain well. To make the vinaigrette sauce, in a medium bowl, mix the remaining ingredients. Add the beans, mix, and serve.

## Red Peppers with Anchovies

S e r v e s   8     ( b l u e )

2 large red peppers

4 garlic cloves, peeled and thinly sliced

4 tablespoons olive oil

1 2-ounce can anchovies

Preheat the oven to 400°F.
Place the peppers on a baking sheet and roast them for 15 minutes. Turn the peppers and roast for 15 minutes more, until both sides are done. Put the peppers in a brown paper bag and set aside to cool.

Peel and seed the peppers, then cut them into ½-inch-wide strips. In a sauté pan over low heat, sauté the garlic in the olive oil until it is golden brown, about 3 minutes. Add the pepper strips and sauté for 10 minutes, shaking the pan a little, or until the garlic has infused the peppers with flavor. Serve cold or warm, with the anchovies wrapped around the peppers.

# Tuna Tapas  Serves 4 to 6   (purple)

1 10 to 12-ounce tuna steak, not too thick

Salt

1 tablespoon extra-virgin olive oil

4 garlic cloves, peeled

Red wine vinegar

1 small onion, finely chopped

½ cup chopped Italian parsley

Wash the tuna steak, drain it, and sprinkle it with salt. In a frying pan over medium-high heat, add the olive oil and garlic, and sauté until it just begins to brown, about 3 minutes. Add the tuna and sauté for 2 to 3 minutes on each side. Remove the tuna to a shallow dish. Add a teaspoon of vinegar to the oil and garlic in the pan. Mix well and pour over the tuna. Cover in plastic and refrigerate for 4 to 8 hours.

To serve, break the tuna into bite-sized pieces. Transfer to a clean serving dish, top with the chopped onion and parsley, and pour the marinade juices over all.

# Spanish Tortilla  Serves 4   (green)

2 large potatoes, peeled and thinly diced

Olive oil

4 cage-free eggs

Salt

In a sauté pan over low heat, sauté the potatoes in enough olive oil to cover them completely. When the potatoes are soft, nearly "boiled" in the oil but now brown, drain them well. In a large bowl, mix the potatoes, eggs, and salt.

In a nonstick sauté pan coated with a very thin film of olive oil, spread the mixture with a pancake turner and shape the edges. Cook over low heat for 3 minutes, or until the egg has hardened around the edges, then invert the tortilla in the pan with the help of a dish or the lid of a pot. Cook the tortilla another 3 minutes, or until it is golden brown on the outside, well shaped, and juicy in the center. Serve immediately. (Traditionally the tortilla is served cold, but you may heat it up if you prefer.)

## Patatas Bravas Serves 4 (green)

3 tablespoons olive oil

1 onion, chopped

1 bay leaf

2 red chili peppers

2 teaspoons garlic

1 tablespoon tomato purée

½ tablespoon Sucanat (a little more if the sauce is too spicy for your taste)

1 tablespoon soy sauce

4 roma tomatoes, chopped

1 cup white wine

Salt and black pepper

8 medium potatoes, washed, peeled, and cubed

3 tablespoons soy margarine, melted

In a medium sauté pan, heat 2 tablespoons of the olive oil over medium-low heat. Add the chopped onion and bay leaf and sauté until soft, about 3 minutes. Stir in the chili peppers, garlic, tomato purée, Sucanat, and soy sauce and turn the heat to medium. Let the mixture simmer until it is almost boiling, then add the chopped tomatoes and white wine. Bring the sauce to a boil, stirring continuously, and then reduce the heat to low and let the sauce simmer for 10 to 15 minutes. Add salt and pepper to taste.

Preheat the oven to 450°F. Grease a baking pan with the remaining olive oil and set aside.

Brush the potatoes with the margarine and season to taste with salt and pepper. Bake the potatoes for 15 to 20 minutes, or until they are golden. Put the potatoes in separate dishes, tapas style. Pour the sauce over each dish and serve.

## Shrimp with Garlic Serves 4 (blue)

6 tablespoons olive oil

2 garlic cloves, thinly sliced

1 small red pepper, crushed by hand

1½ pounds medium shrimp, peeled and deveined

Salt

In a large sauté pan over low heat, heat the oil and sauté the garlic until it is golden brown, about 4 minutes. Add the crushed hot red pepper and shrimp, and sauté for 1 minute, or until the shrimp is pink and cooked thoroughly. Sprinkle with salt and serve immediately.

# Shrimp in Green Sauce  Serves 4  (green)

1½ pounds small shrimp

2 peppercorns

1 bay leaf

1 fresh parsley sprig

¼ teaspoon dried oregano

¼ cup plus 1½ tablespoons flour

Salt and pepper

6 tablespoons olive oil

1 cup minced fresh parsley

2 garlic cloves

¼ cup dry white wine

3 tablespoons finely chopped onion

In a medium saucepan over medium heat, combine the shelled shrimp in 2 cups water with the peppercorns, bay leaf, parsley, and oregano and simmer for 20 minutes, or until the shrimp are almost completely pink. Strain through a sieve, reserving ¾ cup of the liquid. Sprinkle the shrimp with ¼ cup flour and salt and pepper to taste. In a large sauté pan over medium-high heat, sauté in 2 tablespoons of oil until the shrimp look pink, about 2 minutes.

To make the green sauce, in a food processor, blend the parsley, garlic, and ¼ teaspoon salt until smooth. With the machine running add the reserved broth and wine. In a sauté pan over medium heat, add the remaining 4 tablespoons of oil and onion, and cook until soft, about 4 minutes. Add the remaining 1½ tablespoons flour and stir until smooth. Gradually add to the pan and cook until thickened. Add the shrimp and heat through before serving.

# Caramel Custard (Flan de Huevos)

Serves 6    (yellow)

12 tablespoons Sucanat

4¼ cups soy milk

Zest of 1 lemon, torn in pieces

2 cage-free eggs

10 egg yolks

To make the caramelized Sucanat, heat 6 tablespoons of the Sucanat in an ovenproof flan mold over low heat, stirring constantly, until the Sucanat has melted and is golden brown. Tilt the pan to coat the bottom and sides. Remove from the heat and let cool for at least 30 minutes, tilting the pan occasionally to coat the sides.

Preheat oven to 350°F.

To make the custard, in a medium saucepan, mix 2 cups of the soy milk with 3 tablespoons of the Sucanat and the lemon zest. Cook slowly over low heat for 30 minutes, stirring constantly. Remove the lemon pieces and discard. In a large bowl, beat the eggs and egg yolks lightly. Blend 3 tablespoons of the Sucanat and the remaining milk. Gently add the boiled soy milk and stir. Pour the custard mixture into the mold on top of the caramelized Sucanat. Place the mold in a pan of hot water. (The water should come halfway up the sides of the mold) Cook over medium heat for 30 minutes. Transfer the flan mold, still in the pan of water, to the oven and bake for 30 minutes, or until a knife inserted comes out clean. Immediately remove from the pan of water and cool, covered, at room temperature. Refrigerate, covered, until ready to serve. Unmold by loosening the sides of the custard with a knife and place a serving plate over the mold. Turn the mold over onto the serving plate.

## BEVERAGES

## AUTUMN SANGRIA

1 bottle Cabernet Sauvignon or
   nonalcoholic red wine

8 ounces orange juice

3 ounces organic fruit juice–sweetened
   lemonade (I recommend R. W. Knudsen's
   or Santa Cruz lemonade)

1 sliced orange

8 ounces sparkling mineral water, like
   Pellegrino or Perrier

½ apple, sliced

½ cup sliced grapes

In a large pitcher or punch bowl, pour the wine, orange juice, lemonade, and sliced orange over ice. Just before serving, stir in the mineral water. Garnish with the apple and grapes.

## INVITATIONS

- Write the invitation on a map.
- Include an interesting historical note or fact about Christopher Columbus with the invitation.

## DECORATIONS

Maps, sailboats, compasses, sailor hats, telescopes, sacks of spices, telescopes

## SCENTS

Ocean breeze
Exotic spices
Cinnamon
Apples
Pumpkin
Autumn leaves

## ACTIVITIES AND GAMES

- Hold a scavenger hunt around your neighborhood and/or city. Give out explorer maps before your guests arrive and have them find the items before coming to the party, or you can make the hunt part of the evening. Do it the usual way, or make it like the show *Amazing Race* and have someone from your family waiting at each destination.
- Do a variation on Pin the Tail on the Donkey. Tape a map of the world on the wall. With the kids' help, cut lots of small boats (no more three inches wide) out of construction paper. One at a time, blindfold the kids and have them try to place their boat as close to Hispaniola (Haiti) or the East Indies as possible. You could give them three boats (tries) each, just like the three boats Columbus had. The closest boat gets a fun prize.
- Using an atlas, map, or globe as a gameboard, ask questions about geography or the history of America. The correct answer moves each boat inch by inch (or whatever scale you choose) toward the New World. The first one to discover America becomes Columbus and wins.

## PRIZES, GIFTS, AND PARTY FAVORS

Sauces, recipes, spices, compasses, magnifying glasses, maps, globes, an atlas, tub toys, a ship in a bottle, history books, Columbus's diary from the first voyage (widely available online)

## MUSIC

| | | |
|---|---|---|
| *Gypsy Kings* | Gypsy Kings | Album |
| *Waiting for Columbus* | Little Feat | Album |
| *Columbus Stockade Blues* | Willie Nelson | Album |
| *Sailing Toward Home* | The Oak Ridge Boys | Album |
| *Inspirational Journey* | Randy Travis | Album |
| *Maiden Voyage* | Herbie Hancock | Album |

Columbus Day

## MOVIES

| | |
|---|---|
| *America, America* | (1963–NR) |
| *Coming to America* | (1988–R) |
| *Christopher Columbus* | (1949–NR) |
| *1492* | (1992–PG) |

## EXERCISE AND CALORIE CHART

| Activity | Calories Burned/Hour |
|---|---|
| Sailing | 211 |
| Swimming | 394 |
| Rowing | 669 |

## FOR THE KIDS

Set up a craft table with white construction paper for sails, Popsicle sticks for masts, and plenty of bars of Ivory soap for the boats (remember, Ivory floats), along with the usual items you see on a craft table: paste, ribbon, multicolored string, nontoxic paint, glitter, markers, crayons, etc. Let the kids construct their own *Niña*s, *Pinta*s, and *Santa Maria*s that they can play with during their next bath.

## FOR COUPLES

Take extra time tonight to explore and discover. You might find a whole new world.

# Halloween

Halloween is a tricky time of year because we assume that all we have to do is keep the kids from going overboard with the Snickers bars and we'll be okay. But there's a bigger issue here. When the weather gets colder, people unconsciously relax their efforts to stay slim and healthy. They know they can get away with a little more as their clothes get bigger and they can cover up. Colder weather also means more eating because food tends to warm us. Add to this the fact that it's a busy time of year for everyone, which allows less time for exercise, and you've got the makings of a winter weight gain.

I talk about awareness throughout this book, and the awareness I want you to focus on for this holiday revolves around two questions:

1.  Am I starting to wear baggier clothes?
2.  Am I starting to let my exercise regimen slip?

Keep those questions in mind during the month of October, the starting month of the big holiday season. Remember, the routine you follow during Halloween week builds like a snowball rolling down a hill by the time you get to New Year's Day. The eight pounds the average person puts on by January 1 begin with habits established in October. Start on the right foot for the first of the big four holidays, and the other three (Thanksgiving, Christmas, and New Year's) will be a piece of cake (a piece of sugarless, dairyless, chemical-free cake, that is!).

Now let's talk about the usual Halloween problem—candy and kids. Here's a checklist of things to do before sending your kids out trick-or-treating.

1.  Make sure they are well hydrated. Being well hydrated is always important, but even more so on Halloween because it will help their bodies metabolize all that candy. (That is, if you are allowing them to eat it.) Candy is very dehydrating and constipating, and wet food and water will keep their digestive systems hydrated and operating smoothly. It's all about taking out the garbage, and water is the transportation system for the garbage in your body. You may want to give kids whole fruit, too. Fruit hydrates and satisfies their sweet tooth, making it less tempting for them to indulge later as their bags fill up with candy.

2.  Make sure they have something warm in their bellies, especially if it's cold out. Consider hot soup or the healthy pizzas found on page 282.

3.  Make sure that they're dressed appropriately for the weather. This may seem obvious, but I am always amazed every year when I see kids under- or overdressed in their costumes. It's almost as if the look of the costume matters more than the comfort of the child. It doesn't! If it's going to be chilly in your climate, buy their costumes a size larger to make room for thermal wear underneath.

If you're walking around with your kids, make sure you have water or a natural, sweet, hot beverage like hot apple cider in a thermos. This will warm them, rehydrate them, and satisfy their sweet tooth before they dig into their candy. Make it a cool beverage if you've got Indian summer. And you grown-ups should go easy on the candy yourselves. As I suggested for Valentine's Day, if you must pig out on candy, just say to yourself, "Tomorrow it's over and I promise I'll throw the remaining candy in the garbage." And make sure you stick to that promise!

## HISTORY, FACTS, AND FOLKLORE

The word *Halloween* means "eve of All Hallow," or eve of All Saints' Day in the Catholic Church. In the Celtic calendar, summer officially ended on October 31 and the New Year started. On that day the Celts believed all people who had died during the year returned to find a living body to reside in for the next year. To keep this from happening, the Celts turned out the lights, dressed in ghoulish costumes, and paraded disruptively around the village. Today this custom is interpreted as egging, toilet-papering a house, and knocking on doors to demand sweets. This demand for sweets is also a centuries-old custom called souling; if you received a cake at a stranger's door, you would say prayers for their deceased loved ones, moving them along into heaven.

The custom of Halloween came to America with the Irish in the 1800s. The jack-o'-lantern, which has a distinct Irish lilt to its name, was originally a turnip, but pumpkins were more common in America and better to use for lighting one's way through the limbo between heaven and hell. This was the fate of a man named Jack, who mistakenly tricked the devil off his trail and so was not allowed into heaven or hell.

## HENNER HOLIDAY TRADITIONS AND STORIES

Halloween was thrilling at St. Johns Berchmans, our Catholic elementary school. Every classroom was decorated to the hilt, and we all talked about which costumes we were going to wear. Anything but our boring uniforms! The funny thing is that thanks to Britney Spears, the Catholic schoolgirl look is now a popular costume—but not necessarily for Halloween!

My costume was usually a kid's version of the exciting, fashionable, and always hip costume that my mother wore at her annual Halloween bowling league party. She had a great figure and usually showed it off with some kind of leotard and tights outfit. You could say she added a touch of Cyd Charisse to Fireside Bowl, while my knockoff version made me come off more like a Hayley Mills wanna-be. But my brother Tommy looked the best every year because our uncle, the artist, always made superextravagant costumes for him. One year he went as the Tin Man. His costume was perfection, right out of MGM. He looked like a mini-me edition of Jack Haley from *The Wizard of Oz.* He was paraded around the school after winning the award for most outstanding costume. I went as a cannibal that year, and the two of us went trick-or-treating together. I must have looked like the Dorothy from Papua New Guinea.

Back then, we would start trick-or-treating right after school and not stop until our bags were stuffed with candy. We usually used grocery shopping bags, which were much larger than the average trick-or-treat bag today. Sometimes we'd go home, drop our load, and start a new one.

People would put some odd things in your bags back then. You would get stray apples or home-baked brownies, a handful of unwrapped candy corn, or loose change (especially from taverns). Every kid would try to stop in as many taverns as possible. We knew they had no candy but figured everyone inside would be drunk and generous with their pocket change.

When I was tired of trick-or-treating, I would go home and sort my candy based on what I liked and didn't like. Charleston Chews, Whoppers, Bulls Eyes, Slow Pokes, Snow Caps, Chuckles, Good & Plenty, Milk Duds, Mary Janes, Dots, Bit-O-Honey, Bonomo's Turkish Taffy, and Boston Baked Beans on one side; Jaw Breakers, Snaps, Hot Dog bubble gum, wax lips, Razzles, bubble gum cigars, Sweetarts, and wax milk bottles on the other side. We would sometimes give all the candy we didn't like to the trick-or-treaters who came by for the late shift. I don't think that was so terrible; I'm sure everyone recycled their least favorite stuff. I think some of that candy corn has been circulating since the Depression.

Anyway, every year we got more than enough candy to keep us sick for months. I used to think the nuns gave us the following school day off not for All Saints' Day (the Catholic holy day of obligation) but to recover from all the junk. I'm sure Halloween was created just to prepare kids for hangovers later in life. Kids learn all about being sick, bloated, wired, and tired on Halloween. It's a kiddie New Year's Eve.

There was one person in our neighborhood who kept the spirit of Halloween alive year-round: the bubble gum lady. You could go to her house any time of the day, 365 days a year, and she would give you bubble gum or candy just for knocking on her door. Either she was a very sweet, eccentric old woman who loved to see bright-eyed, happy children, or her son was the neighborhood dentist. Anyway, I have mentioned this to friends over the years who told me they had similar experiences. It turns out there were year-round candy-dispensin' spinsters in just about every neighborhood. It must have been a franchise!

I really enjoy trick-or-treating with my kids now, but I do miss that crisp midwestern autumn air. I live in the hills, where it's not very good for walking door to door because there are no sidewalks, so my kids and I usually go to my friend MaryAnn's very safe neighborhood, where kids can walk freely in packs while we parents follow behind. After trick-or-treating, MaryAnn usually throws a fantastic Halloween potluck dinner. In fact, most of the recipes in this chapter have been served at her parties.

When my sons and I get home, we sort through their trick-or-treat bags. You probably think I pat them down for hidden Snickers bars and Reese's Pieces while playing the soundtrack of *Midnight Express.* But no, I'm not that bad. I let them have some candy, but they swap most of it for little toys or healthy candy that I buy ahead of time. I know from my own kids' experience that it's spending time with other kids, showing off your costume, and seeing what people give you that makes it special, not the candy. Also, the trend here in Los Angeles is to give away toys. One house in Beverly Hills gave watercolor sets. I thought that was really nice, even though it's rather expensive. Come to think of it, we got little toys when I was a kid, too, like yo-yos or colored pencils. Even as a child, I preferred toys to candy.

I have been to some great Halloween parties in my life, although I must admit that finding the right costume can be a challenge. This was true especially for the *Taxi* Halloween parties. Whenever I had a crush on somebody, I would dress in something sexy, and whenever I felt fat, I would pick a costume that was ideal for eating and concealing. One year I went as a pregnant leprechaun. I stuffed a pillow under my blouse (not that I needed it) and wore a green turtleneck with leggings, goofy hair, and freckles. It's the perfect look if you plan on sitting at the buffet table.

If you want to be ultracomfortable at a Halloween party, go as I did last year. I wore pajamas, applied several dots of zit medication, put my hair up in pigtails, and carried a stuffed animal. You guessed it: a teenager at a pajama party! I was comfortable all night and already dressed for bed when I got home!

# Skeleton Fingers Dipped in Blood

Serves 4 (green)

- 5 to 6 ounces (³/₄ cups) soy potato chips
- 1 organic egg
- 2 tablespoons soy milk
- 1 organic boneless, skinless chicken breast, cut into finger-size pieces

Preheat the oven to 400°F. In a Ziploc bag, crush the potato chips with the back of a wooden spoon. In a small bowl, whisk together the egg and soy milk. Dip the chicken pieces into the egg mixture, then into the bag of crushed potato chips. Shake gently to coat. Place the chicken pieces on an ungreased cookie sheet and bake for 20 minutes or until chicken is golden, flipping once during the cooking time. Serve with your favorite "bloody" barbecue sauce for dipping.

## Bugs on a Log Makes 6 pieces (blue)

*Fill celery with a crunchy mix, and you'll be snacking healthy all night.*

- 2 stalks organic celery, washed and dried
- 6 tablespoons organic peanut butter
- ¼ cup organic raisins

Cut each celery stalk into three even lengths. Spread 1 tablespoon of peanut butter on each of the celery pieces and press raisins into the peanut butter.

## Creepy Spiders Makes 1 spider (green)

For each spider:

- 2 round organic crackers
- 2 teaspoons creamy organic peanut butter
- 8 small organic pretzel sticks
- 2 organic raisins

Spread the peanut butter on the cracker and put another cracker on top to make a sandwich. Insert the pretzel "legs" into the filling. Top the cracker sandwich with a dab of peanut butter and set raisin eyes into the peanut butter.

## Goblin's Crunch Makes 3³/₄ cups (yellow)

- 1 cup popped organic popcorn
- ³/₄ cup mini pretzels
- ½ cup grain-sweetened chocolate chips
- ½ cup organic raisins

Combine all the ingredients in a large bowl.

## Vegetable Bones with Brains

Serves 15   (purple)

*Choose the freshest vegetables you can find.*

½ head organic cabbage

4 stalks organic celery, cut into 4-inch pieces

1 organic green zucchini, cut into 2-inch rounds

1 organic yellow squash, cut into 2-inch rounds

6 organic cherry tomatoes

20 organic baby carrots (for fingers and toes)

2 organic broccoli florets

2 organic cauliflower florets

Scoop out the inside of the cabbage, leaving a shell to hold the brain (peanut) dip (recipe follows). On a large platter, placing the cabbage at one end as the head, use the vegetables to create a skeleton shape. Place the peanut dip in the cabbage head.

## Brain Dip   (blue)

½ cup organic natural style peanut butter or soy nut butter

⅓ cup reduced-fat organic firm silken tofu

3 tablespoons maple sugar

2 tablespoons fresh organic lime juice

2 tablespoons low-sodium soy sauce

2 cloves organic garlic, crushed

Place all the ingredients in a blender and process until smooth, scraping the sides. Place inside the hollowed-out cabbage head of the vegetable skeleton.

# Witches' Hands 12 cups (yellow)

8 cups popped organic popcorn

3 cups mini pretzel twists

1 cup roasted peanuts

2 tablespoons soy margarine

½ cup Sucanat

1 tablespoon pure maple syrup

Clear plastic gloves

Spider rings (optional)

In a large bowl, mix the popcorn, pretzels, and peanuts. To make a toffee syrup, in a saucepan over low heat, melt the margarine. Use a wooden spoon to stir in the Sucanat, and continue stirring until the mixture bubbles. Remove from the heat and stir in the maple syrup until the toffee is smooth. Drizzle the toffee onto the popcorn mixture, tossing to glaze evenly. Cool the mixture. Distribute the mixture into the plastic gloves, put a spider ring on the middle finger of each hand, and tie the gloves at the top.

# Chicken Mummies Serves 6 (green / yellow)

*MARY BETH BORKOWSKI*

3 whole skinless, boneless organic free-range chicken breasts, split to make 6 pieces

12 teaspoons Earth Balance margarine, softened

1 cup Italian seasoned bread crumbs

Preheat the oven to 350°F.
Lay 1 chicken breast piece on a plate. Spread 1 tablespoon of margarine across the breast, sprinkle the chicken with 1 tablespoon bread crumbs, and roll it up, jelly-roll style. Place the roll seam side down in a 9×11-inch baking dish. Repeat with the remaining chicken. Dot the top of each chicken roll with 1 tablespoon of margarine and sprinkle with the remaining bread crumbs. Bake for 25 to 30 minutes, or until golden.

# Warlock Legs Serves 8 (yellow)

⅔ cup honey

1¼ cups low-sodium soy sauce

1 cup water

2 organic garlic cloves, crushed

2 dozen organic chicken drumettes

Combine the honey, soy sauce, water, and garlic in a large baking dish. Set aside ¾ of the sauce for dipping. Toss in chicken drumettes in the remaining sauce and marinate for at least 2 hours. Broil in a pan or grill for 10 to 15 minutes on each side, allowing the drumettes to char slightly. Serve with the reserved sauce.

Halloween

## Mystical Spell Soup Serves 8 (blue)

1 medium organic onion, chopped

1 large organic carrot, peeled and chopped

1 organic celery stalk, chopped

½ pound soy sausage, broken into small
   pieces

1 tablespoon olive oil

1 medium organic zucchini, chopped

4 cup organic chicken or vegetable broth

⅓ cup broken spaghetti (1-inch pieces)

½ teaspoon dried oregano

1 28-ounce can organic peeled and crushed
   tomatoes

1 tablespoon salt

In a large saucepan over medium-high heat, add the onion, carrot, celery, soy sausage, and olive oil. Sauté for 5 to 10 minutes, or until the soy sausage is cooked and the vegetables start to become tender. Add the rest of the ingredients and increase the heat to high. Bring to a boil, reduce the heat to low, and simmer for 30 minutes, or until the vegetables are tender.

## Ghostly Corn Bread Serves 6 to 8 (yellow)

1 cup unbleached all-purpose flour

1 cup organic cornmeal

2 teaspoons baking powder

½ teaspoon baking soda

¼ cup maple sugar

½ cup soy milk

½ cup plain soy yogurt
   (Whole Soy is the best)

1 organic egg, lightly beaten

¼ (½ stick) cup soy margarine, melted

Preheat the oven to 425°F.
   Grease an 8-inch-square baking pan. In a large bowl, mix the flour, cornmeal, baking powder, baking soda, and maple sugar. In a medium bowl, whisk together the soy milk, soy yogurt, egg, and soy margarine. Add the wet ingredients to the dry ingredients and stir until just combined. Pour into the prepared pan and bake for 15 to 20 minutes or until the top is golden and a toothpick inserted into the center comes out clean. Serve with Goblin Stew.

# Goblin Stew   Serves 8 to 10   (green)

*Kids will appreciate this not-too-spicy chili.*

1½ pounds organic ground turkey or Gimme
  Lean soy sausage

1½ cups chopped organic onions

3 tablespoons olive oil (plus 2 tablespoons
  optional)

3 crushed organic garlic cloves

2 tablespoons chili powder (or more
  to taste)

1 teaspoon cumin

1 teaspoon oregano

1 teaspoon salt

½ teaspoon black pepper

1 28-ounce can organic crushed tomatoes

1 28-ounce can organic whole tomatoes

2 15-ounce cans organic kidney beans,
  drained

1 28-ounce package frozen organic corn

In a large skillet over medium heat, brown the turkey or soy meat (if using soy meat, add the optional 2 tablespoons of olive oil to the skillet before adding the soy meat). In a large soup pot, sauté the onions over medium heat in the 3 tablespoons of olive oil for about 5 minutes, or until translucent. Add the garlic and cook for a few more minutes. Drain the fat from the turkey or soy meat and add the meat to the onion mixture. Lower the heat and add the seasonings, tomatoes, beans, and corn. Stir well, cover, and simmer for ½ hour, or until it thickens.

# Scary Halloween Pizza Makes 1 pie (green)

### PIZZA SAUCE:

1 tablespoon olive oil

1 small organic onion, chopped

1 large organic garlic clove, minced

1 15-ounce can organic tomato puree, drained

1 4-ounce can organic tomato paste

1/4 cup water

1 1/2 teaspoons Sucanat

1 teaspoon dried oregano

1 teaspoon dried basil

Salt and pepper to taste

### PIZZA DOUGH:

1 1/4-ounce package active dry yeast

1 teaspoon Sucanat

1 cup warm water (tap water that feels
warm on your hand—not hot)

2 tablespoons olive oil

1 teaspoon salt

2 1/2 cups unbleached all-purpose flour, plus
more for rolling the dough

In a large saucepan over medium heat, heat the oil. Add the onion and sauté about 3 minutes, or until translucent, stirring with a wooden spoon. Add the garlic and sauté for 1 minute, stirring constantly. Reduce the heat to low. Add the tomato puree, tomato paste, water, Sucanat, oregano, basil, salt, and pepper. Turn the heat to high and bring to a boil, stirring constantly. Turn heat back to low and simmer the sauce for 30 minutes, stirring occasionally. While the sauce is cooking, make the pizza dough. When the sauce is done, remove from the heat and set it aside.

In a large bowl, mix the yeast, Sucanat, and warm water, stirring with the spoon until the yeast dissolves. Stir in the oil, salt, and flour. When the dough becomes too stiff to stir, flour your hands and a work surface. Transfer the dough to the work surface. Gather the dough together in your hands and knead the dough: gently press the dough with the palms of your hands, pushing part of it away from you. Fold the dough back over the dough nearest you and pat into a loose circle. Turn the circle a quarter turn and knead again. Do this for 8 to 10 minutes, adding a little flour to keep it from sticking. When the dough is kneaded enough, it will feel soft and smooth and no longer sticky. Dust the dough with flour and put it on a plate. Cover with a kitchen towel and let the dough sit and rise in a warm place until doubled in volume, about 1 hour.

**To ASSEMBLE THE PIZZA:**

    10 ounces grated soy mozzarella cheese

    5 tablespoons olive oil

    Cornmeal

    Unbleached flour

Place the oven rack in the lowest position in your oven. If you have a pizza stone, put it on the rack. Preheat the oven to 500°F.

Grease 2 pizza pans with olive oil and dust the pans lightly with cornmeal. Sprinkle your hands with flour. Form the dough into 2 round patties and place each on an oiled pan. Let the dough rest for 5 minutes. With your hands, press the dough over the bottom of the pan, forming a 10- to 12-inch circle. (Or dust a rolling pin with flour and roll the dough into a circle.) With a spoon, spread the pizza sauce (all of it or less, depending on your taste) evenly over the dough circle. Sprinkle the circles with the soy mozzarella cheese. Using a large spoon, drizzle a little (about 1 tablespoon) olive oil over the top of each pizza. If you want to add extra toppings, sprinkle them on now. Place the pans on the lower rack of the oven and bake until the cheese is melted, about 10 minutes.


# Baked Apples  Serves 4  (yellow)

*SUSAN ROMITO*

    4 apples

    ³/₄ cup raisins

    ¹/₄ teaspoon ground cinnamon

    4 teaspoons Earth Balance margarine or 4
       teaspoons apple cider

Preheat the oven to 350°F.

Cut the stem out of each apple in a cone shape so that it can be replaced. Core the apple, making sure not to go through the bottom. Fill each apple with raisins, sprinkle with cinnamon, and top with a pat of margarine or sprinkle with apple cider. Replace the top of each apple and wrap in aluminum foil. Bake for 45 to 50 minutes, or until the apples are tender. Serve warm. In the warmer weather, these can also be made on the grill.


# Gross and Gooey Apple Dip

Serves 1  (yellow)

    ¹/₂ cup plain or vanilla soy yogurt

    ¹/₄ teaspoon cinnamon

    ¹/₄ teaspoon vanilla extract

    1 organic apple, sliced

Combine the soy yogurt, cinnamon, and vanilla extract in a small bowl. Serve with sliced apples on the side.

## Miniature Pumpkin Breads

Serves 6 (yellow)

3 cups raw pumpkin seeds (pepitas)
(about 15 ounces)

3½ cups flour

2 teaspoons baking powder

2 teaspoons baking soda

1½ teaspoons salt

1½ teaspoons ground cinnamon

¾ teaspoon grated nutmeg

3 cups canned pumpkin (about 24 ounces)

1½ cups Sucanat

½ cup maple sugar

1 cup vegetable oil

4 large cage-free eggs

1 teaspoon peeled minced fresh ginger

¾ cup soy milk

Preheat the oven to 350°F. Spray six 5¼×3¼×2-inch baby loaf pans with cooking spray.

Spread the pumpkin seeds on a rimmed baking sheet. Roast until they begin to color, stirring twice, about 20 minutes. Cool the seeds. Set aside ½ cup of whole seeds for topping. Using on/off turns, coarsely grind the remaining seeds in a food processor.

In a medium bowl, whisk together the flour, baking powder, baking soda, salt, cinnamon, and nutmeg. Mix in the ground pumpkin seeds. In a large bowl, using an electric mixer, beat the pumpkin, Sucanat, and maple sugar until blended. Gradually beat in the oil, the eggs, one at a time, then the minced ginger. Stir in a quarter of the flour mixture, then ¼ cup of the soy milk, alternating until all are incorporated. Divide the batter among the prepared pans. Sprinkle with the reserved whole pumpkin seeds. Bake until a tester inserted into the center comes out clean, about 1 hour.

## Fruit and Slime Serves 8 (blue)

Organic apples

Organic bananas

Organic pineapple, fresh or canned

Assorted organic melons

Organic kiwis

Organic strawberries

Organic star fruits

Honey

Cut the fruit into bite-size chunks, slices, or shapes. To make kebabs, carefully push a skewer through the fruits, alternating colors and shapes. Drizzle honey over the kebabs and serve.

# Witches' Fruit Cauldron  Serves 6  (yellow)

½ cup plain soy yogurt

2 tablespoons Vegenaise

1½ tablespoons maple syrup

6 large organic lettuce leaves

1 large organic orange, peeled, and diced

1 large organic apple, cored and diced

1 medium organic pear, cored and diced

⅔ cup organic seedless grapes (use both
    green and red)

3 tablespoons chopped walnuts

3 tablespoons organic shredded coconut

In a small mixing bowl, blend the soy yogurt, Vegenaise, and maple syrup. Set aside. Line each of six small serving bowls with a large lettuce leaf. Put an equal amount of orange, apple, and pear pieces and grapes in each lettuce-lined serving bowl. Top the fruit with the yogurt sauce, dividing the sauce equally among the 6 bowls. Sprinkle each bowl with ½ tablespoon walnuts and ½ tablespoon coconut.

# Frozen Jack-o'-Lantern Pie

Serves 10  (yellow)

*Prepare this pie a day ahead.*

1 quart soy vanilla ice cream, softened

1 cup plain organic canned pumpkin

¼ cup Sucanat

¼ teaspoon cinnamon

¼ teaspoon ginger

1 recipe Graham Cracker Crust

GRAHAM CRACKER CRUST:

6 tablespoons soy margarine

3 tablespoons Sucanat

1½ cups broken organic graham crackers

In a large bowl, stir together all the ingredients except the crust. Pour the mixture into the prepared crust and set it in a level place in the freezer to harden overnight.

Preheat the oven to 350°F. In a small saucepan, gently melt the soy margarine. Combine the Sucanat and graham cracker crumbs in a bowl or food processor. Slowly add the melted soy margarine and mix or process until well blended. Press the crumbs into the bottom and sides of a 9-inch pie plate. Bake the crust for 8 to 10 minutes, just until it begins to brown. Cool on a wire rack before filling with Jack-o'-Lantern pie mixture.

Halloween

## Mud Cup serves 1 (yellow)

2 paper muffin cups

2 tablespoons grain-sweetened chocolate
   chips

2 heaping tablespoons organic creamy
   peanut butter

Place 1 tablespoon of the chocolate chips in a double paper muffin cup. Microwave on high for 1 minute. Stir, then microwave for about 30 seconds more, or until the chips are completely melted. Place the cup in the freezer for 10 minutes, or until the chocolate has hardened. Spoon the peanut butter on top of the chocolate, then sprinkle with the remaining chips. Microwave on high for another 1 minute. Stir and swirl with a butter knife. Microwave for 30 seconds more, or until chocolate melts. Set aside to cool.

### BEVERAGES

- Apple cider—Serve hot with a cinnamon stick.
- Pumpkin shake—Make with soy ice cream, fresh pumpkin, and cinnamon.
- Orange juice ice cream float—Use Soy Dream ice cream.
- Count Dracula's Drink—cranberry juice and cherry juice served warm, with a pair of fangs for garnish
- Ghostly Gulp—vanilla shake made with soy ice cream
- Mummy Milkshake—vanilla shake served with chocolate and maple syrup with a dingy cloth napkin.
- Frankenstein Freeze—limeade and crushed ice with a scar garnish made from Panda all-natural licorice.
- Witches' Brew—Mix apple cider, cranberry juice, and chocolate soy milk, and make a frown.

For more grown-up tastes, with or without the alcohol:

### BLOODCURDLING MARY

4 ounces R. W. Knudsen's Very Veggie

1½ ounces vodka (optional)

½ ounce organic natural lemon juice

2 dashes of Tabasco sauce

Pinch of black pepper

¼ teaspoon horseradish

Sea salt

Celery stick or lime wedge for garnish

Over ice, combine the Very Veggie, vodka (if using), lemon juice, Tabasco, pepper, horseradish, and salt to taste over ice. Stir and serve in a highball glass. Garnish with a celery stick or lime wedge.

## Tom Ghoulins

4 ounces organic fruit juice–sweetened lemonade (I recommend R.W. Knudsen's or Santa Cruz)

1½ ounces gin (optional)

Sparkling mineral water

Orange slice and fresh cherry for garnish

Over ice, pour the lemonade and gin, if using. Shake or blend and pour into a Collins glass. Top with mineral water and garnish with the orange slice and fresh cherry (not maraschino).

## THM Zombie

2 ounces natural pineapple juice

2 ounces orange juice (without pulp)

2 ounces Knudsen's organic fruit juice–sweetened lemonade

2 ounces natural fruit punch

3 ounces light or dark rum (optional)

Orange slice and fresh cherry for garnish

Over ice, combine the juices, lemonade, fruit punch, and rum, if using. Shake or blend, then pour into a tall Collins or pint-size glass. Garnish with an orange slice and a real cherry (not maraschino).

## THM White Russian
*Warning: not lo-cal!*

2 ounces Silk Coffee Soylatte

2 ounces Silk Soy Creamer or regular soy milk

1½ ounces vodka (optional)

Combine all the ingredients over ice. Shake or stir, pour into a rocks glass, and serve.

Halloween

## PARTY IDEAS

- Kids' party
- Family dress-up
- Adult party
- Couples party—Invite couples and ask them to dress up as famous or unlikely couples in history or show business.
- Walk around the neighborhood—Invite families before trick-or-treating and load up on healthy food before following your kids around the neighborhood.
- Have a séance party and try to contact friends and relatives who are no longer with us. You never know—Harry Houdini might even show up.
- Select one of the following costume party themes and tell your guests to come as his or her favorite—
    - —Movie character
    - —Monster
    - —Cartoon character
    - —Sex symbol
    - —Characters found in famous artwork
    - —Sitcom star
    - —Comedian
    - —Musician
    - —Athlete
    - —Famous couple
    - —Politician
    - —Person in uniform

## INVITATIONS

- Ghost shapes, bat shapes, pumpkin shapes, or haunted houses
- A photo of your own house with added ghosts, bats, spiderwebs, witches, and goblins
- A CD or cassette tape with all the information told in an ominous voice (think Boris Karloff) with creepy organ music playing in the background
- Hand-deliver small pumpkins with all the party details written on them with a Sharpie pen. Draw creepy jack-o'-lantern faces on them if you want.
- Make a collage with scary creatures, movie characters, cartoon monsters, or other scary images you find in magazines. Or use the Halloween clip art on your computer. Place the party details somewhere in your collage, photocopy, and send.

## DECORATIONS

- Skeletons, bats, cobwebs, black lights, spiders and snakes, Indian corn, pumpkins, gourds, autumn leaves, haystacks
- Display one or two dummy scarecrows, witches, or ghosts to lull your guest into thinking that all the decorations are dummies. Then have someone (child or adult) dress up in a similar costume and scare the guests as they arrive.

- If you have an overhead ceiling fan, tape a paper witch on a broom or a ghost onto one of the blades. It will appear to fly around the room when the fan is on. Put it at the slowest setting.
- This one requires some artwork. Paste together sheets of white tissue paper and drape them over a fresh helium balloon on a string. The ghost will appear to be suspended and floating in air. Be sure to go light on the glue and tissue paper, or the ghost will sink and ruin the effect!

## SCENTS

Pumpkin
Licorice
Apple
Cinnamon
Candy corn
Chocolate

## ACTIVITIES AND GAMES

- Grab bag costume party—Have your guests bring a costume in an unmarked paper bag. Put all the bags in the middle of the room, have everyone grab a bag, and watch what happens! Provide tables of makeup and props to add to the merriment. This is the perfect party for people who don't want to spend a lot of time finding the perfect costume or who hate riding public transportation dressed as Little Bo Peep—especially the guys!
- Famous people *Dating Game*—Have everyone dress as a celebrity and then play the *Dating Game* as the character. This leads to some very interesting matchups and role-playing.
- Halloween charades—Set up a black light and play charades in the dark using scary titles from movies and books. Charades is much harder this way, and it adds a spookiness to the game.
- Haunted house—Turn your entire house into a haunted mansion, inside and out. Use the ideas from the "Decorations" section and buy lots of fiberfill. Pull it apart and drape it around picture frames, couches, and lighting fixtures. Tape some of it to the ceiling corners. Put some in the windows so you can see it from the outside, too. Place old-looking thick white candles strategically throughout the house. The more they melt, the better they look. Converting your house into a haunted mansion is challenging, but it is also a blast! Don't forget to take lots of pictures.

## PRIZES, GIFTS, AND PARTY FAVORS

Mystery novels, trick-or-treat bags filled with little toys or healthy treats, soundtrack to a horror film; video or CD of a classic horror film or anything from the "Music" section below; scary stickers, scary puzzles, face-painting kits, passes to the wax museum or Ripley's Believe It or Not.

## MUSIC

| | | |
|---|---|---|
| *Rocky Horror Picture Show* | Various | Soundtrack |
| "Monster Mash" | Bobby Pickett | Song |
| "Werewolves of London" | Warren Zevon | Song |
| *Scary Monsters* | David Bowie | Album |
| *Monster* | REM | Album |
| *New Wave Halloween* | Various | Album |

## MOVIES

| | |
|---|---|
| *E.T.* | (1982–PG) |
| *Halloween* | (1978–R) |
| *Legend of Sleepy Hollow* | (2000–R) |
| *Nightmare Before Christmas* | (1993–PG) |
| *House on Haunted Hill* | (1958–NR) |
| *Fight Night* | (1985–R) |
| *Nightmare on Elm Street* | (1984–R) |
| *Carrie* | (1976–R) |
| *Hocus Pocus* | (1993–PG) |
| *Witches of Eastwick* | (1987–R) |
| *Escape from Witch Mountain* | (1975–G) |
| *Beetlejuice* | (1988–PG) |

## EXERCISE AND CALORIE CHART

| Activity | Calories Burned/Hour |
|---|---|
| Walking | 176 |
| Walking in costume | 226 |
| Watching a scary movie | 119 |
| Bobbing for apples | 174 |

## FOR THE KIDS

- One of the traditions I've started in my house is to take a picture of my kids in their costumes, mount the pictures in little cardboard frames from the art store, and then let the boys decorate the frames and write anything they want. We have done this the last three years. I think this will make a great collection and visual log. I wish I had photos of all the costumes I wore when I was a kid, or for that matter, throughout my teens and adult life.
- Offer to take individual pictures of your children's classmates in costume, and have the kids make cards or frames using construction paper and Halloween art supplies.
- Have a magic talent show—tell kids to prepare magic tricks to bring to the party. Who knows? You might find the next Houdini!
- Here's something I do with my boys that's fun, takes the focus away from the candy, and provides a healthier treat. When we're carving our pumpkins, we save the seeds and roast them. It's really easy and a lot of fun.

# Roasted Pumpkin Seeds

2 cups pumpkin seeds

1½ tablespoons nonhydrogenated soy margarine

1¼ teaspoons sea salt (or 1¼ teaspoons Bragg's Liquid Aminos)

Preheat the oven to 250°F. In a large, shallow baking pan combine the pumpkin seeds, melted soy margarine, and salt or Bragg's. Bake approximately 2 hours, stirring occasionally, or until seeds are crisp, dry, and golden brown. You can also lightly spray the Bragg's on after, rather than before, baking the seeds, for a stronger flavor.

## FOR COUPLES

This is the perfect opportunity to use your imagination and have some fun. Every fantasy role you have ever wanted to play with each other can be explored, whether it's the Emperor and the Slave Girl, Elvira meets Raggedy Andy, or whatever works for you. Tonight there are no boundaries! I suggest you don't reveal your identity to each other until the moment before you . . .

# Thanksgiving

Keeping Thanksgiving healthy is...definitely a challenge! It is the beginning of the big holiday season, so your mindset (and belt buckle) are ready to let loose. And it's the one holiday of the year that is *all* about *food*! Mention Thanksgiving and people immediately think of only two things: *turkey* or *stuffing.* That's it—and it's usually both! If you love turkey and stuffing and overeating is a problem for you, make an extra effort this Thanksgiving holiday to keep from looking like a Butterball turkey in your Christmas card photo. The problem is not just Thanksgiving dinner, it's the additional three or four days of eating leftovers that follow. You need a plan—a *healthy* Thanksgiving plan!

Here's a THM plan that will start your holiday season right and keep you looking your best till New Year's without sacrificing anything you love—even the leftovers! The plan involves three key points I want you to remember: 1) eat light, 2) eat right, 3) muscles tight!

## 1. Eat light

Let's face it. You're not going to skip the things you love most on Thanksgiving, so don't even try. But here's where I want you to exercise some discipline. Before you take even one bite of your Thanksgiving dinner, decide exactly how much you're going to eat. Make it a reasonable amount, and place only that specific amount on your plate. When you're done, stop! That's all there is to it. Most of us get into trouble because once we start, we have a hard time stopping, especially on Thanksgiving, when the food is so luscious. Our brain is always twenty minutes behind our stomachs, so we end up eating twenty minutes of food we really don't need. And it's that twenty extra minutes that add about two or three hours to our digestion time. Keep it light, and you might actually get through the NFL game without moaning like a beached whale.

## 2. Eat right

Let's talk about leftovers. They can get you into big trouble because of bad food combining and all the naughty extras like gravy, butter, and mayonnaise that are often added to bring the juicy flavor back. Well, I suggest you enjoy leftovers as usual, but make a few adjustments. First, go easy on the extras—the mayo, the margarine, and especially the gravy. Pick only one per meal, and limit it to one tablespoon. The more you add those heavy fats, the more you'll crave them. And you really don't need them. Your taste buds will adjust, and you'll better appreciate the real turkey and stuffing flavors you started with.

## 3. Muscles tight

I'm always saying, "Try to break a sweat every day." Well, during Thanksgiving weekend, I want you to focus more on resistance training and good posture with tight abdominals. A good exercise program should involve both aerobic training *and* resistance training. Now, I don't know what kind of physical shape you're in, and resistance training can be serious business for anyone who doesn't do it on a regular basis. When it comes to exercise, nothing is more important than safety. That is why I am giving you a list of three suggested levels of resistance training. Only you know what level is right for you. If all this is completely new to you, consider taking a basic class in resistance training so that you will be doing it on a regular basis by the next holiday, Christmas. If you already have some experience with resistance training, consider buying or renting a video. I recommend any videos by Karen Voight or Kari Anderson. Kari is known more for her aerobic videos, but she also makes some great body-sculpting videos.

Here's a mini-workout that you can do while the turkey is in the oven.

### Beginner

- 2 minutes of stepping up and down to warm up. (March in place if you don't have a brand-name step or staircase. Footstools can be dangerous.)

- 5 minutes of stretching
- 1 minute of abdominal crunches
- 1 minute of side leg lifts (½ minute on each leg)
- 1 minute inner leg lifts (½ minute on each leg)
- 1 minute back leg lifts (½ minute on each leg)
- 3 to 10 male or female push-ups (broken up into 3 sets)

### Intermediate

- 3 minutes of stepping up and down to get warmed up
- 5 minutes of stretching
- 2 minutes of various abdominal crunches
- 10 to 20 male or female push-ups (broken up into 3 sets)
- 2 minutes of side leg lifts (1 minute on each leg)
- 2 minutes of inner leg lifts (1 minute on each leg)
- 2 minutes of back leg lifts (1 minute on each leg)

### Advanced

- 3 minutes of stepping up and down to get warmed up
- 5 minutes of stretching
- 4 minutes of various abdominal crunches
- 15 to 50 male or female push-ups (broken up into 3 sets)
- 2 minutes of side leg lifts (1 minute on each leg using a Resist-A-Band)
- 2 minutes of inner leg lifts (1 minute on each leg using a Resist-A-Band)
- 2 minutes of back leg lifts (1 minute on each leg using a Resist-A-Band)

And make sure you drink plenty of water throughout the day, because with so many wonderful smells, you'll think you are hungry most of the time when in fact you may just be thirsty because your mouth is salivating.

## HISTORY, FACTS, AND FOLKLORE

Did you know that about one-third of the people who arrived on the Mayflower in 1620 were Puritans or Separatists? I would like to believe that they were called Separatists because they were the first food combiners, separating their proteins and carbohydrates. But they were in fact members of the English Separatist Church, seeking religious tolerance and a better life. Their food-combining habits may have been out of necessity, but I'll bet they were some of the few Americans to feel great after a Thanksgiving feast.

Why?

They ran out of flour, so there were no pastries of any kind. Their consumption of nightshade plants (peppers and potatoes) was limited. And even better, there were no cows to produce butter or milk. So no pumpkin pie—but boiled pumpkin, yes. They had what they called "turkey," but that meant wild (organic!) fowl. The original table probably had berries, watercress, fish, lobster, dried fruit, and plums. Not bad.

"Thanksgiving" then disappeared from the calendar for many years. It wasn't until October

1777 that the thirteen colonies designated a day for celebrating and giving thanks—but this time, it was to honor a victory in the battle at Saratoga. As the nation grew stronger, many citizens felt the Pilgrims should not be remembered for their overcoming adversity. Even Thomas Jefferson said the whole concept of Thanksgiving was "the most ridiculous idea I've ever heard."

So how did it happen?

A woman.

Who probably wanted to throw a party.

Her name was Sarah Josepha Hale, and she was a magazine editor hell-bent on making Thanksgiving a national holiday—so much so that she launched, through the pages of her magazine, a forty-year campaign that would stop only at triumph. Finally, in 1863, President Lincoln declared the last Thursday in November a national day of Thanksgiving. The date was rearranged a few times—once by President Roosevelt, who wanted a longer Christmas shopping season. (My kind of president!) But it was eventually moved to the fourth Thursday of November, and in 1941, Thanksgiving Day was declared a legal holiday by Congress.

## HENNER HOLIDAY TRADITIONS AND STORIES

I will always remember the Thanksgivings I had growing up in Chicago. I loved going shopping with my mom right after school on Wednesday. We would run into lots of friends from our parish, and you could just feel the warmth and friendliness that people naturally exude when they're happy with holiday anticipation. After shopping, we would unload the grocery bags and start sorting the goods according to the dishes we'd be cooking—the turkey and dressing (my mom always called the stuffing "dressing"), the green bean casserole (with mushroom soup and fried onion rings), and the pumpkin pie (usually prebaked from the Jewel Supermarket bakery). I loved waking up really early on Thursday morning to help my mom prepare the stuffing and clean the turkey. I'd chop the celery and onions and get them cooking on the stove. No matter how many times I've made turkey as an adult, the smell of onions and celery cooking together takes me right back to our kitchen on Logan Boulevard. It is one of the strongest sense memories ever. Helping my mom prepare Thanksgiving dinner is when I first fell in love with cooking. My mother became so famous for her surefire crowd-pleasing turkey and dressing that not only has it been passed around to every relative and friend, but it even beat out Wolfgang Puck *and* the Butterball Turkey lady in a Celebrity Turkey Cook-Off. Can you imagine?

After our dinner, the family tradition was that we would each thank my mother for making a wonderful dinner (à la *Little House on the Prairie*). Then my older sisters, Jo Ann and Melody, would help her clean up and do the dishes, while my father (to get us out of their way) would take us four Little Rascals to the only place that was open for business in the entire city of Chicago on Thanksgiving—Union Station. In reality, it was just a boring old train depot, but to us, it was like Disneyland! There was a gift shop, a little quarter photograph stall, and best of all, an actual recording booth for making 45 rpm records. All four of us would pile into the photograph booth and take all kinds of crazy composite shots. Then, for two dollars, we'd cut a record and say things like "We love you, Mommy!" "Thank you for a great dinner!" "We really loved the dressing!" We'd usually end with a Christmas song (à la Alvin and the Chipmunks). My younger brothers, Tommy and Lorin, would always plan to come back and cut a demo record in hope of becoming the next Lennon and McCartney. (Too bad they had no talent!)

Before leaving, we would always buy our mom the best gift the fabulous Union Station had to offer: an aluminum Chinese checker set (with carrying case!), a Buckingham Fountain snow globe, or even a LEAVE YOUR BUTT IN CHICAGO ashtray—"Now she'll know we love her for sure!"

These childhood memories only reinforce the notion that Thanksgiving has always been my absolute favorite holiday. The entire week is wonderful, no matter what age you are—the preparation, the shopping, the cooking, the smells, the stuffing, the pumpkin pie, watching classic movies, playing games, the foliage, the crisp fall air. I even like the football. I love Thanksgiving most of all because it's about my two favorite things—family and *eating*! And it all starts on Thanksgiving eve, the night that officially kicks off the holiday season. Just knowing that Christmas is right around the corner, especially when you're a kid, helps you enjoy those few weeks of school before Christmas break—the best two weeks of the school year. Weeks full of festivities, from caroling and candlelight ceremonies to shopping and Secret Santas. Even the crabbiest of nuns were happy during those few weeks between Thanksgiving and Christmas.

Another thing that separates Thanksgiving from the rest of the holidays is that adults tend to love it just as much as they did as children, perhaps even more. That's not something you can say about most other holidays. Christmas and Halloween don't have quite the same joy factor for adults as they do for kids, and birthdays can be almost depressing after thirty-nine. But Thanksgiving consistently appeals to every age. Kids look forward to candy on Halloween and Easter, and toys on Christmas and birthdays. On Thanksgiving, *everyone* looks forward to *food*! Thanksgiving dishes were my favorite growing up, and now that I've removed the chemicals, meat, sugar, and dairy, they are still my favorite holiday dishes as an adult as well.

The average American gains seven pounds between Thanksgiving and New Year's.
—*LOS ANGELES TIMES*

We all know that we are going to overeat on Thanksgiving. It goes with the territory. It is the one holiday that is designed around food and very little else. Of course, you are supposed to count your blessings and express gratitude on this day, but you're usually counting your helpings and thanking someone for passing the yams. I can think of only one Thanksgiving in my life when I didn't pig out, and that's only because I was shooting a bedroom scene the next day. I had half a veggie burger until the director yelled "That's a wrap!" on Friday night, and then I ate my way through the rest of the weekend.

This Thanksgiving will be different, I promise you. You will overeat, sure, but if you eat healthier food and exercise even a little, it will make a huge difference. As I am always saying, "If you improve the quality of your food, the quantity will take care of itself!"

# RECIPES

Columbus thought that the land he discovered was connected to India, where peacocks are found in considerable number. And he believed turkeys were a type of peacock (they're actually a type of pheasant). So he named them tuka, which is "peacock" in the Tamil language of India.

Turkeys have been around for a long time. In fact, fossil evidence shows that turkeys actually roamed the Americas 10 million years ago. They probably survived natural selection only because every animal (including *Homo sapiens*) wanted them around to eat! In fact, the first meal eaten on the moon by astronauts Neil Armstrong and Buzz Aldrin was roasted turkey and all the trimmings. And even if you don't eat turkey, other dishes associated with Thanksgiving are stars in their own right. I have not eaten turkey since 1981, but I never feel deprived of a total Thanksgiving experience. In fact, my Thanksgiving dinner feels even more complete because I am not loading up solely on turkey, stuffing, and mashed potatoes. I am filling my plate with eye-pleasing, palate-pleasing, digestion-pleasing, and colorful vegan dishes.

This is only a small sampling of the Thanksgiving dishes my friends and I have enjoyed over the years. I am even including my mother's famous dressing/stuffing recipe. If you do eat turkey, make sure you buy a fresh, organic turkey. It really does make a difference, not only in flavor but in the way you will feel afterward. Hens are more tender, but they usually only go up to twenty pounds. For large groups of people, you may want to cook two hens rather than buying a very large tom turkey.

## Chestnut Fennel Soup   Serves 6   (green)

- 2 cups roasted, shelled, and skinned chestnuts
- 1 shallot, chopped
- 2 leeks, chopped, white and pale green parts only
- 6 tablespoons (¾ stick) soy margarine
- 2 tablespoons dry white wine
- ½ fennel bulb (sometimes called anise), stalks and core discarded, bulb coarsely chopped
- 1 cup vegetable broth
- ¼ cup soy cream
- Salt and pepper

Coarsely chop the chestnuts and reserve ⅓ cup for garnish. In a 5-quart heavy pot over moderate heat, cook the shallot and leeks in 2 tablespoons of the soy margarine, stirring, until softened, about 4 minutes. Add the wine and simmer until almost all the liquid is evaporated, about 1 minute. Stir in the fennel, broth, chestnuts (excluding garnish), and 2½ cups water, then simmer, covered, 20 minutes. Stir in the soy cream and cool the mixture slightly. Purée the soup in batches in a blender until smooth, transferring to a bowl. (Use caution when blending hot liquids.) Return the soup to the pot and bring to a simmer, thinning with water if desired. Season to taste with salt and pepper.

While the soup is reheating, in a 10-inch heavy skillet over moderately high heat, heat the remaining 4 tablespoons soy margarine until the foam subsides. Sauté the reserved chestnuts with salt and pepper to taste, stirring constantly, until crisp, about 4 minutes. Serve the soup topped with the chestnuts and drizzled with the browned soy margarine.

# Beet Soup in Acorn Squash s e r v e s   8  (b l u e)

8 1¼-pound acorn squashes

3 tablespoons vegetable oil

1 tablespoon kosher salt

1 large red onion, chopped

1½ tablespoons olive oil

5 medium beets (2 pounds without greens),
   peeled and cut into 1-inch pieces

1 red apple, such as Gala, peeled, cored,
   and cut into 1-inch pieces

2 garlic cloves, minced

6 cups vegetable broth

1 teaspoon maple sugar

Pepper

To roast the squash, preheat the oven to 375°F. Cut off the tops of the squash (about 1 inch from the stem end) and reserve. Scoop out the seeds and discard. Cut a thin slice off the squash bottoms to create a stable base, but do not make an opening in the bottom of the squash. Brush the vegetable oil inside and on top of the squash and sprinkle the kosher salt inside. Arrange the squash bowls, with tops alongside, stem ends up, in two large, shallow baking pans. Roast the squash in the upper and lower thirds of the oven, switching the positions of the pans halfway through baking, until the flesh of the squash is just tender, about 1¼ hours.

While the squash is roasting, make the soup. In a 5-quart heavy saucepan over medium heat, cook the onion in the olive oil, stirring occasionally, 5 minutes, or until the onion is softened. Add the beets and apple and cook, stirring occasionally, 5 minutes. Add the garlic and cook, stirring, 30 seconds, or until well combined. Add the broth and 2 cups water, then simmer, uncovered, until the beets are tender, about 40 minutes. Stir in the maple sugar. Purée the soup in 3 batches in a blender until very smooth, at least 1 minute per batch, transferring the soup to a large bowl. (Use caution when blending hot liquids.) Return the soup to the pan, season to taste with salt and pepper, and reheat. If the soup is too thick, add enough water to thin to the desired consistency. Serve the soup in the squash bowls.

# Watercress Salad s e r v e s   4  (p u r p l e)

1 bunch watercress, torn

½ head of romaine lettuce, torn

3 tablespoons olive oil

3 teaspoons red wine vinegar

Soy Parmesan cheese (optional)

In a large serving bowl, toss together the watercress and romaine. Sprinkle the oil and vinegar over the salad. Garnish with the soy Parmesan cheese, if desired, and serve.

## Mixed Green Salad Serves 4 (blue)

1 bunch organic watercress, torn

1 bunch organic arugula, torn

1 head of organic romaine lettuce, torn into
   bite-sized pieces

½ bunch fresh basil, cut into chiffonade

2 tablespoons soy Parmesan cheese

4 tablespoons olive oil

4 tablespoons balsamic vinegar

Combine the watercress, arugula, romaine, basil, and cheese in a large bowl. In a small bowl, whisk together the olive oil and balsamic vinegar. Toss the salad with the dressing and serve.

## Roast Turkey Serves 8 (blue)

¼ cup (½ stick) soy margarine

1 teaspoon kosher salt

1 teaspoon freshly ground black pepper

1 tablespoon chopped fresh rosemary

¼ cup dry vermouth

1 10- to 12-pound turkey

Preheat the oven to 450°F.

In a small bowl, combine the soy margarine, salt, pepper, rosemary, and vermouth. Rub or brush into the flesh and skin of the turkey. Loosely fill the cavity with stuffing and place the bird on a rack in a roasting pan in the oven. Roast, uncovered, for 30 minutes. Reduce the oven heat to 350°F. and cook for 3 to 4 hours, or about 15 to 20 minutes per pound. If desired, baste with pan drippings every 30 minutes.

Begin testing the turkey for doneness after it has cooked for 2½ hours. If you are using a thermometer, place it deep in the inner thigh. The turkey is done when the internal temperature reaches 180°F. If you do not have a thermometer, you can tell that the turkey is done when the juices run clear from the breast and the leg moves easily in the joint.

# Roast Turkey Giblet Stock Serves 6 (blue)

1 tablespoon olive oil

Neck and giblets (excluding the liver) from
  the turkey

1 celery stalk, coarsely chopped

1 carrot, coarsely chopped

1 onion, quartered

3 cups chicken broth

1 bay leaf

1 teaspoon black peppercorns

Heat the oil in a 3-quart saucepan over moderately high heat until hot but not smoking. Sauté the neck and giblets until browned, about 6 to 8 minutes. Add the remaining ingredients with 3 cups water and simmer until reduced to about 4 cups, 45 minutes to 1 hour. Pour the stock through a fine sieve into a bowl. Skim off and discard any fat. The stock can be used for any soup dish or any recipe that requires a light soup base.

# Henner Holiday Dressing Makes enough to stuff a 20-pound turkey (green)

8 ounces soy margarine (preferably Earth
  Balance)

2 bunches celery, cut in $1/2$- to 1-inch chunks

2 large onions, chopped

2 pounds turkey sausage (such as Shelton
  Farms Breakfast Sausages)

2 loaves whole grain bread, torn into 1-inch
  pieces

2 packages seasoned croutons

1 packet poultry seasoning, or 1 teaspoon
  each of parsley, sage, rosemary, and thyme

2 cups Rice Dream, or to taste

Preheat the oven to 350°F.
  In a large skillet over medium-high heat, add the margarine, celery, and onions and cook for about 5 to 7 minutes, until the onions are translucent. Add the turkey sausage to the mixture and continue cooking for 15 minutes, or until the sausage is cooked.

In a large bowl, combine the bread, croutons, and seasoning. Add the sausage mixture to moisten the dry ingredients. Stir in $1/2$ cup of the Rice Dream at a time, until the dressing reaches the desired moistness. Stuff the inside cavity of the turkey. Place the leftover dressing in tinfoil and bake alongside the turkey for $1\frac{1}{2}$ hours.

Thanksgiving

## Wild Rice Dressing Serves 8 (green)

1½ cups uncooked wild rice

6 cups 1-inch cubes country-style bread
(from ½ pound bread)

½ pound sliced turkey bacon, coarsely
chopped (optional)

2 Spanish onions, chopped

2 tablespoons olive oil

4 celery stalks, cut crosswise into ¼-inch-
thick slices

½ cup chopped Italian parsley

Salt and pepper

1 cup organic chicken broth or turkey stock
(page 301)

Preheat the oven to 325°F.
Rinse the rice in a sieve under cold water. Place the rice in a 4-quart saucepan, and cover with cold water by 2 inches. Simmer over low heat, covered, until tender, 50 minutes to 1 hour. Drain the rice in the sieve and cool 10 minutes.

In a large, shallow baking pan in the middle of the oven, toast the bread until golden and dry, about 30 minutes.

In a large skillet over medium heat, cook the bacon, if using, stirring until crisp. Transfer with a slotted spoon to a large bowl. In the same pan, cook the onions in the remaining fat, or in the olive oil, if not using the bacon, stirring until softened, about 3 minutes. Add the celery and cook, stirring, 1 minute. Add the onions and celery to the bacon. Stir in the parsley, bread, rice, and salt and pepper to taste.

Increase the oven temperature to 375°F. Transfer the dressing to a greased 3- to 4-quart baking dish and drizzle the chicken broth over the top. Stuff the turkey with the dressing. If cooking separately, bake the dressing covered, 20 minutes, then uncover and bake 20 minutes more, or until the bread is golden brown and the dressing is heated through.

## Orange Zest Cranberry Sauce

Serves 10 (yellow)

2 12-ounce bags fresh cranberries

½ cup organic orange juice

2 cups Sucanat

1 tablespoon orange zest

1 tablespoon fresh organic lemon juice

In a medium saucepan over medium heat, bring the cranberries, ¾ to 1 cup water, and the orange juice to a boil. Cook until the cranberry skins burst, about 15 minutes. Add the Sucanat, orange zest, and lemon juice and return to a boil, then simmer until the proper jellylike consistency is achieved, 25 to 30 minutes more. If the mixture is too dry, add more orange juice. The mixture will thicken even more upon cooling.

# Mary Beth's Stuffing

- 1 onion, chopped
- 2 celery stalks, chopped
- 1 cup (2 sticks) Earth Balance margarine
- 1 loaf white spelt bread, cut into 1-inch cubes
- Salt and pepper
- 2 to 3 tablespoons rubbed sage (not dried)
- 2 pounds chestnuts, roasted or boiled, then hulled and chopped

Preheat the oven to 350°F.

In a large frying pan over medium heat, sauté the onion and celery in the margarine until slightly softened and the onion becomes opaque, about 3 to 5 minutes. Add the bread a bit at a time and stir until it browns slightly. As you add more bread, you won't be able to brown it as easily, but patience is the key. Add salt and pepper to taste, the sage, and a little water as you go along. Add as much as a cup to a cup and a half, a bit at a time to moisten the stuffing. When the bread is browned, put the stuffing in a large bowl and stir in the chopped chestnuts to taste. Bake in a 9×11-inch pan for 20 minutes, or until firm on top.

# Cranberry Chutney Serves 10 (green)

- 5 shallots, coarsely chopped (6 ounces)
- 1½ tablespoons vegetable oil
- 1 12-ounce bag fresh cranberries
- ⅔ cup Sucanat
- ¼ cup cider vinegar
- 1 teaspoon peeled minced fresh ginger
- ½ teaspoon salt
- ½ teaspoon black pepper

In a 3-quart heavy saucepan over moderate heat, cook the shallots, stirring occasionally, until softened, about 3 to 4 minutes. Stir in the remaining ingredients and simmer, stirring occasionally, until the berries just pop, 10 to 12 minutes. Cool before serving.

# Cranberry Orange Relish Serves 6 (yellow)

*SUSAN ROMITO*

- 2 cups fresh cranberries
- 1 cup orange juice
- ⅓ cup maple syrup
- Zest of 1 orange

In a medium saucepan, combine all the ingredients. Bring to a simmer over medium heat and cook for 20 to 30 minutes, or until the berries are tender and a syrup has formed. Chill or serve at room temperature.

## Pecan Sweet Potatoes   Serves   8   (yellow)

8 medium sweet potatoes or yams (about 3
  pounds)

¼ cup (½ stick) soy margarine

⅓ cup maple sugar

¾ teaspoon salt

⅓ cup chopped pecans

Heat the oven to 350°F.
Scrub the sweet potatoes thoroughly with a vegetable brush; do not peel. Pierce the potatoes on all sides with a fork to allow steam to escape while they bake. Place the potatoes directly on the oven rack. Bake for about 1 hour, or until tender when pierced with a fork. Be sure to use a potholder to remove the potatoes; they will be very hot. When the potatoes are cool enough to handle, gently peel off the skins using a paring knife. Cut the potatoes into ½-inch slices.

In a large saucepan over medium heat, heat the margarine, maple sugar, ¼ cup water, and salt about 2 minutes, stirring constantly, until the mixture is smooth and bubbly. Add the potatoes and pecans and stir gently until the potatoes are coated with the sauce.

## Butternut Squash and Carrot Purée with Maple Syrup   Serves   8   (yellow)

3 tablespoons soy margarine

1 onion, chopped

3 carrots, peeled and thinly sliced

1 3½-pound butternut squash, peeled,
  seeded, and cut into ½-inch pieces

1 cup fresh organic orange juice

3 tablespoons pure maple syrup

Salt and pepper

In a large sauté pan over medium heat, melt 2 tablespoons of the soy margarine. Add the onion and sauté until just tender, about 8 minutes. Stir in 1 tablespoon of the margarine. Add the carrots and sauté until coated with margarine, about 1 minute. Add the squash and sauté until it begins to soften, about 8 minutes. Pour the orange juice over the vegetables. Cover and simmer until the vegetables are soft, about 25 minutes. Uncover and simmer until all the liquid evaporates, about 5 minutes. Stir in the maple syrup and cool slightly. Working in batches, purée the mixture in a food processor until smooth. Season to taste with salt and pepper. Transfer to a serving bowl.

# Mashed Potatoes with Rosemary

Serves 4     (green)

- 2 pounds Yukon Gold or Yellow Finn potatoes
- 3 fresh rosemary sprigs, plus extra
  for garnish
- Salt
- 1 tablespoon mild extra-virgin olive oil
- 1 cup soy milk, warmed
- Freshly ground black pepper
- 1 lemon

If you will be mashing the potatoes with a ricer, simply cut them into 1- to 1½-inch pieces. If you will be using a food mill or a hand masher, peel the potatoes, then cut into 1- to 1½-inch pieces.

Place the potatoes in a medium saucepan and add water to cover by 1 inch. Place the 3 rosemary sprigs in a square of cheesecloth (muslin) and gather the cloth with a kitchen string. Add to the pan along with 1 tablespoon salt. Bring to a boil over medium-high heat. Reduce the heat slightly, cover partially, and gently boil until the potatoes are just tender when pierced with the tip of a sharp knife, 15 to 20 minutes.

Remove the rosemary pouch and discard. Drain the potatoes, return them to the saucepan, and mash them with a potato masher until they are free of lumps.

Return the saucepan to very low heat, add the olive oil, and beat vigorously with a wooden spoon until well blended. Add the warm soy milk, a little at a time, continuing to beat and scraping the sides and bottom of the pan each time, until the potatoes are smooth and fluffy. You may not need all the milk. Add salt and pepper to taste and continue to stir over low heat until very hot.

Spoon the potatoes into a warm serving dish. Using a zester or fine-holed shredder, shred the zest from the lemon directly onto the potatoes. Garnish with fresh rosemary and serve immediately.

# Roasted Asparagus     Serves 8     (purple)

*MARY BETH BORKOWSKI*

- 2 bunches fresh organic asparagus, cut into
  1½-inch pieces
- 2 tablespoons extra-virgin olive oil
- 2 tablespoons balsamic vinegar
- Sea salt

Preheat the oven to 350°F.

Place the asparagus on a baking sheet and drizzle with the olive oil. Stir the pieces to coat. Roast the asparagus for 7 to 10 minutes, or until they are firm but tender, checking for doneness by piercing with a fork. Drizzle the asparagus with the vinegar and a little sea salt. Stir to coat.

## Brussels Sprouts with Marjoram and Pine Nuts Serves 8 (green)

3 tablespoons soy margarine

½ cup pine nuts

1½ pounds fresh brussels sprouts, halved, or 1½ pounds frozen brussels sprouts, thawed and halved

1 cup canned vegetable broth

2 shallots, minced

1 tablespoon chopped fresh marjoram

⅓ cup soy cream

Salt and pepper

In a large, heavy skillet over medium heat, melt 1 tablespoon of the margarine. Add the pine nuts and stir until golden, about 3 minutes. Transfer the nuts to a small bowl. Add 1 tablespoon of the margarine to the skillet, then add the sprouts, and stir 1 minute. Add the broth; cover and simmer until the sprouts are almost tender, about 7 minutes. Uncover and simmer until the broth evaporates, about 5 minutes. Using a wooden spoon, push the sprouts to the sides of the skillet. Melt the remaining 1 tablespoon margarine in the center. Add the shallots and sauté until tender, about 2 minutes. Stir in the marjoram, then the cream, and simmer until the sprouts are coated with soy cream, stirring frequently, about 4 minutes. Season to taste with salt and pepper.

Transfer the sprouts to a serving platter. Mix in half the pine nuts and sprinkle the remaining pine nuts on top.

## Overnight Biscuits

Makes 30 biscuits (green)

*SUSAN ROMITO*

1 package dry yeast

2 cups soy buttermilk

3 tablespoons Sucanat

1 teaspoon sea salt

5 cups whole wheat pastry flour

1 tablespoon baking powder

1 teaspoon baking soda

¾ cup soy margarine

In a small bowl, dissolve the yeast in 2 tablespoons water. Add the buttermilk substitute, Sucanat, and salt and set aside. In a large bowl, mix the flour, baking powder, and baking soda. Cut in the margarine. Add the liquid ingredients and mix lightly—don't knead. Store in a large covered bowl in the refrigerator overnight.

When you are ready to bake the biscuits, preheat the oven to 450°F. You can either pinch off pieces of the dough and form them like hamburger patties, or you can knead the dough, roll it out, and cut out biscuit shapes. Place the biscuits on a baking sheet and bake for 10 minutes, or until lightly browned on the bottom.

# Pilgrim Pumpkin Pie <small>Serves 10 (yellow)</small>

Pastry Dough (recipe follows)

1 16-ounce can organic pumpkin or 2 cups mashed cooked pumpkin

1 12-ounce container soy cream

2 large cage-free eggs

¼ cup maple sugar

½ cup Sucanat

1 teaspoon ground cinnamon

½ teaspoon ground ginger

¼ teaspoon grated nutmeg

½ teaspoon salt

Soy whipped cream (optional)

Prepare the dough as directed through the chilling. Roll out the dough and line a 9-inch pie plate; make a turret edge. Refrigerate or freeze 10 to 15 minutes to firm the dough.

Preheat the oven to 425°F.

Line the pie shell with foil and fill with pie weights, dry beans, or uncooked rice. Bake 15 minutes. Remove the foil and weights and bake 5 to 10 minutes longer, until golden. If the crust puffs up during baking, gently press it to the pie plate with the back of a spoon. Cool on a wire rack. Turn the oven temperature down to 375°F.

In a large bowl, combine the pumpkin, soy cream, eggs, maple sugar, Sucanat, cinnamon, ginger, nutmeg, and salt and beat until well mixed. Place the pie plate on the oven rack and pour in the pumpkin mixture. Bake 50 minutes, or until a knife inserted 1 inch from the edge comes out clean. Cool on a wire rack about 1 hour. Serve with soy whipped cream, if you like.

## Pastry Dough for Pumpkin Pie

Makes crust for 1 pie    (yellow)

- ¼ cup whole wheat flour
- 1 cup unbleached white flour
- ¼ teaspoon salt
- 6 tablespoons (¾ stick) cold soy margarine, cut up
- 3 to 5 tablespoons ice water

In a large bowl, mix together the flours and salt. With a pastry blender or two knives used scissor fashion, cut in the soy margarine until the mixture resembles coarse crumbs.

Sprinkle in the ice water, 1 tablespoon at a time, mixing lightly with a fork after each addition, until the dough is just moist enough to hold together.

Shape the dough into a disk. Wrap in plastic and refrigerate for 30 minutes or overnight. If chilled overnight, let stand at room temperature for 30 minutes before rolling.

On a lightly floured surface, with a floured rolling pin, roll the disk into a 12-inch round. Roll the dough round gently onto the rolling pin and ease into the pie plate. Trim the edge, leaving a 1-inch overhang. Make the desired decorative edge. Refrigerate or freeze 10 to 15 minutes to firm the pastry before baking. Fill and bake the pie as directed in the recipe.

## Apple Bars Makes 1 dozen bars    (yellow)

*SUSAN ROMITO*

*Great served warm with a side of Soy Delicious vanilla ice cream!*

- 2 cups whole wheat pastry flour
- ½ cup soy margarine
- 1 cup Sucanat
- 1 teaspoon organic vanilla extract
- 1 organic eggs or 1 egg's worth of egg replacement
- 4–5 organic apples, peeled, cored, and sliced thin
- 2½ tablespoons soy margarine
- 1 teaspoon cinnamon
- ⅓ cup date sugar

Preheat the oven to 350°F and lightly grease a 9 × 13-inch pan. In a large bowl, combine the flour, margarine, Sucanat, and vanilla. Mix well with a pastry blender or hand mixer until it resembles small crumbs. Press the mixture into the pan.

In a large bowl, toss the apples with the date sugar and cinnamon. In a small saucepan over medium heat, melt the margarine and drizzle it over the apple mixture. Toss until well combined. Spread the apple mixture evenly over the crust with a spatula. Bake for 45 to 55 minutes, or until the fruit bubbles. Cut into bars while still warm.

## BEVERAGES

### COFFEE CHAI Serves 4

4 cups low-fat rice or soy milk

1 tablespoon instant coffee

1/8 cup Sucanat or 1/3 cup maple sugar

3 cinnamon sticks

6 cardamom pods (available in the spice
    section at most supermarkets)

1/8 teaspoon grated nutmeg

1/8 teaspoon ground allspice

4 sticks cinnamon (optional)

Combine all the ingredients (except the 4 cinnamon sticks) in a medium saucepan. Simmer over low heat for 5 minutes, stirring to dissolve the Sucanat and instant coffee. Do not let the mixture boil. Heat and let steep for 20 to 30 minutes. Pour the mixture through a clean sieve or strainer. Serve hot or cold. Use cinnamon sticks as stirrers, if desired.

### HOT LATTE Serves 3

3 cups low-fat rice or soy milk

2 cups water-processed decaf coffee

Cocoa powder or ground cinnamon
    (optional)

In a microwave oven or a small saucepan over low heat, heat the milk just until it starts to steam and a few bubbles appear; do not let it boil. Divide the coffee and milk equally among three mugs. Sweeten to taste and dust with cocoa powder or cinnamon, if desired.

## PARTY IDEAS

A traditional Thanksgiving Dinner.

## INVITATIONS

- Write the invitations as thank-you notes to your guests.
- Include your favorite Thanksgiving memory or recipe and ask the person to bring his or hers.
- Ask each guest to bring a toy or canned good, and donate the bounty to a local homeless shelter.
- Iron a leaf onto wax paper.
- Have the children make a turkey out of their handprints.

## DECORATIONS

You don't have to go out of your way to make a Thanksgiving centerpiece that is natural and healthy, there are so many beautiful fruits, vegetables, flowers, and leaves that naturally make you feel healthy, even when you're overeating.

Thanksgiving decorations should have a harvest theme: Fill a large cornucopia with natural produce (which can always be eaten by starving guests while they wait). Write your guests' names on gourds and use as place cards. Make donations to various charities in your guests' names; write the particular charity on each person's place card.

## ACTIVITIES AND GAMES

The Pilgrims who had survived the difficult year at Plymouth would never have called their celebratory feast Thanksgiving, because to the Puritans, Thanksgiving was actually a religious holiday instead of a celebration. The first "Thanksgiving" was not a solemn religious observance, but rather a traditional English harvest festival with dancing, the singing of secular songs, and the playing of games. Therefore you can keep to the spirit of the original holiday by dancing after dinner, singing popular songs, and playing charades.

You can also start a family tradition by videotaping each family member and guest saying what they are thankful for. If you do this every year, over time you can see what changes—and what remains the same.

## PRIZES, GIFTS, AND PARTY FAVORS

Thanksgiving is not a big party favor holiday because it is not about being acquisitive, except for the thank-yous, memories, and until now, an expanding waistline. However, if you want to leave your guests with something besides a tryptophan hangover, here are some suggestions:
- recipe cards,
- pumpkin pie spices tied up in seasonal fabric,
- apple cider mulling spices
- savory spices, such as sage, rosemary, thyme, and basil, papaya enzymes for better digestion,
- faux Plymouth Rock paperweights.

## MUSIC

The following music selections are intended to inspire you throughout the weeks prior to Thanksgiving, while preparing the meal, and throughout the feast itself.

| | | |
|---|---|---|
| *Thanksgiving* | George Winston | Album |
| *Thanks a Million* | Louis Armstrong | Album |
| *Beggars Banquet* | Rolling Stones | Album |
| *Gratitude* | Earth, Wind, and Fire | Album |
| *Grace* | Jeff Buckley | Album |

# Toasts

There is something moving about raising our glasses, especially during a family holiday that brings us all together. Thanksgiving is a perfect opportunity to go around the room and have each person to say what he or she is thankful for. This works well for a small dinner party, but if a large group follows the toast rules (one sip per toast), then too much drinking goes on before anyone has had a chance to start eating. Therefore the following all-encompassing toasts are my favorites for Thanksgiving, including the one toast my family is sure to say every time we all get together:

To health, wealth, love, and time to enjoy them all.
—JOSEPH HENNER

To the life we love with those we love.

From what we get, we can make a living; what we give, however, makes a life.
—ARTHUR ASHE

Thanksgiving dinner is truly a magical meal. It keeps reappearing for days.
—LINDA PERRET

To temperance—in moderation.
—LEM MOTLOW

"Say grace, Pa."

"Much obliged, Lord."
—MA AND PA KETTLE

Women, the better half of the Yankee world—at whose tender summons even the stern Pilgrims were ever ready to spring to arms, and without whose aid they could not have achieved the historic title of the Pilgrim Fathers. The Pilgrim Mothers were more devoted martyrs than were the Pilgrim Fathers, because they not only had to bear the same hardships that the Pilgrim Fathers endured, but they had to bear with the Pilgrim Fathers besides.
—JOSEPH CHOATE

| | | |
|---|---|---|
| *Thanks, I'll Eat It Here* | Lowell George | Album |
| *Thank You* | Duran Duran | Album |
| *Thank You in Advance* | Boys II Men | Album |
| *Thank You Folks* | Perry Como | Album |
| *My Thanks to You* | Connie Francis | Album |
| *The Food Album* | Weird Al Yankovic | Album |
| (anything by) | Smashing Pumpkins | Band |
| (anything by) | Grateful Dead | Band |

## MOVIES

The following films were chosen because they are either about Thanksgiving, have a Thanksgiving scene, or embody the spirit of Thanksgiving. You can watch these films to get ideas for your dinner party, or you can always pop one in to avoid getting cornered by Uncle Louie and his Bic lighter trick.

| | |
|---|---|
| *What's Cooking* | (2000—PG-13) |
| *Planes, Trains and Automobiles* | (1987—R) |
| *Hannah and Her Sisters* | (1986—PG-13) |
| *Home for the Holidays* | (1995—PG-13) |
| *Vegas Vacation* | (1997—PG-13) |
| *Soul Food* | (1997—R) |
| *Pilgrim's Progress* | (1942—NR) |
| *Friendly Persuasion* | (1956—NR) |
| *Drums Along the Mohawk* | (1939—NR) |
| *Plymouth Adventure* | (1952—NR) |
| *Mayflower: The Pilgrim's Adventure* | (1979—NR) |

## EXERCISE AND CALORIE CHART

"A spooked turkey can run at speeds up to 20 miles per hour. They can also burst into flight approaching speeds between 50 and 55 mph in a matter of seconds."

| Activity | Calories Burned/Hour |
|---|---|
| Shopping for groceries | 192 |
| Eating while shopping for groceries | 0 |
| Cleaning house for guests | 246 |
| Cleaning house for in-laws | 492 |
| Walking | 176 |
| Running | 363 |
| Touch football | 573 |
| *Friends* version | 62 |

But be careful . . .

Turkeys have heart attacks. When the air force was conducting test runs and breaking the sound barrier, fields of turkeys would drop dead.

## ETHNIC TRADITIONS

### German Thanksgiving

Long before our Pilgrim forefathers celebrated the first Thanksgiving in 1621, harvest celebrations were held all over Europe. They were called *Erntefests* and were great community gatherings celebrating the harvest of locally grown produce. Today these festivals are traditionally held in early October, on the Sunday after the full moon closest to the autumnal equinox. Although many of these Thanksgiving celebrations have their origins in pagan ritual, most are celebrated in conjunction with a special church service. In Germany, in fact, it is an official holiday called Erntedanktag (literal translation "Harvest–Thanksgiving Day"). All over Germany, festivals that include dancing, parades, games, banquets, and pageants help mark the end of the heavy labor it takes to bring in the harvest. What better way to commemorate a lot of hard work than with a big party!

### Canadian Thanksgiving

Thanksgiving Day in Canada is celebrated in much the same way as in the United States except that it is celebrated the second Monday of October because the Canadian harvest season ends earlier. Thanksgiving was brought to Canada by explorers from various countries and became a national holiday in 1879. My Canadian friends had two important things to say about their Thanksgiving: first, "It is less about the settlers and more about the harvest," and second, "We don't eat as much as you do in America." (Maybe that's why they celebrate it on a Monday. They don't need a whole weekend to recover!)

## FOR THE KIDS

Thanksgiving is even better for me now that I am a mom, and it is still my favorite meal of the year to cook. I usually prepare about fifteen dishes and about six or seven desserts with help from my boys, siblings, nieces, friends, and whoever else offers to chip in. I have cooked Thanksgiving dinner almost every year since I was six, even the years that I hosted or performed in the Macy's Thanksgiving Day Parade in New York City. Three years ago, while I was cleaning and preparing a twenty-eight-pound turkey with my boys, I let them discover the giblet bag stuffed inside. I said, "We have to clean out the turkey now, so go ahead. Put your hands in there."

They couldn't believe it. They were shocked. "What's this?" "What happened? Did he swallow his lunch?" They thought the poor turkey died from swallowing the giblet bag. They couldn't believe there was this paper bag inside containing his heart and liver and stomach. Nicky got a little squeamish, but Joey loved it! He wanted to take the heart and stomach to his room to play for a while. That's when I realized he was becoming a little *too* fascinated. I can already see him grossing out girls in his biology class. I was thinking, "Oh no! My kid's going to turn out like Jeff Spicoli in *Fast Times at Ridgemont High.*"

I know this sounds a little like *Six Feet Under* meets *Sesame Street,* but don't get the wrong idea. It was a great experience. I normally can't stand to handle animal meat, but for some reason, I never mind cleaning and preparing a turkey, I guess because it is connected to so many wonderful childhood memories. Getting the kids involved really helps build their appreciation for helping and sharing and holidays and family. It does a lot for moms, too. Seeing it through their eyes rekindles so many beautiful and warm moments and feelings.

Another way to engage your children in Thanksgiving is to make all the crafty things children love to make. Last year I set up a crafts table for my boys and their friends, and they spent hours making napkin holders, place mats, and even a centerpiece. They were so proud of their work that they even cleaned up afterward! They then reset and decorated the table with their handiwork and, for the first time, created a kids' table so they could all sit together. There's nothing like pride of ownership! Best of all, it gave them something to do during the kitchen ballet that takes place every year during the last hour and a half before dinner is ready.

## FOR COUPLES

If you're preparing Thanksgiving dinner for two: think of your partner as the turkey. Spend the day appreciating his/her individual body parts—legs, thighs, breasts, and so on. Between courses, make some time for "dressing" (or undressing) and/or "stuffing." If the two of you are celebrating your Thanksgiving dinner alone, there's no limit to how far you can go. (You can even dress like John Smith and Pocahontas if you want.) Use your imagination. But remember—whoever gets the wishbone earns an hour of "Your wish is my command."

# Hanukkah

Hanukkah is known as the holiday of miracles, but it doesn't take a miracle to get healthy. It takes dedication, which is what the word *Hanukkah* actually means. What better gift to give yourself and your family than to dedicate yourself to your health? It takes only four days to make something a habit. Why not use the eight days of Hanukkah as an opportunity to incorporate a healthy habit that could change your life?

You may want to start small. Take a few baby

steps in the right direction—but choose steps that will be effective. Let's say you want to begin an exercise program, but you don't have a lot of time because of shopping and preparing for the Hanukkah celebrations. You could walk for ten minutes on day one, long enough to get your heart rate up. If you increase it by five minutes every day, or even every other day, by the end of the eight days of Hanukkah you will be up to twenty-five to forty-five minutes at a time!

You could even use the eight days of Hanukkah and what they stand for as an opportunity to do something healthy for yourself. For example, on day one, which stands for freedom, get into the mind-set that you are going to free yourself from the tyranny of bad eating habits. On day two, which honors family, you could study your family's health history to determine a plan of action. Day three is about the Torah. After reading the holy book for inspiration, you may want to create a daily journal where you keep a log of what you eat every day, how much you exercise, and how you are feeling.

Day four is all about hope. There is always hope, because you are never too old or too young to feel better than you do right now. You just have to make the commitment to do something one day at a time, and then live up to it. Charity, which is the theme of day five, is an easy one. Give the gift of health to someone else. Buy a membership to a health club, new exercise gear, or even a copy of this book as one of your Hanukkah gifts. Or if you don't want to spend money, how about getting someone you care about to go on a walk with you? That's true charity and love. Share your newfound knowledge as you walk and talk.

Day six is about peace. This is a perfect opportunity to learn to meditate. Learning to relax and put your body in a neutral state is an integral part of any health program. You may also want to take this day as an opportunity to improve your sleeping habits. Day seven focuses on brotherhood. Part of being healthy is communicating with others. This is a great day to call someone and ask them about their health. A little interest from you may encourage them to arrange a health-related appointment. The eighth and final night of Hanukkah commemorates faith. What better way to celebrate your faith than by truly believing that this time you will do whatever it takes to live a healthier life?

Let's say that after reading this book, you've decided to try giving up dairy products. Traditionally, dairy dishes are popular at Hanukkah time. The origin of this custom is the legend of Judith, the daughter of the high priest. It is told that she entertained the leader of the enemy and served him great quantities of cheese to make him thirsty. He then drank excessive amounts of wine and passed out. This gave her the opportunity to slay him. When his soldiers found him dead, they ran away. In honor of Judith's bravery, dairy dishes are served.

I don't know about you, but that's enough to make me want to give up dairy—for life! Why not truly honor Judith and do what she did—skip the dairy altogether!

## HISTORY, FACTS, AND FOLKLORE

If you're wondering about the different spellings (Hanukkah, Chanukah, and Channukah), they're all correct, and pronounced the same (hah'-nu-ka). Hanukkah, also known as the Festival of Lights, is celebrated for eight days. It begins on the twenty-fifth day of the month of Kislev

(November/December) and honors the victory of the Jews over the Hellenist Syrians in 165 B.C. After their victory, sons of the priestly Hasmonean family, the Maccabees, who led the Jews in their revolt against the Syrian leaders, entered the Holy Temple in Jerusalem defiled by the Syrian invaders, cleaned it, and rededicated it to the service of God. Then, in memory of their victory, the Maccabees celebrated the first Hanukkah.

The Talmud, the body of Jewish law, relates how the Judean heroes were making ready to rededicate the Temple and were unable to find enough undefiled oil to light the lamps. However, in one of the Temple chambers, they finally came upon a small container of oil, which under normal circumstances would have lasted only a short time. Miraculously, this small amount of oil kept the Temple lights burning not for one night but for all the eight nights, until new oil worthy of being burned in the temple could be obtained. This is the miracle commemorated by the kindling of the Hanukkah lights.

## RECIPES
# Healthy Potato Latkes Serves 6

( green w/o applesauce / yellow w/applesauce )

*BETH EVIN HEFFNER*

2 tablespoons plus 6 teaspoons canola oil

1 medium organic Spanish onion

6 medium organic baking potatoes

2 large cage-free eggs

2 tablespoons matzo meal

½ teaspoon garlic powder

1 teaspoon salt

½ teaspoon freshly ground black pepper

Traditional Applesauce (recipe follows)

Preheat the oven to 350°F.

In a heavy nonstick saucepan over low heat, put 2 tablespoons of the oil. Add the onion and sauté until softened, about 10 minutes. Cool. Coarsely grate the potatoes into a mixing bowl. Squeeze out the excess liquid or drain in a colander. Transfer the potatoes to a bowl and mix in the sautéed onion, eggs, matzo meal, garlic powder, salt, and pepper. Grease a 12-cup nonstick muffin pan well and pour ⅓ cup potato mixture into each muffin tin. Smooth the tops lightly and spoon ½ teaspoon oil over each. Bake about 45 minutes, or until firm and brown at the edges. Remove from the oven and run a small, sturdy rubber spatula around the edges of the latkes to release them. You can leave them in the pan 15 to 30 minutes to keep hot. Serve the latkes hot with the applesauce.

## TRADITIONAL APPLESAUCE

Serves 8    (purple/blue)

- 4 pounds organic apples, cored, peeled, and quartered
- 1/2 cup Sucanat
- 1/2 teaspoon ground cinnamon
- 1 tablespoon strained fresh organic lemon juice

In a large saucepan, combine the apples, Sucanat, cinnamon, and 1/2 cup water and bring to a boil over medium-high heat. Cover and simmer 10 minutes over medium-low heat. Uncover and cook, stirring frequently, about 15 minutes, or until the apples are very tender. Cool. Use a slotted spoon to transfer the apples to a food processor. Purée the apples. Return the purée to the saucepan and simmer a few more minutes, stirring, until it is the desired thickness. Add the lemon juice and more Sucanat, if needed, stirring to blend.

## Moroccan Pepper Salad Serves 6    (blue)

- 1 organic yellow bell pepper
- 2 organic red bell peppers
- 3 medium organic tomatoes, peeled, seeded, and diced into 1/2-inch pieces
- 1/4 cup finely chopped organic flat-leaf parsley
- 3 tablespoons chopped fresh organic mint
- 1 garlic clove, minced
- 2 tablespoons extra-virgin olive oil
- 1 1/2 tablespoons red wine vinegar
- 1/2 teaspoon sweet paprika
- 1/2 teaspoon ground coriander
- 1/4 teaspoon ground cumin
- Salt and freshly ground black pepper

Preheat the grill or broiler to high. Char the peppers until the skins are black all over, about 3 to 4 minutes per side. Place the charred peppers in a brown paper bag and set aside to cool for 10 minutes. When the peppers are cool, peel and seed with a knife and cut into 1/2-inch pieces. In a large salad bowl, combine the peppers, tomatoes, parsley, mint, garlic, olive oil, vinegar, spices, and salt and pepper to taste and toss to mix. Season with any additional spices to taste.

# Bulgur Pilaf Serves 4 (blue)

- 2 tablespoons olive oil
- 1 medium organic Spanish onion, finely chopped
- 2 garlic cloves, minced
- 2 tablespoons pine nuts
- 1/4 cup finely chopped organic flat-leaf parsley
- 1 cup bulgur wheat, rinsed in a strainer and drained
- 1/2 cup cooked chickpeas
- 2 cups vegetable broth
- Salt and freshly ground black pepper

In a nonstick sauté pan over medium heat, heat the oil. Add the onion and sauté for 3 minutes, or until soft. Add the garlic, pine nuts, and 3 tablespoons of the parsley and sauté until the onion and nuts are lightly browned, 2 to 3 minutes more. Stir in the bulgur and cook until the grains are shiny, about 1 minute. Add the chickpeas, broth, and salt and pepper to taste and bring to a boil. Reduce the heat to low, cover the pot, and cook until the bulgur is tender, about 20 minutes. The broth should be completely absorbed; if it isn't, cook the pilaf uncovered for a few minutes. Remove the pan from the heat, remove the lid, cover the pan with a dish-towel, cover with the lid, and let the bulgur stand for 5 minutes to steam. Fluff the bulgur with a fork and add salt and pepper to taste. Transfer to a serving dish and sprinkle with the remaining parsley.

# Kasha Serves 6 (blue)

- 1 cup uncooked kasha
- 1 cage-free egg white
- 2 cups vegetable broth
- 1 tablespoon soy margarine
- Salt and freshly ground black pepper

In a large mixing bowl, combine the kasha with the egg white and stir until all the grains are coated with egg and shiny. Transfer the kasha to a large non-stick frying pan and cook over medium heat, stirring with a wooden spoon. Cook the kasha until the grains no longer stick together, about 2 to 3 minutes. Stir in the broth, soy margarine, and salt and pepper to taste. (I use 1 teaspoon salt and 1/4 teaspoon pepper.) When the mixture boils, reduce the heat to low and tightly cover the pan. Cook the kasha until tender and all the liquid has been absorbed, 8 to 10 minutes. Remove the pan from the heat and fluff the kasha with a fork.

## Swordfish Portuguese Serves 6 (blue)

3 pounds swordfish steaks

Salt and freshly ground black pepper

1/4 cup fresh organic lemon juice (optional)

3 tablespoons olive oil

1 large yellow onion, chopped

4 garlic cloves, minced

3 large ripe tomatoes, seeded and cut into
   1/4-inch dice

1/2 cup tomato paste

2 tablespoons maple sugar

1/2 cup dry sherry

3/4 cup dry white wine

1/2 cup chopped fresh organic parsley

Arrange the swordfish steaks in a single layer in a lightly oiled shallow baking dish. Sprinkle with salt and pepper and rub all over with the lemon juice, if using.

Heat the oil in a medium saucepan over medium-high heat. Add the onion and garlic and cook, stirring frequently, for 10 minutes, or until translucent. Stir in the tomatoes, tomato paste, maple sugar, sherry, and wine. Simmer uncovered for 15 minutes. Stir in the parsley and season to taste with salt and pepper.

Preheat the oven to 375°F. Pour the sauce over the fish in the baking dish and cover the dish tightly with aluminum foil. Bake just until the fish is cooked through, 25 to 30 minutes.

# Henri's Hanukkah Chicken  Serves 6  (blue)

1½ to 2 pounds free-range skinless, boneless chicken breast halves (6 pieces)

2 cups vegetable oil

5 tablespoons whole wheat flour

½ teaspoon salt

½ teaspoon cracked black pepper

3 medium cage-free eggs

2 teaspoons olive oil

½ cup chopped shallots

2 teaspoons chopped garlic

3 cups sliced organic portobello mushrooms

3 cups sliced organic shiitake mushrooms

1 cup sliced organic cremini mushrooms

¼ cup white wine

2 cups organic chicken stock

1 14-ounce can artichoke hearts, drained and quartered

Salt and pepper

½ cup organic chopped parsley

Preheat the oven to 350°F.

Gently pound the chicken; set aside. In a large sauté pan over medium-high heat, warm the vegetable oil. On a large plate, mix together 4 tablespoons of the flour, the salt, and pepper. In a medium bowl, lightly beat the eggs. Dredge each chicken breast in the flour mixture, shake off the excess, and then dip into the beaten eggs. Place the chicken in the hot oil and cook for 3 minutes on each side, or until golden brown. Place the chicken in a roasting pan and roast until cooked through, about 40 minutes. Transfer the chicken to a serving platter, drain the oil from the pan, add the olive oil and shallots, and sauté over medium-high heat for 2 minutes, or until soft. Add the garlic and mushrooms and sauté until golden brown, about 5 minutes. Sprinkle with the remaining tablespoon of flour and continue to cook for 30 seconds. Deglaze the pan with the wine and stock; stir in the artichokes. Bring to a boil, reduce the heat to low, and simmer until the sauce has thickened slightly, about 8 minutes. Season to taste with salt and pepper. Serve the sauce over the chicken and sprinkle with parsley.

## Mandelbrot  Makes 36 pieces  (yellow)

1 cage-free egg, plus 2 egg whites

1 cup Sucanat

1/3 cup vegetable oil

2 teaspoons vanilla extract

1/2 teaspoon almond extract

2 1/2 cups flour

2 teaspoons baking powder

Pinch of salt

1/2 cup skin-on sliced almonds

Combine the egg, egg whites, and Sucanat in the bowl of a mixer and mix at high speed until pale yellow, thick, and mousselike, about 10 minutes. Reduce the speed to low and mix in the oil and the extracts. Sift in the flour, baking powder, salt, and almonds and beat just to mix. Transfer the dough to a mixing bowl, cover, and refrigerate for at least 6 hours, or preferably overnight.

Preheat the oven to 350°F.

Wet your hands. Lightly spray a non-stick baking sheet with oil. Turn the dough onto the sheet and pat it into a rectangle about 18 inches long, 3 inches wide, and 1/2 inch high. Using a sharp knife (dip the blade in cold water), make a series of parallel, 1/2-inch-wide widthwise cuts through the top of the dough, each about 1/4 inch deep. Bake until lightly browned, 20 to 30 minutes. Transfer the loaf to a cutting board. Cut all the way through the cuts you made earlier. Return the slices to the baking sheet, keeping them 1/2 inch apart. Bake until firm and lightly browned, 5 to 10 minutes more. Let the mandelbrot cool to room temperature.

## Carrot Purée  Serves 8  (blue/green)

1 1/2 pounds carrots, peeled and cut into 2-inch pieces

4 tablespoons (1/2 stick) soy margarine

1 teaspoon maple sugar

Salt and pepper

Freshly grated nutmeg

Pinch of dried thyme

In a heavy saucepan over medium-high heat, boil the carrots, margarine, and maple sugar. Cook until very tender, about 30 to 40 minutes. Drain and purée in a blender or food processor until smooth. Season to taste with salt and pepper, nutmeg, and thyme. Serve hot.

# Basic Challah Makes 4 loaves (yellow)

4 packages dry yeast

3½ cups warm water

½ cup milled cane sugar

1¼ teaspoons salt

13 or 14 cups unbleached flour

6 cage-free eggs

1 cup vegetable oil

1 teaspoon honey

Poppy seeds (optional)

Preheat the oven to 350°F.

In a large bowl, sprinkle the yeast over the warm water and let it sit until it dissolves. Add the sugar, salt, and half the flour and mix well. Beat 5 eggs and stir in with the oil. Add in the remaining flour, 1 cup at a time. Turn the dough onto a floured board and knead for 10 minutes. If the dough is too moist, add a little more flour. When it becomes smooth, the dough is ready to rise. Place it in a large bowl, smear the top with oil, cover with a kitchen towel, and let rise for 1 hour. Set the raised dough on a baking sheet. In a small bowl, beat the remaining egg and blend with the honey. Brush this mixture on top on the dough. Separate the dough into 4 smaller portions. Braid each section of the dough into a loaf and let rise for 1 hour. Brush each with egg glaze; sprinkle with poppy seeds if desired. Bake for 1 hour, or until golden brown.

# Lemon (or Orange) Deluxe Bars

Makes 1 dozen bars (yellow)

*DEANNA LITTLE*

**CRUST:**

1 cup sifted whole wheat pastry flour

½ cup powdered Sucanat (grind it really fine in a coffee grinder)

1 cup (2 sticks) soy margarine

**FILLING:**

4 eggs, beaten

2 cups Sucanat

⅓ cup lemon or orange juice

¼ cup whole wheat pastry flour

½ teaspoon baking powder

Preheat the oven to 350°F.

To make the crust, in a large bowl, sift the flour and Sucanat together. Blend in the soy margarine until the mixture clings together. Press the mixture into a 13×9×2-inch pan. Bake for 15 to 20 minutes, or until lightly browned.

To make the filling, in a medium bowl, beat together the eggs, Sucanat, and lemon or orange juice. Sift together the flour and baking powder and stir into the egg mixture. Pour over the baked crust and bake for 25 minutes, or until the top has set. Cool and cut into bars.

## BEVERAGES

Kosher wines from Israel or France.

## PARTY IDEAS

A traditional Hanukkah observance—Hanukkah is primarily a home celebration, with the candle lighting and blessings at the center of the event. When the candles are burning, no work should be done. It is customary to have a dinner for relatives on the fifth night.

## DECORATIONS

Blue and white streamers with paper symbols of Hanukkah: Star of David, dreidel candles, flames, coins shields, latkes, Israeli flag, and so on. Menorah surrounded by Maccabee figures—Lion of Judah, Star of David, Mattathias, and so on.

## SCENTS

The smell of latkes cooking.

## ACTIVITIES AND GAMES

- Pin the Candle on the Menorah—Set up the game the same way as you would Pin the Tail on the Donkey.
- Hanukkah Says—A twist on the game Simon Says, in which orders given by Judah the Maccabee are obeyed and orders given by the king are ignored.

## MUSIC

| | | |
|---|---|---|
| *Music for Hanukkah and Purim* | Cantor Nathan Lam | Album |
| *Chanukkah Song Parade* | Various | Album |
| *Debka* | Various | Album |
| *Back from Israel* | Various | Album |
| "Eight Days a Week" | The Beatles | Song |
| "The Hanukkah Song" | Adam Sandler | Song |

## EXERCISE AND CALORIE CHART

| Activity | Calories Burned/Hour |
|---|---|
| Spinning the dreidel | 177 |

## ETHNIC TRADITIONS

- Spain and Portugal—Cheese pancakes are served, most often using pot cheese or cottage cheese.

# Toast

Blessed art Thou oh Lord our God, King of the universe, who created the fruit of the vine.
— T R A D I T I O N A L

- Poland—*Ratzelach,* a plain pancake using confectioner's sugar, is made.
- Israel—Fruit fritters and jelly-filled doughnuts or *sufganiyot* are quite popular.
- Middle East—They make couscous and a fruit compote.
- Holland—The favorite Dutch dish is known as *hutspot* (a vegetable stew), and they also make Holland brown beans, which are beans baked with goose fat and syrup.
- Italy—Sweet and sour chestnuts have been introduced into the cuisine.

# Christmas

Christmas is never about just one day. December 25 is only the peak. It's more like a month—the weeks leading up to Christmas and the week or two following it. If you've been following my advice throughout the year, your healthy habits should be second nature by this point and you are well prepared for the whole Christmas season. However, if this is your first attempt at having a healthy holiday, there are baby steps you can take to start you on your road to health. Good health practices must be as routine as brushing your teeth for you to have any hope of surviving Christmas, the biggest holiday of all. To recap and simplify, I'm going to break these healthy practices down to three basic habits to execute throughout the Christmas holiday season.

1. *Use movement to break a sweat (or at least elevate your heart rate) for several minutes every day.* It's probably cold outside, so this can be a challenge. I suggest you incorporate exercise into your regular activities. For example, wear comfortable shoes while you're Christmas shopping. I have always regretted the times I've worn high-heeled boots or fashionable shoes while shopping. Not only was I tired within a couple of hours, but the extra weight of shopping bags really took its toll on my back, since higher heels throw off your balance. Shop in an outfit that makes you feel like an athlete—think sneakers and a sweat suit. If you feel like an athlete, you will move like one, and you'll actually get a nice workout while you're shopping. Hey! You're multitasking! Also, carry your packages evenly distributed by weight, and make sure your body is aligned properly as you hold those packages. Think of the posture of a dancer: stomach in, lower back flat, pelvis pressed forward, shoulders pressed down, and head held high. Imagine a string being pulled through the top of your head.

   To find your center and proper alignment before you go out shopping, lie on your back with your knees bent and feet elevated on the seat of a chair while pressing your lower back against the floor. Feel the position your stomach muscles should be in while you are standing, and remember this alignment while you're walking throughout your day. This will improve your posture, and all those tiny muscles your body recruits to hold this alignment will get a workout as well. Professional body builders always tell you to think about the specific muscle, or muscles, you're working during every set while weight lifting. When your mind is focused on a muscle, the muscle responds more intensely. I know it sounds a little crazy, but try incorporating this kind of workout in your daily activities. Even holding your stomach tight while you're driving provides a fitness benefit in your day. You can slip these mini-workouts into any part of your day, but they work especially well with an activity like shopping. Think of it as your Christmas shopping workout. Don't wait for the video! Do it yourself today! And with sneakers on, it's a lot easier to zip in and out of crowds, too. You'll always be the first in line when a sale breaks out.

2. *Start your day with a fruit breakfast.* I know I have said this before, but it is especially important during this season. With dinner parties and other events this month, you're probably going to be eating some heavier foods at night. Heavier foods will pass through your system much more easily if your system is well hydrated and flowing freely. Unfortunately, there aren't as many fruits in season as in summer, but there are enough to satisfy you and get the job done, especially pears and apples. If you live in a warmer climate, like Southern California or Florida, you can also get fresh oranges and grapefruit. You can, of course, get tropical fruits in northern states, too, but they won't be as fresh, since they will have traveled a great distance. But do not eat melons during the winter. They are not very hardy fruit and cannot withstand traveling a great distance without losing their flavor and vitamins.

3. *Try to food-combine properly at least one or two meals a day.* Don't mix everything together at *all* your meals. During this season, you'll be staring at many party spreads and holiday buffet tables. You're probably going to miscombine Christmas dinner and most of the dinner parties you'll be attending, so do your best to properly combine your every-day nonfestive meals. That way your more indulgent meals won't do as much damage. The biggest mistake people make is that once they go off their program for one meal, they feel derailed and overindulge at every meal.

And one last thought, definitely *don't* starve all day. That is the worst mentality that you can adopt during this holiday. It's common for people to assume they can pig out at night after fasting all day. This may be the best way to pack on weight and store fat. It's much better to pace yourself and have small meals throughout the day so that your metabolism is regulated and balanced. If you arrive famished at a party, the party table becomes nothing more than gut fill, and you pay no attention to what you're eating and how you're chewing and digesting. Your brain (always twenty minutes behind your stomach) finds out much too late that you're stuffed.

If you follow just these three habits throughout the Christmas holiday, I promise you'll still enjoy yourself (perhaps more than ever), and you won't gain weight. You might even lose a few pounds!

## HISTORY, FACTS, AND FOLKLORE

Okay, here's the truth about Christmas. Jesus might not have actually been born on December 25. (Shhhhh. It's too late to rearrange the last two thousand years.) Passages in the Dead Sea Scrolls give details about the flora and fauna of Bethlehem that place Jesus' birthdate in late September or early October. (I always knew Jesus was the Libra type: balanced, just, and easily adored.) Thankfully, old habits die hard, even in the face of scientific knowledge. Plus, Rudolph would be out of a job, Santa Claus would need a cardigan, and "White Christmas" would need some serious editing. So let's all agree that Christmas is still December 25.

The Christmas tree originated in Germany in pre-Christian times. It symbolized the Garden of Eden or a tree of paradise and was decorated with gems, baubles, fruit, candles, and so on. Eventually other cultures and Christians took on the tree motif.

As for mistletoe and holly, these plants were believed to keep away goblins and bring peace—hence the kissing under the mistletoe. Though these too have their roots in a pagan traditionalism, they were adopted as symbols by Christians.

## HENNER HOLIDAY TRADITIONS AND STORIES

Ah . . . Christmas! Wonderful Christmas! It's the most important holiday of the year for many kids and adults, and the one everybody remembers most from childhood. It's the holiday that brings tons of joy—and the one most likely to leave us depressed. Throughout December Christmas is everywhere; you can't avoid it even if you don't celebrate it. Every year I still begin counting down the days to Christmas, starting in early November, just like I did when I was seven. And now I have my boys to count down the days with me.

# Christmas

Christmas at St. John Berchmans was truly special, full of anticipation, preparation, and religious ritual. Best of all was the beautiful candlelight ceremony held on the morning of our last day in school before the two-week holiday. The girls loved it because it was elegant and emotional, and the boys loved it because it meant vacation time was just around the corner. Two representatives were chosen from every grade to parade to the altar to light a candle. During the lighting, the grade being represented would sing a carefully chosen and well-rehearsed Christmas carol. The little first graders would start, and each grade took its turn until the eighth graders lit the final candle. Being chosen to be the candle person was a huge honor. It was like being picked prom king and queen, because your classmates did the voting. So I was excited when in sixth grade I was picked, and our chosen Christmas carol was "O Holy Night," to me the most sophisticated and beautiful Christmas carol of all.

When you're a child, nothing compares to waking up Christmas morning to see what Santa brought. I remember leaping out of bed to find my own little pile of toys every year. Santa had a specific spot for each of the six of us. Mine were always placed on the chair to the right of the Christmas tree. Santa never wrapped any of our presents; they were just laid out in separate piles. And there were no signs or labels; each of us just *knew* which was our pile. This made total sense to me because I figured Santa had enough to do without having to wrap and label everything. In fact, I think this made Santa more believable. I totally bought the chimney entrance, the flying reindeer, and his ability to hand-deliver 3 billion toys in one night—as long as they weren't wrapped.

By the time I was in my teens, my Christmas focused less on Santa and more on boys—the Logan Boys. My family was very popular in our neighborhood, which we called Logan Square, and it became a tradition for many of our friends from the parish to come to our house right after Midnight Mass for a late night/early morning Christmas party. Most of the guys were in a wholesome neighborhood gang called the Logan Boys—think Justin Timberlake, not Eminem.

It's hard to talk about any holiday, especially Christmas, without mentioning my eccentric bohemian uncle who lived upstairs. He was the Michelangelo of Logan Square, and everyone knew him, or knew of him, even though he rarely left his apartment except to teach art at St. John's. From years of studying at the Art Institute and experience acquired while designing windows at Marshall Field's department store downtown, he sculpted the most beautiful lifelike (and life-size) Madonna and child out of chicken wire and plaster of Paris. He encased the holy pair in a huge round pastel blue frame about six feet high and three feet deep. It was really special! The Virgin Mary was gorgeous, with soft, fleshy, porcelain-smooth skin and chiseled runway model features. My uncle would place the sculpture out on our front lawn every year and decorate it with Christmas wreaths and lights. But he was such a crazy perfectionist that he would put it out only after a light, billowy snowfall. He needed perfect weather conditions to display his perfect work of art. The whole neighborhood was familiar with it, especially the church. The pastor blessed it, and the nuns often knelt before it to say rosaries, even in the snow. He stored the sculpture year-round in the dark hallway outside his apartment door, and it was always a little scary to stare into Mary's eyes while waiting outside his door. I always expected her to come to life and grab me.

Buying presents for everyone in the family has always been a lot of fun, no matter how old we are. In 1983 I started the Henner Family Survey, which you'll find on page 354. At that time, we all lived in different parts of the country and met in Chicago for Christmas. I got the idea for the survey when I realized that we were all still buying each other presents based on our childhood understanding of each other's likes and dislikes. We needed to get reacquainted with each other's current interests and tastes. The survey is a great guide for shopping so that everybody gets presents they really want. Best of all, the surveys have become a great family record of how our styles, curiosities, and credos have evolved over the years. I've saved every single one since 1983.

The survey has grown and changed over the years. At first I designed it to focus mostly on clothing styles, colors, sizes, likes, and dislikes, and it also asked lifestyle questions: which current events, locations, films, art, and music each person was into that year. By the second year, I thought it would be fun to let everyone submit a soul-revealing kind of question, and those twenty-five or so questions have become the second (and definitely most interesting) part of the survey.

Along with changes in the survey, we have also changed the way we give each other gifts over the years. We usually do a grab bag now because there are thirty-five of us (and growing!) in the immediate family. It's especially fun to do a grab bag with the kids—they get so excited when they pick a name and look for the right gifts, and they love the secrecy of it all. We've also done themed gifts like travel and toys from childhood, and a few years ago we did recycled gifts. This is the best choice when your family wants to save money. You do all your shopping in your own house by looking through your wardrobe, bookcase, or CD collection and picking out items you no longer use that might be perfect for someone else, based on their surveys. This way of gift-giving takes the pressure off family members who may not have the money or time to shop for Christmas. It also inspires creativity because it takes investigation and ingenuity, and it can lead to some heartfelt moments as you give away something you once loved.

One year we did a grab bag called the White Elephant Christmas Grab Bag. It led to some of the funniest gift exchanges ever. My brother Lorin was finally able to dump his twenty-pound plaster bear claw imprint from Yosemite on Rob. Obviously Lorin didn't read Rob's survey that year, because I'm pretty sure Rob didn't mention anything about wanting grizzly prints. Lorin saved the bear claw after he found that Rob had tossed it in the garbage right after the party. He patiently waited for seven months, rewrapped it, and gave it to Rob again for his birthday in July. It's become their "old maid" present. You never know which event it's going to pop up at next.

Christmas in my family has gone through four periods. When we were little kids, it focused on Santa. During our teen years, it was all about boyfriends and dating. Then Christmas seemed to be one big sophisticated adult's party. It was like the show *thirtysomething* with my siblings and their spouses. And now we have children of our own, and the focus is on Santa again. It's come full circle. I love seeing Christmas through my children's eyes. It's like reliving my childhood, but now it's a retro version. Many things are the same, but much is different, too. I have them sit on Santa Claus's lap, but I also have them fill out little surveys.

Christmas is a never-ending source of family memories and love. I don't care how much energy it takes, it's always worth it. I love Christmas, and I always will!

## RECIPES
# Salad of Fall Greens with Persimmons

Serves 10    (green)

3/4 cup fresh tangerine juice

1 tablespoon grated tangerine zest

1/2 cup vegetable oil

1/4 cup walnut oil

2 tablespoons balsamic vinegar

1/2 teaspoon salt

1/4 teaspoon ground cinnamon

Pepper

1 head escarole (about 12 cups)

1 large bunch watercress, stems removed
(about 6 cups)

1 5-ounce package mixed baby greens

2 Fuyu persimmons, peeled, halved, and
thinly sliced

1/2 cup hazelnuts, toasted, skin rubbed off,
and coarsely chopped

In a heavy small saucepan over medium-high heat, boil the tangerine juice and zest until reduced to 1/4 cup, about 5 minutes. Transfer to a medium bowl. Whisk in the oils, vinegar, salt, and cinnamon and season to taste with pepper. Place all the greens and half of the persimmon slices in a large bowl. Add the dressing and toss to coat. Divide among ten plates and top with the hazelnuts and the remaining persimmon slices.

# Harmony Holiday Delight

Serves 8 (blue/green)

*This hearty dish can stand in for the turkey.*

3 tablespoons vegetable oil

1 cup coarsely chopped organic shiitake
mushroom caps

1½ tablespoons peeled minced fresh organic
ginger

4 organic garlic cloves, minced

2 cups fresh or thawed frozen shelled organic
edamame (green soybeans)

1 cup frozen organic whole kernel corn

½ cup fat-free organic soy milk

1 tablespoon rice vinegar

2 teaspoons low-sodium tamari sauce

⅛ teaspoon ground white pepper

16 English cucumber slices

16 organic plum tomato slices

2 tablespoons toasted organic black sesame
seeds (optional)

In a large nonstick skillet over medium-high heat, heat the oil. Add the mushrooms, ginger, and garlic, and sauté in the oil for 2 minutes, mixing well. Add the edamame and stir-fry 1 minute. Stir in the corn, soy milk, and vinegar and cook until the liquid almost evaporates (about 3 minutes). Remove from the heat, and stir in the tamari and white pepper.

Spoon the edamame mixture into the center of a large platter; arrange the cucumber and tomato slices alternately around the mixture. Garnish with the sesame seeds, if desired.

# Roast Turkey with Apples, Onions, and Apple Cider Gravy

Serves 8 (green)

1 12- to 14-pound turkey, neck and giblets (but not the liver) reserved for stock

Salt and freshly ground black pepper

1 pound pearl onions

2 pounds Lady apples, peeled, cored, and cut into 2-inch cubes (16 to 20 apples)

6 tablespoons (3/4 stick) soy margarine, melted

Pan juices from turkey

4 cups Roasted Turkey Giblet Stock (page 301)

1 cup apple cider

2 tablespoons apple cider vinegar

1/4 cup whole wheat flour

Preheat the oven to 425°F.

Rinse the turkey well inside and out and pat dry. Season inside and out with salt and pepper. Fold the neck skin under the body and secure with a small skewer. Tie the drumsticks together with kitchen string and secure the wings to the body with small skewers. Put the turkey on a rack set in a large roasting pan. Roast the turkey in the middle of the oven for 20 to 30 minutes; this helps crisp the skin later. Then reduce the heat to 350°F. While the turkey is roasting, in a medium saucepan of boiling water, blanch the onions 1 minute. Rinse under cold water. Peel the onions. In two separate bowls, toss the onions and apples with 1 tablespoon melted margarine each and salt and pepper to taste. Brush the remaining 4 tablespoons melted margarine over the turkey and roast 30 minutes more. Baste the turkey and scatter the onions around it, then roast 30 minutes more. Baste the turkey and add the apples to the roasting pan. Roast another 1 to 1½ hours, or until a thermometer inserted into the fleshy part of a thigh registers 180°F. Transfer the turkey, onions, and apples to a heated platter, leaving the juices in the pan. Remove the skewers and discard the string. Let the turkey stand at least 30 or up to 45 minutes.

While the turkey stands, make the gravy. Skim the fat from the pan juices and reserve ¼ cup of fat. Pour the pan juices into a 2-quart glass measure and add enough turkey giblet stock to make 4½ cups total. Set the roasting pan to straddle two burners. Add 1 cup of the stock mixture and deglaze by boiling over moderately high heat, stirring and scraping up the brown bits. Add the remaining 3½ cups stock mixture, cider, and vinegar and bring to a simmer. Transfer to a glass measuring cup.

Whisk together the reserved ¼ cup of fat and the flour in a large heavy saucepan and cook the roux over medium-low heat, whisking, 3 minutes, until the flour dissolves. Add the hot stock mixture in a fast stream, whisking constantly to prevent lumps, and then simmer, whisking occasionally, until thickened, about 10 minutes. Stir in additional turkey juices from the platter and season the gravy with salt and pepper to taste. Pour the gravy through a fine sieve into a gravy boat.

# Rosemary Roast Chicken Serves 4 (blue)

1 3- to 3½-pound organic free-range chicken, rinsed, giblets removed

4 organic garlic cloves

6 fresh organic rosemary sprigs, plus a few more for garnish

3 tablespoons extra-virgin olive oil

2 teaspoons kosher salt

Freshly ground black pepper

Preheat the oven to 400°F.

Pull the fat from inside the chicken and discard. Set the chicken in a small roasting pan and put the whole garlic cloves under the skin in the meatiest part of the chicken. Stuff the chicken with 3 rosemary sprigs. Pour the oil over chicken and sprinkle it with the salt and pepper to taste. Rub the oil and seasonings into the chicken. Tuck 3 rosemary sprigs under the chicken. Roast the chicken, uncovered, basting occasionally, about 1 hour, or until the chicken juices run clear. Remove the rosemary from the chicken and from the pan. Carve the chicken and put the pieces on a platter. Garnish with fresh rosemary sprigs. Skim the excess fat from the roasting juices and add salt and pepper to taste. When serving, spoon a little of the pan juices over the chicken.

# Salt-Baked Fish Serves 4 (purple)

1 pound red snapper fillet

Cracked black pepper

14 fresh organic flat-leaf parsley sprigs

10 pounds coarse rock salt

Preheat the oven to 425°F.

Wash the fish and pat it dry. Sprinkle the inside cavities of the fish well with pepper and stuff with the parsley sprigs. Spread two baking trays with half the salt. Place the fish on the baking trays and cover with the remaining salt. Press the salt firmly around the fish and sprinkle with a little water. Bake for 15 minutes, remove the trays from the oven, and let the fish sit for 5 minutes before serving. Remove the salt in large pieces and place the fish on serving plates.

# Cornish Game Hens with Juniper Berries and Beets Serves 4 (green)

- 4 medium beets with greens, beets peeled and cut into ½-inch pieces, greens finely chopped
- 1 tablespoon coarsely chopped juniper berries
- Salt and pepper
- 4 1½- to 1¾-pound Cornish hens, giblets removed
- 2 tablespoons olive oil

Position one rack in the top third of the oven and the second rack in the bottom third of the oven. Preheat the oven to 375°F.

Mix 1½ cups of the chopped beet greens and the juniper berries in a medium bowl. Season to taste with salt and pepper. Fill the hens' cavities with the greens mixture, dividing equally. Tie the hens' legs together. Place the hens in a heavy large roasting pan and rub 1 tablespoon of the olive oil over them. Sprinkle the hens with salt and pepper. (This can be prepared 8 hours ahead; cover and refrigerate.)

Roast the hens on the bottom oven rack until golden and the juices run clear when the thickest part of the thigh is pierced, about 1 hour 15 minutes. Meanwhile, toss the chopped beets with the remaining tablespoon of olive oil on a large, heavy baking sheet. Season to taste with salt and pepper. Arrange the beets in a single layer. Roast the beets on the top rack until tender and beginning to caramelize, stirring occasionally, about 45 minutes.

Transfer the hens to plates and remove the string. Scrape up any browned bits from the bottom of the roasting pan. Pour the pan juices through a sieve into a 2-cup glass measuring cup. Spoon the fat off the top of the pan juices. Spoon the beets around the hens, drizzle the pan juices around the hens, and serve.

Due to the time zones, Santa has thirty-one hours to deliver gifts. This means visiting 832 homes each second! I suggest saving him some time. Leave out just one cookie and serve the soy milk in a shot glass.

# Whole Roasted Yams with Maple-Allspice Butter Serves 8 (green)

1 cup (2 sticks) soy margarine, at room
   temperature

¼ cup maple syrup

½ teaspoon salt

½ teaspoon ground allspice

½ teaspoon ground black pepper

8 small yams (red-skinned sweet potatoes),
   lightly pierced all over with a fork

In a medium bowl, mix the margarine, maple syrup, salt, allspice, and pepper. (This can be made up to 3 days ahead; cover and refrigerate, but bring back to room temperature before using.)

Preheat the oven to 375°F.

Set the yams directly on the oven rack and roast until tender when pierced with a skewer, about 1 hour. Cut a cross on the top of each yam. Using oven mitts to protect your hands, squeeze the yams gently in from the sides, forcing the crosses to open. Spoon 1 tablespoon of the soy margarine mixture onto each potato. Serve, passing the remaining margarine mixture separately.

# Honey-Baked Winter Vegetables

Serves 6 (green)

3 tablespoons honey

2 tablespoons (¼ stick) soy margarine,
   melted

¼ teaspoon salt

1 pound organic carrots, cut into 4 × ½-inch
   sticks

1 pound organic rutabagas, cut into
   4 × ½-inch sticks

Preheat the oven to 375°F.

In a large bowl, combine the honey, melted margarine, and salt. Stir well. Add the carrots and rutabagas and toss to coat the vegetables. Spray a 15 × 10 × 1-inch jelly roll pan with cooking spray and arrange the carrot and rutabaga sticks in a single layer. Bake for 1 hour, or until golden. Serve.

## Carrots and Rutabagas with Lemon and Honey  Serves 8    (green)

*Lemon juice adds a refreshing flavor to earthy root vegetables.*

1¼ pounds rutabagas, peeled and cut into
   matchstick-size strips

1 pound carrots, peeled and cut into
   matchstick-size strips

¼ cup (½ stick) soy margarine

¼ cup fresh organic lemon juice

3 tablespoons honey

1 teaspoon grated lemon zest

Salt and pepper

½ cup chopped fresh chives

In a large pot of boiling salted water, cook the rutabagas for 2 minutes. Add the carrots and cook until the vegetables are tender, about 6 minutes. Drain.

In a large pot over medium-high heat, melt the margarine. Add the lemon juice, honey, and lemon zest. Bring to a boil. Add the vegetables and cook until glazed, stirring occasionally, about 6 minutes. Season to taste with salt and pepper and mix in the chives.

## Roasted Asparagus with Garlic

Serves 4    (blue)

2 bunches organic asparagus (about 2
   pounds)

4 tablespoons extra-virgin olive oil

5 organic garlic cloves, finely chopped

½ teaspoon coarse sea salt

Freshly milled black pepper

Preheat the oven to 450°F.

With a vegetable peeler, peel off the last inch of tough stalk on each asparagus spear. Arrange the spears on a baking sheet in a single layer. In a small bowl, mix the oil, garlic, salt, and pepper. Add to the asparagus and roll to coat. Roast about 10 minutes, or until crisp and tender.

Americans produce 5 million extra tons of trash each year between Thanksgiving and New Year's Day.

# Roasted Cauliflower and Sweet Peppers

Serves 4 (green)

4 tablespoons freshly squeezed organic
lemon juice

3 tablespoons extra-virgin olive oil

2 tablespoons Bragg's Liquid Aminos

1 teaspoon salt

1 teaspoon ground cumin seeds

1 teaspoon ground coriander

1/2 teaspoon hot red pepper flakes

1 organic cauliflower (about 2 pounds),
cored and separated into florets

1 large organic red bell pepper, halved,
seeded, and sliced into 1-inch-wide strips

1 large organic yellow bell pepper, halved,
seeded, and sliced into 1-inch-wide strips

1/2 cup fresh organic cilantro leaves

Preheat the oven to 450°F.

In a large bowl, whisk together the lemon juice, oil, Bragg's, salt, ground cumin, coriander, cumin seeds, and red pepper flakes. Add the cauliflower and bell peppers and toss well. In a large baking dish, spread out the vegetables and roast for 45 minutes, or until well browned, stirring every 15 minutes. Transfer the vegetables to a serving dish, garnish with fresh cilantro leaves, and serve.

Three years after Thomas Edison invented the electric light bulb in 1879, Edward H. Johnson, who worked for Edison's company, had Christmas tree bulbs especially made for him. He proudly displayed his electric tree lights at his home on Fifth Avenue, New York City. They caused a sensation, although some years were to pass before mass-manufactured Christmas tree lights were widely available.

The custom of trimming and lighting a Christmas tree had its origin in pre-Christian Germany, the tree symbolizing the Garden of Eden. It was called the "Paradise Baum," or tree of paradise. Gradually, the custom of decorating the tree with cookies, fruit, and eventually candles evolved. Other countries soon adapted the custom. Charles Dickens called it the "pretty German toy." — d i d y o u k n o w . c o m

Christmas

## Herbed Shallot Stuffing Serves 10 (green)

*This stuffing goes great with Roast Turkey with Apples, Onions, and Apple Cider Gravy (page 334).*

2 cups finely chopped shallots

1 cup (1 stick) soy margarine

10 cups fresh bread crumbs (from 2 long baguettes; 1 pound total)

3 tablespoons chopped fresh tarragon

3 tablespoons chopped fresh chives

3 tablespoons chopped fresh Italian parsley

1 tablespoon kosher salt

1 teaspoon ground black pepper

3 tablespoons vermouth

1 to 1½ cups organic chicken broth

Preheat the oven to 325°F.

In a large, heavy skillet over medium-low heat, sauté the shallots in the margarine until the margarine is melted and the shallots are slightly softened, about 5 minutes. In a large bowl, combine the bread crumbs, tarragon, chives, parsley, salt, and pepper and stir in the margarine mixture. Drizzle with the vermouth, tossing to combine, and gently stir in the broth. (Use 1½ cups broth if you like a moist stuffing or 1 cup if you prefer it drier.) Transfer the stuffing to a buttered shallow 3-quart baking dish. Cover with foil and bake in the middle of the oven for 30 minutes, then uncover and bake until the top is crisp and the stuffing is heated through, about 30 minutes more.

## Garlic Mashed Potatoes Serves 4 (green)

*When garlic is added, this classic comfort food thrills both the squealing child and the sophisticated adult lurking within.*

2 pounds small red potatoes, unpeeled, or Yukon Gold, peeled and quartered

2 garlic cloves, smashed

1 teaspoon salt

½ cup soy cream

½ teaspoon paprika

2 tablespoons soy Parmesan cheese

Pepper

Place the potatoes in a medium pot over medium-high heat, and cover them with water. Add the garlic and salt. Bring to a boil and simmer for 15 to 20 minutes, or until the potatoes are tender. Drain the potatoes and garlic and return them to pot. Add the soy cream, paprika, soy Parmesan cheese, and salt and pepper to taste. Mash all the ingredients together. For a creamier texture, use a whisk.

# Baking Powder Biscuits Serves 8 (green)

2 cups flour

1 tablespoon baking powder

1/2 teaspoon salt

4 tablespoons (1/2 stick) cold soy margarine

3/4 cup soy milk

Preheat the oven to 450°F.

In a large bowl, stir together the flour, baking powder, and salt. With a pastry blender or two knives used scissor fashion, cut in the margarine until the mixture resembles coarse crumbs. Stir in the soy milk just until the mixture forms a soft dough that leaves the sides of the bowl. Turn the dough onto a lightly floured surface; knead 6 to 8 times, just until smooth. With a floured rolling pin, roll the dough 1/2 inch thick for high, fluffy biscuits or 1/4 inch thick for thin, crusty ones. Using a biscuit cutter or a glass dipped in flour, cut out biscuits from the dough. Place them on a baking sheet and bake for 12 minutes, or until golden.

# Sweet Potato Biscuits Serves 8 (yellow)

*SUSAN ROMITO*

1 pound sweet potatoes (about 2 medium)

2 1/4 cups all-purpose baking mix

1/4 to 1/2 cup Sucanat

3 tablespoons soy milk

Preheat the oven to 425°F. In a medium saucepan over high heat, cook the potatoes until tender, about 20 to 25 minutes. Drain, cool, peel, and mash the potatoes. Transfer the potatoes to a large bowl and add the baking mix and Sucanat. Add enough soy milk to form a soft dough. Turn the dough out onto a lightly floured surface and pat it to make a 1/2-inch-thick round. Using a 2 1/2-inch round biscuit cutter, cut out biscuits. Transfer to a greased baking sheet and bake until golden brown, about 18 minutes. These biscuits are best served warm with a little Earth Balance margarine!

Eighty-four percent of Americans would prefer a less materialistic holiday, but Christmas retail sales increased 7 percent in the year 2000— *Eugene Weekly*

It takes an average of six months for a credit-card user to pay off holiday bills.

The total U.S. credit card debt is more than $450 billion and is growing at a rate twice that of wage increases. The number of personal bankruptcies has quadrupled in the last fifteen years.

## Caramel Walnut Tart  Serves 10    (yellow)

SWEET PASTRY CRUST:

> 1 cup unbleached flour
>
> ¼ teaspoon salt
>
> 7 tablespoons cold soy margarine, cut up
>
> 2 to 3 tablespoons ice water

TART:

> 1 cup Sucanat
>
> ¼ teaspoon fresh lemon juice
>
> ¾ cup soy cream
>
> 1 tablespoon soy margarine
>
> 1 large cage-free egg
>
> ½ teaspoon vanilla extract
>
> 1 cup toasted walnuts

To make the pastry crust, in a large bowl, mix the flour and the salt. With a pastry blender or two knives used scissor fashion, cut in the soy margarine until the mixture resembles coarse crumbs. Sprinkle in the ice water, 1 tablespoon at a time, mixing lightly with a fork after each addition, until the dough is just moist enough to hold together.

Shape the dough into a disk, wrap in plastic, and refrigerate 30 minutes or overnight. If chilled overnight, let stand at room temperature 30 minutes before rolling.

Roll the dough into an 11-inch round and fit into a 9×1-inch round tart pan with a removable bottom. Fold the overhang in and press against the side of the tart pan to create a ⅛-inch rim above the edge of the pan. Refrigerate or freeze 10 to 15 minutes to firm the pastry before baking.

Preheat the oven to 375°F.

Line the tart shell with foil and fill with pie weights, dry beans, or uncooked rice. Bake 15 minutes. Remove the foil and weights and bake 8 to 10 minutes longer, or until golden brown. Transfer to a wire rack. Lower the oven heat to 350°F.

To make the tart, in a heavy 2-quart saucepan, stir the Sucanat and lemon juice together. Cook over low heat, stirring gently, until the Sucanat melts. Increase the heat to medium and cook until amber in color. (With a pastry brush dipped in water, occasionally wash down the sides of the pan to prevent the Sucanat from crystallizing.) Remove the saucepan from the heat. Add the soy cream to the pan gradually, stirring constantly; the mixture will bubble vigorously. Add the margarine, return the pan to low heat, and stir until the caramel dissolves. Cool.

In a large bowl, whisk the egg and vanilla until smooth. Add the cooled caramel mixture and whisk until blended. Sprinkle the walnuts over the cooled shell and pour the caramel mixture on top. Bake 30 to 35 minutes, until bubbly at the edges but still slightly jiggly in the center. Cool on a wire rack 10 minutes. Carefully remove the side of the pan; cool completely.

# Chocolate Almond Toffee Crunch

Makes 20 to 24 pieces     (yellow)

*SUSAN ROMITO*

- 1 sleeve all-natural saltine or graham crackers
- 1 cup (2 sticks) Earth Balance margarine
- ½ cup Sucanat
- 3 ounces sliced almonds
- 12 ounces Tropical Source semisweet chocolate chips (or espresso roast for a more decadent taste)

Preheat the oven to 375°F.

Line a cookie sheet with foil, making sure it goes up the sides. Place a single layer of crackers on the sheet, covering it completely. In a medium saucepan, melt the margarine and Sucanat, whisking the whole time, just until it starts to get frothy and the slightest golden brown. Do not caramelize and do not let the Sucanat dissolve completely. Pour the mixture over the crackers, using a spatula to cover as evenly as you can. Bake immediately for 7 minutes, or until caramel colored. Sprinkle the crackers with the almonds, then the chocolate chips, and bake for 2 to 3 minutes more, until the chips are soft. Swirl the chips with a butter knife to spread the chocolate over the surface. Cool, then refrigerate about 30 minutes until the chocolate is set. Cut into bars or break into pieces. Store in the refrigerator.

# Sweet Christmas Nuts   Serves 12     (green)

- 1 teaspoon canola oil
- ¾ tablespoon soy margarine
- ½ cup Sucanat
- ¾ teaspoon salt
- ⅛ teaspoon ground cinnamon
- 1 teaspoon vanilla extract
- ¾ cup almonds
- ¾ cup pecans
- ¾ cup walnuts

Coat a baking sheet with the canola oil and set aside. In a large skillet over medium heat, melt the margarine. Add the Sucanat and salt and stir constantly until it starts to caramelize, about 10 minutes. Remove from the heat and add the vanilla, almonds, pecans, and walnuts. Stir just until the nuts are coated. Transfer to a baking sheet. When completely cooled, break apart and store in an airtight container.

# Lumberjacks Makes 72 to 96 cookies (yellow)

*MARY BETH BORKOWSKI*

- 1 cup evaporated cane juice crystals, plus
  - ½ cup for rolling the dough
- 1 cup (2 sticks) Earth Balance margarine
- 1 cup blackstrap molasses
- 2 organic cage-free eggs
- 4 cups flour
- 1 teaspoon baking soda
- 2 teaspoons ground cinnamon
- 1 teaspoon ground ginger

Preheat the oven to 350°F.

In a large bowl, cream together the cane juice crystals and margarine. Add the molasses and eggs and blend completely. In another large bowl, blend the flour, baking soda, cinnamon, and ginger. Add the dry ingredients to the molasses mixture and mix completely.

Have at hand a small bowl of cane juice crystals. Pinch off a ball of dough the size of a walnut. Roll it in the crystals and place on a cookie sheet. Repeat with the rest of the dough. Bake for 12 to 15 minutes, or until golden.

## BEVERAGES

- Hot apple cider—with cinnamon sticks
- Hot cocoa made with Rice Dream
- Soy Dream eggnog by Imagine Foods

For grown-up tastes, with or without the alcohol:

## THM EGGNOG

- 4 ounces Silk Vanilla Creamer or Soymilk
- 1 whole egg or 2 egg whites
- Pinch of salt
- ¼ teaspoon pure vanilla extract
- 1½ ounces brandy or rum (optional)
- Grated nutmeg

Blend together well the creamer, egg, salt, and vanilla. Slowly add the liquor, if using. Pour into a highball or Collins glass, sprinkle with the nutmeg, and serve.

# CINNAMINT CAPPUCCINO Serves 3

- 3 cups low-fat soy milk or rice milk
- 2 cups water-processed decaf coffee
- 1 bunch fresh mint leaves, about ½ cup tightly packed, plus 6 to 9 leaves for garnish
- 4 cinnamon sticks or ½ teaspoon ground cinnamon
- Sucanat
- 1 teaspoon mint syrup or 2 tablespoons white crème de menthe (optional)

In a medium saucepan or a microwave-safe bowl, combine 2 cups of the soy milk, the coffee, mint, and cinnamon. Heat over medium heat or in the microwave just until the liquid starts to steam and a few bubbles appear; don't let it boil. Set aside and let steep for at least 15 minutes and as long as 1 hour.

For the foamed milk, heat the remaining 1 cup of soy milk in the microwave or in a small saucepan over low heat. Place the milk and Sucanat to taste in the blender and cover with a vented lid. Switch the blender on and off quickly to avoid splashing overflows, and then continue blending until frothy, about 30 seconds.

Pour the coffee-mint mixture through a clean strainer into a pitcher or larger measuring cup; if it has cooled, reheat without letting it come to a boil. Stir in the optional mint syrup or crème de menthe. Divide the coffee among three mugs and spread foamed milk over each one. Garnish with 2 or 3 mint leaves.

# HOT TODDY

- 2 ounces R.W. Knudsen's unsweetened Cider and Spice (or similar all-natural product)
- 1½ ounces whiskey or rum (optional)
- 4 ounces boiling water
- Cinnamon stick (optional)

Pour the cider and spice and whiskey, if using, into a coffee mug. Add the boiling water and garnish with a cinnamon stick, if desired.

# POLAR BEAR

*Warning: not lo-cal!*

- 2 ounces Silk French Vanilla Soylatte
- 2 ounces Silk Soy Creamer or regular soy milk
- 1½ ounces vodka (optional)

Combine the soylatte, creamer, and vodka, if using, over ice. Shake or stir, pour into a rocks glass, and serve.

## THM MOCK KAHLÚA AND CREAM
*Warning: not lo-cal!*

2 ounces Silk Coffee Soylatte

2 ounces Silk Vanilla Creamer or soy milk

1½ ounces vodka (optional)

Grated nutmeg or ground cinnamon
  (optional)

Combine the soylatte, creamer, and vodka, if using, over ice. Shake or stir, pour into a rocks glass, and serve. Sprinkle with nutmeg or cinnamon, if you like.

## PARTY IDEAS
- Pre-Christmas party—a great way to celebrate the holiday with friends, especially if you're going to be out of town on the big day
- Caroling party—An opportunity to gather friends who are game and dressed warmly
- Christmas Eve dinner—A tradition in my family, usually cooked by the men while the women wrap and prepare the gifts
- Christmas Day dinner—A big sit-down feast with all the trimmings

## INVITATIONS
- Print the information on a special Christmas card or ornament that can be assembled and hung on the tree.
- Send a small booklet of traditional Christmas carols, which can be sung at the party or while caroling around the neighborhood. I have done this a few years in a row at a friend's house, and it's a lot of fun. She passed out candles, and the entire party made its way around the neighborhood.
- Design your own Christmas cards that tell something about you.
- Create personalized cards that are unique to each person, saying something special about them.
- Send a special photo that tells someone about your year.

## DECORATIONS
The usual Christmas decorations, of course, but you may also want to add something at each person's table setting to make your guests feel special. My friends Barbara and Marvin Davis throw the best Hollywood Christmas party, complete with carolers, strolling violinists, ice skaters, and snow (in LA!). The first time I went to one of their Christmas parties, I had just given birth to Joey three weeks earlier. I went there alone because Rob was out of town, and the whole party was swirling around me. I'd never seen a party like this in my life, but when I got to my place and saw my name written on a personalized ornament, it made me feel special and like I really belonged. Barbara always manages to make you feel important and connected by adding a personal touch. Believe me, anything that does this for your guests will be greatly appreciated.

# Toasts

Christmas is the perfect time of year to celebrate with your family, especially if it's the only time you all get together. Why not start a dinner ritual that's inspired by a Polish tradition? Go around the room and have each person say something brief but meaningful about each other person. If there are too many people, have each person say something about the person to their right. You'll be amazed how warm, cozy, and funny this becomes.

It is Christmas in the heart that puts Christmas in the air.
—W. T. Ellis

I will honor Christmas in my heart, and try to keep it all year.
—Charles Dickens

God bless us every one.
—Charles Dickens

## SCENTS

Pine
Peppermint
Holly berry
Bayberry
Cranberry
Gingerbread
Christmas cookie
Cinnamon
Chocolate
Vanilla
Pecan
Orange and clove

## ACTIVITIES AND GAMES

- Organize a Christmas grab bag.
- Make personalized tree ornaments for each family member as a gift, then hang them on your tree every year.
- Special stockings—Take a sock from each family member and decorate it with sequins, glitter, cotton, yarn, and whatever else would make it personal.
- Christmas caroling—Practice singing your favorite tunes together (in simple harmony, too, if possible). If you're feeling creative, write your own special lyrics and make your own arrangements of songs. Each child who can play an instrument should bring one. Try to coordinate your caroling outfits, with matching scarves and hats, or you can even go Dickensian if you have the wardrobe. Going to a local hospital or retirement home with a large group can be very rewarding.

Christmas

- Make a meal for the homeless, or grocery-shop for people in need, and surprise them with a package of wholesome goodies at their doorstep.

## PRIZES, GIFTS, AND PARTY FAVORS

- Ornaments for each person to take home to their tree
- Donations to a special charity given in your guest's name
- Kits designed for a person's personal talent: an art kit with paint, clay, crayons, and paper; a photographer's kit of film, a photo book, lenses and batteries; a musician's kit of music, staff notation paper, and pencils
- A box of thank-you cards (if you really want to be generous, prestamp the envelopes)
- A personalized calendar that you design for each person
- An outing with a family member you don't ordinarily spend time with, or a dinner for your parents
- A concert, a play, a dinner, a vacation
- A personalized photo album, or a special engraved souvenir

## MUSIC

| | | |
|---|---|---|
| *The Nightmare Before Christmas* | Danny Elfman | Soundtrack |
| *Once Upon a Christmas* | Kenny Rogers and Dolly Parton | Album |
| *Christmas* | Lynrd Skynrd | Album |
| *Christmas Through the Years* | Louis Armstrong | Album |
| *Christmas and the Beads of Sweat* | Laura Nyro | Album |
| *Christmas Memories* | Barbra Streisand | Album |
| *Mr. Hankey's Christmas Classics* | South Park | Album |
| *A Christmas Celebration of Hope* | B. B. King | Album |
| *Merry Christmas* | Mariah Carey | Album |
| *A Charlie Brown Christmas* | Various | Soundtrack |
| *I Believe in Father Christmas* | Emerson, Lake & Palmer | Album |
| *The Harlem Nutcracker* | Duke Ellington and Billy Strayhorn | Album |
| *Christmas Album* | Four Seasons | Album |
| *How the Grinch Stole Christmas* | Various | Soundtrack |
| *Jackson 5 Christmas Album* | Jackson 5 | Album |
| *Grace* | Jeff Buckley | Album |

## MOVIES

| | |
|---|---|
| *White Christmas* | (1954–NR) |
| *Holiday Inn* | (1942–NR) |
| *A Christmas Carol* | (1938, 1951–NR) |
| *It's a Wonderful Life* | (1946–NR) |
| *A Christmas Story* | (1983–PG) |
| *Miracle on 34th Street* | (1947, 1973–NR; 1994–PG) |
| *How the Grinch Stole Christmas* | (2001–PG) |
| *Scrooge* | (1935–NR; 1970–G) |
| *Scrooged* | (1988–PG-13) |
| *A Christmas to Remember* | (1978–NR) |
| *The Nightmare Before Christmas* | (1993–PG) |
| *The Santa Clause* | (1994–PG) |
| *All I Want for Christmas* | (1991–G) |
| *The Homecoming* | (1971–NR) |
| *Christmas in Connecticut* | (1945–NR) |
| *Desk Set* | (1957–NR) |
| *Die Hard* | (1988–R) |

Two-thirds of Americans say they would be happier if they had more time to spend with family and friends. Only 15 percent say they'd be happier if they had nicer possessions.
—*Eugene Weekly*

Real Christmas trees are an all-American product, grown in all fifty states, including Alaska and Hawaii.

For every Christmas tree harvested, two to three seedlings are planted in its place.

The biggest-selling Christmas single of all time is Bing Crosby's "White Christmas."

## EXERCISE AND CALORIE CHART

| Activity | Calories Burned/Hour |
|---|---|
| Shopping for gifts in dress shoes | 176 |
| Shopping for gifts in sneakers | 320 |
| Wrapping gifts | 160 |
| Opening gifts | 160 |
| Returning gifts | 176 |

Wrapping gifts is not much of a workout, and most people are not interested in group sports on Christmas. The best thing is to find one hearty person who is willing to walk or run while dinner is cooking.

## ETHNIC TRADITIONS
### Poland

- Traditional meal—Polish people celebrate Christmas with a meatless meal (*Wigilia*), on Christmas Eve. After they break and share a white wafer (*Oplatek*), they sing Christmas songs in Polish, such as "Dziasia Betlehem" and "Jesus Christus Rogie." They serve two kinds of pea soups (*grochowka*), one of yellow peas and one of green peas; a mushroom soup called *barszcz* that is fermented in oatmeal for one month; *natacana kasha,* which is roasted buckwheat served with cooked prunes (bathrooms get real busy); herring in wine and cream sauces; smoked fishes; and the favorite, pierogies: dumplings stuffed with sauerkraut, wild mushrooms, potatoes, cheese, and plums. They also serve egg bread with raisins, rye bread, and pumpernickel. And for dessert, babka and *kalachzkis* with apricot and raspberry filling, and poppy seed cakes. Last but not least, a shot of brandy, wine, or vodka is served with the coffee.
- Presents—The Christmas tree is decorated with nuts; apples; ornaments made from eggshells, colored paper, and straw; and hand-blown glass baubles. Carolers walk from house to house, and many families attend a Midnight Mass called Pasterka, the Shepherd's Mass. And the "Little Star" (the first star that's seen that night) brings presents to very small children before Christmas morning.

In 1822 the postmaster of Washington, D.C., complained that he had to add sixteen mailmen at Christmas to deal with cards alone. He wanted the number of cards a person could send limited by law. "I don't know what we'll do if this keeps on," he wrote.
—20ishparents.com

## Greece

- Traditional meal—Christmas in Greece means *kourampiedes, melomakarona, skaltsounia,* baklava, special loaves of bread called *christopsomo* (Christ Bread), and lots of wine. This feast is extra-special considering that it comes after forty days of fasting and eliminating heavy foods. There's lots of music, too.
- Presents—On Christmas Eve, children go door to door giving good wishes and singing Greek carols, aka *kalanda*. Presents are given to children on the morning of New Year's Day (not Christmas) by a jolly and generous guy named Agios Vasilis.

## Finland

- Traditional meal—Casseroles containing macaroni, rutabaga, carrot, and potato are served with cooked ham or turkey.
- Presents—Santa Claus brings presents on Christmas Eve, but he lives in Korvatunturi, above the Arctic Circle in Northern Finland, not at the North Pole like our Santa.

## Belgium

- Traditional meal—An appetizer of seafood is followed by a main course of stuffed turkey. The traditional dessert is Christmas log cake.
- Presents—Saint Nicholas brings presents to children on December 6, Saint Nicholas Day.

## Portugal

- Traditional meal—Salted dry codfish with boiled potatoes is eaten at midnight on Christmas Eve.
- Presents—Father Christmas leaves presents under the Christmas tree or in shoes by the fireplace.

## France

- Traditional meal—Good meat and fine wine.
- Presents—Père Noel (Father Christmas) brings presents on December 25.

## Latvia

- Traditional meal—Cooked brown peas with bacon sauce, small pies, cabbage, and sausage.
- Presents—Father Christmas brings presents on each of the twelve days of Christmas, starting on Christmas Eve.

## Germany

- Traditional meal—Fish (usually carp) or goose is served.
- Presents—Der Weihnachtsmann (Father Christmas) leaves presents by the Christmas tree in the afternoon on Christmas Eve, while everyone is in church.

## Ireland

Traditional meal—Candles are placed in the windows, and after the evening meal, the table is set with bread and milk and the door left unlatched. This is to symbolize a home that is lighting the way and open for Jesus, Mary, and Joseph. And others passing by are also welcome, especially priests, who might say the Christmas Mass, eat dinner, and share the evening with the family.

## Chile

- Traditional meal—Christmas Eve dinner is eaten very late, often after Midnight Mass, and consists of salads, seafood, olives, turkey, and a nice Chilean wine. Dessert is usually *pan de Pascua,* a sweet Christmas bread, along with fruit, cake, and cookies.
- Presents—Viejo Pascuero (Old Man Christmas) delivers the presents with a team of reindeer, which is a little unusual considering it's usually very hot there at Christmastime.

## Guyana

- Traditional meal—On Christmas day they eat pepperpot for breakfast, which is a dish made of meat stewed in a special dark sauce. A late lunch consists of baked chicken or turkey, stuffing, garlic pork, and homemade pickled onions. Dessert is black fruitcake soaked for months in wine and rum. Ginger beer, mauby, and sorrel drink are the traditional Christmas beverages.
- Presents—Gifts are exchanged after breakfast on Christmas Day.

## Egypt

- Traditional meal—Coptic Christian celebrate Christmas on January 7. They eat a strict vegetarian diet (no meat or dairy) for the forty-five days leading up to Christmas, until Christmas Eve, January 6, when they eat a meal called *fatta,* which consists of meat and rice.
- Presents—Sunday school teachers give presents to children on Christmas Day.

## FOR THE KIDS

One of my favorite Christmas rituals started in my first grade classroom. On the first day of Advent, Sister Joseph Leo taught us how to make small Popsicle-stick cribs to be placed at our desks. These cribs were meant for our very own little plastic baby Jesus, which would be given to us the last day before Christmas vacation. Every time any one of us did a good deed or act of kindness, we were allowed to add one piece of straw to Jesus' future crib. It became our responsibility to do enough kind deeds during Advent to make sure that our own little baby Jesus would be comfortable when he was born on Christmas Day. I became an obsessive do-gooder. It was my personal mission to make sure my little baby Jesus would have a nice fluffy crib overflowing with straw.

I loved this idea so much, I introduced it to my son Joey's classroom this year when I was room mom. Instead of adding straw to a crib, we started an "Acts of Kindness Chain." Every time

Epiphany, or Twelfth Night, January 6, is the traditional end of the Christmas holiday and is the date on which we take down the tree and decorations. To do so earlier is thought to bring bad luck for the rest of the year. From the Middle Ages until the mid-nineteenth century, Twelfth Night was more popular than Christmas Day, and even today some countries celebrate Epiphany as the most important day of the Christmas season.

the kids did something nice at home or at school, they got to add a link to a paper chain that was eventually used to decorate the Christmas tree. The great thing about this straw-for-Jesus' crib or kindness chain is that it gets kids thinking about others rather than themselves. Kids spend enough time thinking about what they're going to get from Santa Claus. I know I did!

## FOR COUPLES

Couples are so busy during this time they usually don't have time for each other. How about deciding on a day between Christmas and New Year's for just the two of you? Shop, see a movie, eat in a cozy restaurant, or whatever you like, but no kids, no in-laws, no work. Buy each other gifts throughout the day so that what you receive is what you really want.

# Family Christmas Survey

DATE:

NAME:        FOR:

## I. CLOTHING

### Sizes:

| shirts/blouses | shoes | sweaters |
|---|---|---|
| hats | skirts /pants | gloves |
| T- shirts | sweatpants | |

### Styles:

| preppie | urban | punk |
|---|---|---|
| classic | romantic | vintage |
| sporty | dramatic | eclectic |

### Type:

| dressy | casual | exercise |
|---|---|---|
| office | sleepwear | artsy |

| | I LOVE | I HATE |
|---|---|---|
| Colors: | | |
| Fabrics: | | |
| Accessories: | | |
| Jewelry: | | |

| | NEED MOST | NEED LEAST |
|---|---|---|
| | | |

|  | NEED MOST | NEED LEAST |
|---|---|---|

### BEDROOM

_____
_____
_____
_____
_____

### LIVING ROOM/
### DINING ROOM

_____
_____
_____
_____
_____

### KITCHEN

_____
_____
_____
_____

### BATHROOM

_____
_____
_____
_____
_____

# Family Christmas Survey

PAST YEAR    ALL-TIME

## III. ENTERTAINMENT

### Movies:
(Including videos and DVDs)

### Concerts:

### Events:

### Restaurants:

I LIKE    I HATE

### Appetizers:

### Entrées:

Healthy Holidays

|  | I LIKE | I HATE |
|---|---|---|
| Desserts: | | |
| Beverages: | | |
| Fun Foods: | | |

## V. TRAVEL

Ideal Locations:

Travel Needs:

## VI. Fantasy

# Family Christmas Survey

## PART TWO

## PERSONAL PROFILE

(SAMPLE QUESTIONS FROM MEMBERS OF MY FAMILY)

What interesting discoveries have you made this year?

_____
_____
_____
_____
_____

What is the funniest one-liner or short joke you've ever heard?

_____
_____
_____
_____
_____

If you were forced to change everything in your life, and you could retain only one aspect (e.g. place, person(s), thing(s), etc.), what would that one thing be and why?

_____
_____
_____

How do you clip your toenails?

_____
_____

Healthy Holidays

If you could live during any time period, when would it be, and what would you do?

_____
_____
_____
_____
_____

What do you like best about yourself?

_____
_____
_____
_____
_____

What's the first thing you notice when you visit a new place?

_____
_____
_____
_____
_____

If you had to change places with a member of the opposite sex (past or present), who would it be and why?

_____
_____
_____
_____
_____
_____

# Family Christmas Survey

What was the worst thing your parents did in raising you?

_____

_____

_____

_____

_____

If you could take three people (past or present) out to dinner, who would they be and what would you all talk about?

_____

_____

_____

_____

_____

If you were in the witness protection program, where would you live and what would you do?

_____

_____

_____

_____

_____

What three people (other than family, mates, and so on) have made an impression on you and why?

_____

_____

_____

_____

If you had a two-week, all-expenses-paid vacation, where would you go and what would you do?

_____

_____

_____

_____

Can you love yourself as much as the person you love most in your life?

_____

_____

_____

_____

In what way has your credo changed in the last year?

_____

_____

_____

_____

.

If you could spend one day invisible, where would you go and what would you do?

_____

_____

_____

_____

If you were to invent a game, what would be the objective and what would you name it?

_____

_____

_____

_____

What is your favorite phase of the moon?

_____

_____

_____

# New Year's Eve

New Year's Eve is a big drinking holiday. It's the final blowout of the year, leaving you grasping for Alka-Seltzer and resolutions the morning after. Why not get a head start on a healthy year and skip the drinking? Even better, why not make yourself the designated driver? Spend the evening watching how stupid everyone else gets long before the stroke of midnight. Or if you must drink, pick one type of liquor (beer, wine, sake, or champagne) and don't mix. Drink two glasses of water for every glass of liquor (four ounces of wine, eight ounces of beer, one shot of hard liquor) and nurse each drink for at least two hours if it's going to be a long night.

And how about picking a New Year's resolution that will work this time? No doubt about it, commitment is the secret to a successful New Year's resolution. In the next week or so, about 100 million Americans will venture down a well-traveled path paved with bold and sometimes hastily conceived New Year's resolutions: promises to exercise more, lose weight, stop smoking, cut down on alcohol, eat a healthier diet, and make new friends. But not all these resolutions are broken. According to a new University of Washington survey, 63 percent of the people questioned were still keeping their number one New Year's resolution after two months. The researchers focused on health-related resolutions, because these types of pledges are the most common, and 60 percent of Americans die from illnesses connected to behavior such as overeating, lack of exercise, and smoking.

Consistency brings results, and desire goes a long way. You have to really want to succeed in order to make a resolution stick. But these resolutions will become part of you only if they are accompanied by those same three elements I talked about in the beginning of this book—awareness, discipline, and practice. So—know what you want to change, try it on for size, and most important, stick with it!

## HISTORY, FACTS, AND FOLKLORE

New Year's Day was originally celebrated in the spring with the vernal equinox. However, after several Roman emperors changed the calendar, it eventually fell out of sync with the sun. When this happened, Julius Caesar chose a random date—January 1—and stretched the year out to 365¼ days in order to align the year properly with the sun. This is why we call it the Julian calendar.

As for New Year's Eve indulgences and resolutions, the resolutions originated first. As with Chinese New Year, it is believed that what you do on the first day of the year will influence the entire year ahead. Quit smoking on New Year's Day and you will stick with it. If you have good luck New Year's Day, you will have good luck all year. The bacchanal that has become New Year's Eve is simply a reaction to the stout resolutions that will ensue in the next twenty-four hours. It was the ancient Babylonians who began this tradition of resolutions, although the most common pledge they made was to return a neighbor's farm equipment. "Happy New Year, and thanks for returning my hoe!"

# Sweet Potato Pancakes with Caviar

Makes 48 pancakes     (green/yellow)

2 pounds tan-skinned sweet potatoes, peeled (about 3 medium)

¾ cup chopped green onions

2 large eggs

1½ tablespoons unbleached flour

1½ teaspoons salt

½ teaspoon ground black pepper

3 tablespoons or more vegetable oil

1 cup soy sour cream

1 ounce any brand black caviar

1 bunch fresh chives, cut into 1-inch pieces

In a large pot of boiling, salted water, cook the sweet potatoes until just tender but still firm, about 15 minutes. Drain and refrigerate until cold, at least 2 hours. The potatoes can be cooked 1 day ahead; keep refrigerated.

Line a large baking sheet with parchment paper. Coarsely grate the potatoes into a large bowl. Stir in the green onions. In a small bowl, whisk the eggs, flour, salt, and pepper and gently mix it into the potato mixture. Form the mixture into 48 walnut-size balls and transfer to the prepared baking sheet. The balls can be made 6 hours ahead. Cover and refrigerate.

In a large nonstick skillet over medium-high heat, heat the oil. Place 8 of the potato balls in the skillet, pressing each gently with a spatula to flatten to 1½ inches in diameter. Cook until the pancakes are a rich golden brown, about 2 minutes per side. Transfer to paper towels to drain. Repeat with the remaining potato balls, adding more oil to the skillet if necessary. Transfer the pancakes to a platter. Top each with 1 teaspoon soy sour cream and a scant ¼ teaspoon caviar. Garnish with the chives. Serve warm or at room temperature.

More than 60 percent of Americans will not make a New Year's resolution. More than half of those who do make resolutions will not fulfill those promises.
—American Medical Association

# Salmon Cakes with Soy Dipping Sauce

Makes about 20 cakes    (yellow)

1 pound salmon fillets, skin and bones removed, flesh diced

1 cage-free organic egg white

2 tablespoons fine rice flour

1 tablespoon finely chopped ginger

1 teaspoon wasabi paste

3 tablespoons chopped fresh organic flat-leaf parsley

Vegetable oil for frying

¼ cup rice vinegar

¼ cup soy sauce

⅛ cup mirin

2 tablespoons Sucanat

To make the salmon cakes, in a medium bowl, combine the diced salmon with the egg white, rice flour, ginger, wasabi paste, and chopped parsley. In a large sauté pan over medium-high heat, heat ½ inch of oil hot enough so the cakes sizzle when placed in the oil. Make cakes using 2 tablespoons of the salmon mixture each. Place the cakes in the hot oil and cook for 35 to 45 seconds each side, or until lightly golden. Drain on absorbent paper and keep on a plate in a warm oven while you cook the rest. To make the dipping sauce, in a small bowl, combine the vinegar, soy sauce, mirin, and Sucanat. Serve the dipping sauce with the warm salmon cakes.

# Cucumber Sour Cream Dip

Serves 8    (green)

2 large organic cucumbers, peeled, seeded, and finely grated

2 pints soy sour cream

2 tablespoons chopped fresh organic parsley

2 tablespoons chopped fresh organic chives

2 tablespoons chopped fresh organic tarragon

2 tablespoons chopped fresh organic dill weed

Salt and pepper

Using a strainer, squeeze the excess liquid from the cucumbers. In a medium bowl, mix the cucumbers, sour cream, herbs, and salt and pepper to taste. Refrigerate until ready to use. Serve with cut-up vegetables.

# Lentils with Port-Glazed Shallots

Serves  4    (green)

*MaryAnn Hennings*

1½ cups ruby port wine or mirin

4 small shallots and 1 large shallot, peeled

1½ cups dried lentils rinsed and drained,

(about 12 ounces)

2 tablespoons olive oil

Salt and pepper

In a heavy medium saucepan, combine the port or mirin and the small shallots. Simmer over medium heat until the shallots are tender and glazed, stirring occasionally, about 35 minutes. Set aside. (This can be prepared 8 hours ahead; keep at room temperature.)

Finely chop the large shallot. Combine the chopped shallot, lentils, and 3 cups water in a large heavy saucepan. Bring to a boil over medium heat. Reduce the heat to medium-low, cover, and simmer until the lentils are just tender, about 30 minutes.

Rewarm the shallot mixture over medium-low heat. Stir the oil and the shallot mixture into the lentils. Season to taste with salt and pepper. Transfer the lentils to a bowl and serve.

# Roasted Mixed Vegetables   Serves  4    (blue)

½ pound button mushrooms, cleaned

1 large red onion, sliced

1 yellow squash, sliced diagonally

1 zucchini, sliced diagonally

6 to 8 garlic cloves, unpeeled

1 teaspoon dried rosemary

½ teaspoon kosher salt

¼ teaspoon black pepper

2 tablespoons olive oil

3 tablespoons balsamic vinegar

Preheat the oven to 400°F.

In a large baking pan, mix all the ingredients except the balsamic vinegar. Roast for about 1 hour, or until the vegetables are tender and golden. Place the vegetables in a serving dish and sprinkle with the balsamic vinegar.

## Fettuccine with Tomato-Anchovy-Caper Sauce  S e r v e s  1 2    ( g r e e n )

1 large Spanish onion, chopped

2 organic garlic cloves, finely minced

4 tablespoons olive oil

1 28-ounce can organic peeled plum
   tomatoes, coarsely chopped

1 2-ounce tin flat anchovy fillets

1 9-ounce bottle tiny capers, drained

1/4 cup chopped organic Italian parsley

2 pounds fettuccine

10 Sicilian olives, sliced

Basil leaves

Coarse salt

Freshly ground pepper

Soy Parmesan cheese

In a heavy skillet over medium heat, sauté the onion and garlic in 2 tablespoons of the oil for 3 minutes, or until the onion is soft and golden. Add the plum tomatoes, anchovies, and capers and sauté for 10 minutes, or until the tomatoes are soft. Add the parsley and cook for 3 minutes longer. Boil the fettuccine according to package instructions. Drain the pasta, put it back into the cooking pot, and toss with the remaining 2 tablespoons oil. Place the pasta on a large platter. Spoon the sauce on top, and garnish with the olives and basil leaves. Season to taste with salt, pepper, and soy Parmesan cheese.

The most popular healthy resolutions are: eating a healthier diet (82 percent), exercising more (84 percent), reducing fat in one's diet (62 percent), and reducing stress levels (76 percent). Unfortunately, Americans are ignoring their physicians' advice to reduce alcohol consumption, with 81 percent declining to lower their alcohol intake.—U n k n o w n

# Baked and Raw Endive Salad with Roasted Beets, Walnuts, Carrot, and Lemon serves 4 (green)

*JONATHAN WAXMAN, WASHINGTON PARK RESTAURANT*

*Jonathan Waxman is a brilliant chef. His restaurant, Washington Park, is my very favorite in New York City. He makes every meal feel like New Year's Eve.*

Sea salt

1 pound fresh organic endive

¼ cup extra-virgin olive oil

1 cup walnuts

1 pound beets, unpeeled

1 garlic clove, peeled

Juice of 1 lemon

1 carrot, peeled, cut into long strips with a
   vegetable peeler

Preheat the oven to 350F.

Cut half the endive into quarters, place the endive quarters in a roasting pan, and sprinkle with sea salt and 1 teaspoon of olive oil. Roast the endive for 45 minutes, or until tender. Cool. On a baking sheet, toast the walnuts for 5 minutes, then roughly chop.

In a medium saucepan over medium heat, poach the beets in boiling, salted water for 45 minutes, or until tender. Cool, peel, and cut into rounds, reserving any beet juice.

In a medium bowl, mash the garlic. Mix in the lemon juice and the remaining olive oil. Stir in the beets and juice. Toss the beet mixture, walnuts, and cooked endive together.

Cut the remaining endive into julienne strips and scatter on a platter. Top with the beet mixture and garnish with the carrot strips.

## Jumbo Shrimp, Parsley, Sweet Onions, and Black Caviar Serves 4 (green)

*JONATHAN WAXMAN, WASHINGTON PARK RESTAURANT*

2 Vidalia onions

16 extremely fresh jumbo shrimp, peeled, shells reserved

6 ounces chardonnay

1 bunch parsley, washed and separated into stems and sprigs

2 tablespoons extra-virgin olive oil

Juice from ½ orange

1 ounce American black caviar

Preheat the oven to 400°F.

Roast the onions in their skins for 1 hour, or until tender. Cool the onions, peel them, and slice them into thin rounds.

To make the shrimp stock, in a medium saucepan, place the shrimp shells, chardonnay, and parsley stems. Bring to a boil over medium heat, lower the heat, and simmer for ½ hour. Strain the stock and discard the shells and parsley stems.

In a large sauté pan over medium heat, heat the olive oil, add the shrimp, and cook for 2 minutes on each side, or until pink. Remove the shrimp and reserve. Add the shrimp stock, orange juice, and onions and simmer over low heat until the liquid is reduced to ¼ cup, about 10 minutes. Add the shrimp back into the mixture to warm.

To serve, place the shrimp on a platter and top with caviar and parsley sprigs.

## Scallops Roasted on Yellow Potatoes, Black Olives, Bay Leaf, and Sea Salt

Serves 4 (green)

*JONATHAN WAXMAN, WASHINGTON PARK RESTAURANT*

1½ pounds very fresh extra-jumbo sea scallops from Maine (three scallops per person)

Sea salt

1 pound medium Yukon gold potatoes, washed and sliced into ¼-inch-thick rounds

¼ cup fantastically green! olive oil

1 cup salt-cured olives, washed and dried

8 bay leaves

Preheat the oven to 375°F.

Clean the scallops and season with sea salt.

Place the potatoes in a roasting pan and sprinkle with the olive oil, ¼ cup water, and sea salt. Roast for 30 minutes, or until tender. Raise the heat to 450°F. Add the scallops, olives, and bay leaves and roast for 10 minutes. Remove the bay leaves and serve immediately.

# Spice Cake  Serves 10  (yellow)

1 cup whole wheat flour

1 cup white flour

1½ teaspoons ground cinnamon

1 teaspoon baking powder

½ teaspoon baking soda

½ teaspoon ground ginger

¼ teaspoon grated nutmeg

¼ teaspoon salt

½ cup (1 stick) soy margarine, softened

¼ cup maple sugar

2 large cage-free eggs

¼ cup light (mild) molasses

½ cup soy sour cream

½ cup soy milk

1 pound soy cream cheese

½ cup liquid fruit juice concentrate

½ teaspoon vanilla extract

Preheat the oven to 350°F. Grease two 9-inch round cake pans. Line the bottoms with wax paper; grease and flour the paper.

In a medium bowl, stir together the flours, cinnamon, baking powder, baking soda, ginger, nutmeg, and salt.

In large bowl, with a mixer at low speed, beat the margarine and maple sugar until blended. Increase the speed to medium-high and beat 2 minutes, until creamy. Add the eggs, one at a time, beating well after each addition. Beat in the molasses until combined.

In a small bowl, with a fork, mix the soy sour cream and soy milk. On low speed, mix in a quarter of the flour mixture, then a third of the soy sour cream mixture, alternating until all are combined. Divide the batter between the two prepared pans, spreading it evenly. Bake 25 or 30 minutes, until a toothpick inserted in the center of the layers comes out clean. Cool in the pans on wire racks 10 minutes. With a small knife, loosen the layers from the sides of the pans. Invert the layers onto wire racks. Remove the wax paper and cool completely.

To make the frosting, in a medium bowl with an electric mixer, beat the soy cream cheese until completely smooth, 3 to 5 minutes. Reduce the speed to low and slowly beat in the fruit juice concentrate and vanilla. Blend for 2 minutes. Refrigerate for 30 minutes before frosting.

Did you know that you are more likely to be killed by a champagne cork than by a poisonous spider?—S q u a r e w h e e l s . c o m

New Year's Eve

## BEVERAGES

- Champagne
- Cosmopolitans
- Martinis
- Sake (try to buy organic brands like Kamotsuru and Koikawa)

## PARTY IDEAS

- Make a romantic dinner for two.
- Throw a family party, celebrating New Year's Eve in earlier time zones.
- Have a dessert party.
- Throw an "Around the World in 80 Bites" potluck brunch. Have each of your friends pick a recipe from this book that represents a foreign country, such as Spain, France, Mexico, China, or Ireland. Set up your healthy international buffet using little flags, posters, or souvenirs. Set alarm clocks so you can celebrate when it hits midnight in each country you're tracking. Play lots of international CDs to add to the atmosphere. This is a great party for the whole family, especially if you time it for midnight in Europe, which is late afternoon/ early evening in the United States.
- Have a black-and-white dress code. Tell your guests they can wear anything they want as long as it's black or white.
- Have a BLT party. Tell your guests they have to choose one of the following options: black tie, lingerie, or toga. This theme is probably more appropriate for twentysomethings, but if your guests are a bit older but adventurous, why not?

## INVITATIONS

- Include an RSVP that asks your guests to list their five favorite songs of the past year to be played at the party.
- Send a Top Ten list from the past year based on your guests' interests.
- Compose a song to the tune of "Auld Lang Syne" that includes all the party information in the lyrics; record your song on a cassette tape and mail it as an invitation.
- Cut your invitations in the shape of a champagne cork, bow tie, top hat, glass slipper, balloon, hourglass, or clock.

## DECORATIONS

The usual party hats, noisemakers, balloons, masks, streamers, and so on. Considering using all black-and-white or silver table settings and decorations. If you've chosen an international theme, add travel posters, postcards, and exotic souvenirs.

## SCENTS

Champagne
Wintergreen
Fireplace

# Toasts

Here's to the bright New Year and a fond farewell to the old;
Here's to the things that are yet to come and the memories that we hold.

## ACTIVITIES AND GAMES

- Write your own version of the Dubious Achievement Awards from *Esquire* magazine that includes funny stories about your guests. Present the awards just before the stroke of midnight.
- Have everyone write three predictions for the coming new year. They should write something about themselves, someone at the party, and the world at large. Seal the predictions in an envelope and read them at next New Year's Eve party.

## PRIZES, GIFTS, AND PARTY FAVORS

Calendars, cameras, little notebooks for writing resolutions, diaries, time capsules, *People* magazine's Most Fascinating People of the Year issue, almanacs for the next year.

## MUSIC

| | | |
|---|---|---|
| *Celebration* | Kool & the Gang | Album |
| *Another Year* | Leo Sayer | Album |
| *Newness Ends* | The New Year | Album |
| *Please Come Down* | James Combs | Album |
| *New Year* | Jon Spencer Blues Explosion | Album |

## MOVIES

| | |
|---|---|
| *When Harry Met Sally* | (1989–R) |
| *Ocean's Eleven* | (1960–NR; 2001–PG-13) |
| *200 Cigarettes* | (1999–R) |
| *Go* | (1999–R) |
| *Night on Earth* | (1991–R) |
| *An Affair to Remember* | (1957–NR) |

## EXERCISE AND CALORIE CHART

Make it a point to exercise earlier in the day unless you're going to be dancing your buns off at a New Year's Eve party. And if you are dancing, be sure to wear comfortable shoes so that you'll be able to move well, burn more calories, and most important, be able walk the next day! Let your outfit start with the most stylish, comfortable shoes possible, and build it from there.

| Activity | Calories Burned/Hour |
| --- | --- |
| Dancing | 320 |
| Watching the ball drop | 119 |
| Kissing everyone in the room | 125 |

## FOR THE KIDS

One of the best New Year's Eve parties I've ever attended was in Los Angeles at Scott Bakula and Chelsea Field's house. It was a family party that began at six o'clock with a buffet dinner and dancing, and at 8:45, everyone got out on the front lawn with Silly String, bubbles, and noisemakers. At the stroke of 9:00 (midnight on the East Coast), all hell broke loose! This all happened on our way out the door. The kids were home by 9:30, in bed by 10, and I was off to a dessert party for a grown-up New Year's Eve!

For preteens and older kids, hold an all-night film festival. When I was about eleven or twelve, WGN in Chicago would have all-night film festivals. Each year it would be somebody different: the Marx Brothers, W. C. Fields, Fred Astaire and Ginger Rogers, Sherlock Holmes, or Charlie Chan. I looked forward to it every year and usually planned a pajama party around it. You can easily plan your own party now by renting four or five movies with a theme. Consider the choices above along with the following: James Bond, Monty Python, Abbott and Costello, Mel Brooks, Woody Allen, Frank Capra, Marilyn Monroe, the *Godfather* series, Cary Grant, Hitchcock, Katharine Hepburn and Spencer Tracy, the *Star Wars* trilogy, Billy Wilder, the Rat Pack, the Brat Pack, Audrey Hepburn, Martin Scorsese, Gene Kelly, Meryl Streep, Meg Ryan. The list is really endless. You can't go wrong. Just don't forget the popcorn. But no butter!

## FOR COUPLES

What could be more romantic than spending the entire day ringing in the New Year in different time zones? Every hour, celebrate with something special, whether it's a food, a groove, or a move. You can even stay in bed wearing nothing but party hats, streamers, and a smile. Warning: don't sit on the noisemaker!

# Recipe Index

# Recipe Index

# ◼ ReganBooks

**Books by Marilu Henner:**

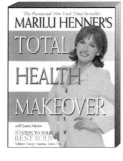

### MARILU HENNER'S TOTAL HEALTH MAKEOVER

ISBN 0-06-098878-9 (paperback); ISBN 0-06-109828-0 (mass market); ISBN 0-694-51927-8 (audio)

With irrepressible enthusiasm and humor, Marilu presents practical advice on diet myths, toxic foods, mood swings, food combining, and her unique, flexible, down to earth 10-step life plan. With *Marilu Henner's Total Health Makeover* you can free yourself from diets and disease-causing toxins, boost your energy, lower and maintain your weight, and change your outlook in as little as three weeks.

### THE 30 DAY TOTAL HEALTH MAKEOVER
*Everything You Need to Do to Change Your Body,*
*Your Health, and Your Life in 30 Amazing Days*

ISBN 0-06-103133-X (paperback)

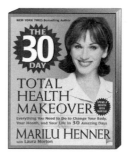

This inspirational how-to guide for total health living and your B.E.S.T body in just 30 days, includes day-to-day goals; strategies for success; recipes for breakfast, lunch, and dinner; shopping lists; exercise ideas; and what to feed the kids.

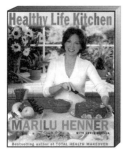

### HEALTHY LIFE KITCHEN

ISBN 0-06-098857-6 (paperback)

Marilu Henner provides a delicious collection of healthy recipes that will help readers change their bodies and their lives forever. Created by Marilu and her favorite chefs from restaurants all over the world, these delectable breakfasts, lunches, dinners, desserts, and snacks will raise healthy cuisine to a new level of taste and ease. There is even a "healthy junkfood" section for converting naughty treats into nutritious recipes.

### I REFUSE TO RAISE A BRAT

ISBN 0-06-098730-8 (paperback); ISBN 0-694-52129-9 (audio)

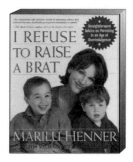

Super-mom Marilu Henner and renowned psychoanalyst Dr. Ruth Sharon provide simple and straightforward advice on how to raise secure, happy and self-reliant children. *I Refuse to Raise a Brat* teaches readers how to distinguish between overg-ratification and love, break the pattern of overindulgence, and offer children the balance of frustration and gratification they need.

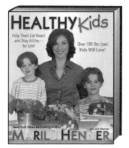

### HEALTHY KIDS

ISBN 0-06-052852-4 (paperback)

Marilu Henner believes that healthy food equals healthy children. In *Healthy Kids*, Marilu shows how the choice of diet for your child will influence his long-term health prospects more than any other action you may take as a parent. This essential guide shows parents that food provides the building blocks for a strong and healthy body, giving your child the energy needed to learn, play, and grow.

**Available wherever books are sold, or call 1-800-331-3761 to order.**